WOMEN'S
MENTAL
HEALTH
SERVICES

WOMEN'S MENTAL HEALTH SERVICES

A Public Health Perspective

Edited by
Bruce Lubotsky Levin
Andrea K. Blanch
Ann Jennings

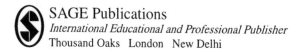

SAGE Publications
International Educational and Professional Publisher
Thousand Oaks   London   New Delhi

For information:

 SAGE Publications, Inc.
2455 Teller Road
Thousand Oaks, California 91320
E-mail: order@sagepub.com

SAGE Publications Ltd.
6 Bonhill Street
London EC2A 4PU
United Kingdom

SAGE Publications India Pvt. Ltd.
M-32 Market
Greater Kailash I
New Delhi 110 048 India

Printed in the United States of America

Library of Congress Cataloging-in-Publication Data

Main entry under title:

Women's mental health services: A public health perspective /
    edited by Bruce Lubotsky Levin, Andrea K. Blanch, Ann Jennings.
        p. cm.
    Includes bibliographical references (p.   ) and index.
    ISBN 0-7619-0508-1 (cloth: acid-free paper).—ISBN 0-7619-0509-X
(pbk.: acid-free paper)
        1. Women—Mental health. 2. Women—Mental health services.
    I. Levin, Bruce Lubotsky. II. Blanch, Andrea K. III. Jennings, Ann, 1936- .
    RC451.4.W6W6665 1998
    362.2'082—dc21   97-45341

98 99 00 01 02 03 10 9 8 7 6 5 4 3 2 1

Acquiring Editor:	Dan Ruth
Editorial Assistant:	Anna Howland
Production Editor:	Diana E. Axelsen
Production Assistant:	Karen Wiley
Indexer:	Ardis Hanson, M.L.S.
Print Buyer:	Anna Chin

Contents

tant ways from women without abuse histories. However, the chapters in this book suggest that the lessons learned from attempting to respond effectively to the needs of trauma survivors may apply equally to all consumers of mental health services.

Through our collaborative work with consumer advocates, we have come to understand that consumers of mental health services, whether in communities, hospitals, nursing homes, or prisons, must play a central role in redefining and shaping services to meet their diverse needs. When consumer voices are not heard, mental health services are likely to be irrelevant, ineffectual, or nonexistent. We want to emphasize that new models for treatment and training must also evolve through a true collaboration between consumer-survivors, clinicians, and policymakers.

The powerful effect of such collaboration has been demonstrated in some recent mental health initiatives. The Dare to Vision Conference in 1994 was unprecedented in its ability to bring together a group of mental health providers, researchers, policymakers, and consumer advocates, and to establish common ground where no dialogue had previously occurred. Out of that dialogue came the impetus for this volume, the development of a task force on the use of restraint and seclusion in Massachusetts, and ongoing policy and planning at the federal level.

As an example of consumer-provider partnerships, the *Report and Recommendations of the Massachusetts Department of Mental Health Task Force on the Restraint and Seclusion of Persons Who Have Been Physically or Sexually Abused*[1] has resulted in new clinical guidelines and policies[2] that have changed mental health assessment and treatment in the public mental health system in Massachusetts. The work of the Massachusetts task force also demonstrates that effective services delivery can occur with only modest changes in mental health policy and practice.

Based on the chapters presented in this volume, as well as our knowledge and experiences in the field, we would like to make the following recommendations about the delivery of mental health services to women that need to be incorporated in any system of care:

1. Adequate assessment and effective treatment of psychological disorders in women of all ages and in all potential mental health treatment settings require that they be asked about histories of physical and sexual abuse.

2. Comprehensive mental health care for women requires the integration of mental health and addiction services, with referrals and linkages to physical health care. It also requires linkages with community-based services such as rape crisis centers and domestic violence shelters.

3. Single-gender inpatient and community residential programs should be available to women diagnosed with concurrent mental illness and abuse histories to provide a safe and therapeutic environment in which recovery can occur. The definition of safety, as it is usually understood in a psychiatric treatment setting, may be quite different from that needed for the therapeutic care of women suffering from traumatic stress syndromes.

4. All state departments of mental health should appoint trauma coordinators who, in collaboration with a consumer/provider network, recommend policy, educational programs and training initiatives, and practice guidelines for the treatment of consumer/survivors.

5. Mental health delivery systems must have in place clear policies and systems for monitoring and reporting human rights violations. Such systems should be user friendly and take into account the different needs that women may have in negotiating allegations of sexual abuse, intimidation, discrimination, and harassment.

6. Advanced mental health care directives should be expanded to include consumer preferences about all aspects of their care, from effective interventions during a crisis or episode of loss of control to drug treatment.

Women's Mental Health Services: A Public Health Perspective addresses the basic elements for understanding women's mental health services delivery issues. It also provides policymakers, administrators, graduate students, and behavioral health services providers with the knowledge base needed to implement improvements and changes in mental health services delivery in the United States.

ELAINE (HILBERMAN) CARMEN, M.D.
PATRICIA PERRI RIEKER, Ph.D.

REFERENCES

1. Carmen E, Crane B, Dunnicliff M, Holochuck, S., Prescott, L., Rieker, P. P., Stefan, S., & Stromberg, N. *Report and Recommendations, Massachusetts Department of Mental Health*

Task Force on the Restraint and Seclusion of Persons Who Have Been Physically or Sexually Abused. Boston: Massachusetts Department of Mental Health, January 25, 1996.
2. *Clinical Guidelines: DMH Clients With a History of Trauma.* Boston: Massachusetts Department of Mental Health, August 6, 1996.

Preface

Women's Mental Health Services: A Public Health Perspective examines major issues in the organization, financing, and delivery of women's mental health services. It combines a discussion of core women's mental health services delivery issues (including epidemiology, service use, management, and the law) with a detailed examination of how mental health problems affect the lives of women who have specific needs (including individuals with severe mental disorders, women with mental disorders who are in jails, and older women with a mental illness). This text also includes chapters that examine the experiences of women who have confronted these illnesses and survived.

The idea for this book originated during the completion of a special issue titled Women's Mental Health Services of the *Journal of Mental Health Administration* (now renamed the *Journal of Behavioral Health Services & Research*). Prior to the publication of this special issue, little attention had been given to women's mental health services delivery issues within the published literature in the field. Furthermore, no single text currently provides an overview of the critical public mental health issues affecting women. We have attempted to respond to this gap in the behavioral health services literature.

This book was developed with three goals in mind: (1) to bring attention to behavioral health issues (including mental health and substance abuse) of particular concern to women; (2) to identify and highlight the unique ways in which women are making important contributions to the organization, management, and delivery of mental health services; and (3) to provide a discussion of these critical services delivery issues within a multidisciplinary public health framework. To accomplish these goals, an editorial decision was made to include chapters based on qualitative research (including descriptive analyses, case studies, and personal observations) as well as more traditional quantitative research and policy studies. Although these editorial decisions challenge many embedded assumptions about what constitutes scientific rigor, the result is an exceptional volume that we hope accomplishes all three stated goals.

This text is particularly timely, since substantial changes in the financing and delivery of health and mental health services have continued to occur, particularly at the state level. Although, more recently, attention has been given to research in women's reproductive health services, overall, women's health and mental health issues have been fundamentally neglected. This book attempts to fill this void.

Nationally recognized experts in the field were invited to prepare the chapters contained in this text. While some of the chapters that appear in this text were originally published in the special issue Women's Mental Health Services (and are used with permission), the majority of the chapters are original contributions written specifically for this volume.

The text is designed for a variety of audiences, including (1) undergraduate and graduate students in public health, health and hospital administration, social work, psychiatric and community health nursing, community and medical psychology, preventive and social medicine, community and social psychiatry, and other graduate students and postdoctoral fellows in the behavioral health care fields; (2) professionals currently employed in mental health and substance abuse programs in hospitals, managed care organizations, substance abuse clinics, and community mental health centers; and (3) policymakers, advocates, consumers, and professionals involved in the fields of mental health and substance abuse services delivery within local, regional, state, and national levels of government.

ORGANIZATION OF THE BOOK

The text is divided into two basic components: an introduction to the major organization, financing, and delivery issues in women's mental health services (Part I), and an examination of special issues and topics in selected at-risk populations (Part II).

The first six chapters, which comprise Part I of this text, present the basic issues in women's mental health services delivery. In Chapter 1, Blanch and Levin summarize the public health (including historical, epidemiologic, legislative, and social) context of mental health services delivery in relationship to women's needs. In Chapter 2, Rhodes and Goering discuss gender differences in the need and use of ambulatory mental health services. Padgett and colleagues (Chapter 3) analyze a large database of insurance claims to identify predictors of ambulatory mental health services use by women of selected ethnicity. In Chapter 4, Scheidt addresses the challenges that women administrators face in management and promoting leadership in a clinical (psychiatric) hospital setting. In the following chapter, Forquer and McDonnell (Chapter 5) describe efforts at the federal level to establish a national database on women's issues in the prevention and treatment of mental disorders and substance abuse. In the last chapter of Part I, Cook (Chapter 6) analyzes whether women and men display differential ability to achieve residential independence when the outcome assessed is living in their own community housing following psychiatric rehabilitation.

Part II of this book (Chapters 7 to 18) explores special issues in women's mental health services via three sections: A. Empowerment (Chapters 7 and 8); B. Severe Mental Illness and Survivors of Trauma (Chapters 9 to 16); and C. At-Risk Populations (Chapters 17 and 18).

Part II of the book begins with two chapters on empowerment. Kalinowski and Penney (Chapter 7) discuss the history and basic principles of the mental patients' movement and its relationship to empowerment and women's mental health services. Ridgway and colleagues (Chapter 8) propose a participatory approach to supportive housing programs, based on the involvement of consumers and consideration of the impact of physical environment on mental health.

The second section of Part II contains eight chapters on women with severe mental disorders and women who are survivors of trauma. Mowbray and colleagues (Chapter 9) examine critical issues and service needs of women with severe mental disorders, and how gender is a barrier to effective mental health treatment. In Chapter 10, Blanch and colleagues discuss the needs of parents diagnosed with serious mental illness who are raising young children. Alexander and Muenzenmaier

(Chapter 11) provide an overview of women with comorbid disorders: severe mental illness, substance use, and victimization histories. Stefan (Chapter 12) examines the impact of the law on women diagnosed with borderline personality disorder who have survived childhood sexual abuse. Newmann and colleagues discuss the effect physical and sexual abuse have on the use of services and the costs of mental health care in Chapter 13. Harris (Chapter 14) also critiques existing mental health care delivery systems for not meeting the needs of women diagnosed with severe mental disorders who are also sexual abuse survivors. Jennings (Chapter 15), using a case study approach, focuses on a group of individuals who have been long neglected by mental health policymakers and administrators: sexual abuse survivors in the mental health system. In the last chapter in this section, Bills and Bloom (Chapter 16) emphasize, from a clinical as well as programmatic perspective, needed treatment modifications for women diagnosed with severe mental illness who have experienced sexual abuse trauma.

The final section of Part II (Section C) contains two chapters (17 and 18) on two special at-risk populations: women in prisons and jails, and older women. In Chapter 17, Veysey describes the characteristics and special needs of women with mental illnesses in correctional settings, drawing our attention to the high prevalence of substance abuse and childhood sexual and physical abuse in the life histories of these women. Padgett and colleagues (Chapter 18) summarize the literature regarding the need, use, and barriers to older women's use of mental health services.

Although space does not permit the examination of all relevant issues in women's mental health services delivery, this text underscores the importance of establishing a multidisciplinary, public health framework for the study of women's mental health services. We hope that this comprehensive framework will assist individuals from various perspectives to join in future policy making and research in women's mental health services.

We would like to thank the many individuals who have provided encouragement, support, and consultation throughout the preparation of this book. In particular, we would like to thank Melodie Peet, Commissioner of Mental Health, Mental Retardation, and Substance Abuse of the State of Maine, and Robert Friedman, Professor and Chair, Department of Child and Family Studies, Louis de la Parte Florida Mental

Health Institute, University of South Florida, for their ongoing support of this work. We also owe a great deal of gratitude to Ardis Hanson, who has made numerous valuable suggestions during the development of this book, and who constructed the comprehensive author and subject indexes. We would also like to extend a special thanks to Ann Taylor and Jamie Waterburg for their assistance in the preparation of this book, as well as express our appreciation to Dan Ruth of Sage Publications for his valuable suggestions during the editing of this text. Finally, we would like to express our deep appreciation and thanks to our families for their love, understanding, and support, particularly through the final preparation of this book.

BRUCE LUBOTSKY LEVIN
ANDREA K. BLANCH
ANN JENNINGS

Part I

Services Delivery Issues

The organization, financing, and delivery of health and mental health services in the United States continue to evolve at a rapid pace. The managed care industry has experienced continued growth and substantial consolidation through mergers and acquisitions, while increased attention to quality, outcomes, and fiscal accountability has forced major changes in the role of hospitals in the health care system. However, despite extensive modifications to health care financing and services delivery, a substantial number of individuals with serious mental disorders receive inadequate treatment, are homeless, and/or remain ignored by society.

Most mental health and substance abuse services in the United States have been delivered within systems of care apart from general (somatic) health care. Nevertheless, the majority of individuals seeking mental health services do so through the general health care sector (e.g., hospital emergency rooms and primary care practitioners). This lack of integration between health and mental health services has contributed to uneven access to specialty services as well as to the underuse of a public health orientation in mental health policy making and services research.

Part I of this book (Chapters 1 through 6) provides a foundation to view women's mental health and substance abuse services from a multidisciplinary, public health perspective. Many of the women affected by the mental health problems discussed in this book are poor, are members of cultural/ethnic minority groups, or have been victims of trauma.

Many of these women have serious mental disorders that have not been adequately treated within the current array of public and private, for-profit and not-for-profit mental health services delivery systems. In addition, these women have not been well represented by administrators, policymakers, interest groups, or other political constituencies.

In their introductory chapter on organization and services delivery, Blanch and Levin (Chapter 1) present the history, legislation, epidemiology, and organization of mental health services for women. They highlight the complex structural array of women's mental health services as well as the major social obstacles experienced by women in seeking treatment for mental disorders.

In Chapters 2 and 3, the authors examine the need for and use of outpatient mental health services by women. Rhodes and Goering (Chapter 2) review epidemiologic studies of gender differences in the need for outpatient mental health services, concluding that women's higher rates of service use exist primarily within the primary health care sector. They discuss the implications for treatment planning and services delivery for women, and they suggest that future surveys of needs assessment should include measures of disability and functioning.

In Chapter 3, Padgett and colleagues analyze insurance claims of more than a million nationally insured female employees (and their families) to assess differences in the use of outpatient mental health services. Their results indicate that White women had a significantly greater likelihood of using outpatient mental health services and used significantly more visits than did Black or Hispanic women, even after controlling for predisposing, enabling, and need factors. The fact that this discrepancy exists even in a generously insured population suggests that cultural and attitudinal barriers may substantially interfere with access to mental health services. The authors suggest that under state (mental) health care reforms, ensuring that women of color receive equal access to mental health services will require more than just liberalizing health benefits.

Scheidt (Chapter 4), through a case study of women's leadership in a psychiatric program at a general teaching hospital in California, discusses the challenges women face as mental health administrators. The author describes a women-focused inpatient team located at San Francisco General Hospital that specializes in treating women diagnosed with severe mental disorders, many of whom also contend with ongoing conditions of poverty and violence. Scheidt explores four challenges to women leaders and administrators: the stereotypes women have about each other as leaders, the expectations and biases of staff and trainees, the relationship between patients and women leaders, and women's leadership in relationship to department administration. The author concludes with specific suggestions regarding how to overcome these challenges.

In Chapter 5, Forquer and McDonnell describe efforts at the federal level to establish a data set of both qualitative and quantitative descriptors of six critical issues related to women's mental health and substance abuse services: (1) physical/sexual abuse of women, (2) women as mothers and caretakers, (3) women with mental and addictive disorders, (4) women with HIV/AIDS/sexually transmitted diseases (STDs) and/or tuberculosis, (5) older women, and (6) women involved in the criminal justice system. The authors conclude that current databases lack critical indicators in these six areas. Future data collection instruments should include specific data elements reflecting these six selected issues in women's mental health and substance abuse services.

Cook (Chapter 6) analyzes outcome data from 650 clients who received services at a large, urban psychosocial rehabilitation agency. Results of the study showed that although there are no gender-related differences in independent living status at the time of entry into the program, a significantly higher proportion of women than men are living independently by the time they leave the program. However, gender itself is not a major differentiator once other variables in the model were controlled. Cook's data suggest that at least in the case of independent living, gender affects outcomes indirectly, mediated by level of functioning, program tenure, independence from ongoing agency support, parental status, and community participation. Cook's analysis also leads to the interesting observation that mental health programs may inadvertently weaken factors that are correlated with independent living, at least for women.

1

Organization and Services Delivery

Andrea K. Blanch, Ph.D.
Bruce Lubotsky Levin, Dr.P.H., FABHM

This book presents women's mental health issues from a public health perspective. While the development of public health concepts and health care delivery dates back to 18th-century Europe and late-19th-century America, few have advocated on behalf of this interdisciplinary approach for examining issues in women's mental health. A public health perspective provides a framework for understanding the role of social factors (such as poverty, discrimination, and interpersonal violence) in women's mental health, a framework that is critical to the development of coherent health and social policy and cost-effective intervention strategies.

In the past decade, the costs of the nation's health and mental health programs have grown unmanageable. U.S. health care expenditures in 1994 totaled just under $950 billion, or 13.7 percent of the nation's gross domestic product.[1] Today, mental disorders and substance abuse cost the U.S. economy more than $450 billion, including behavioral health treatment costs, related health care costs, housing assistance, law enforcement and public safety, and productivity lost due to injury, illness, or premature death.[2] The total cost to society for mental disorders and substance abuse exceeds the cost of heart disease ($128 billion), cancer ($104 billion), Alzheimer's disease ($100 billion), and diabetes ($92 billion).[3]

The exponential growth in health and mental health care expenditures has spawned a series of attempts at health care delivery reform. All of these reforms, including changes in welfare and disability income supports, managed health and behavioral health care, incremental changes in health care coverage (mental health parity legislation and expanded coverage for children), and the shift of a wide range of responsibilities from the federal government to the states, focus on the organizational structure and financing of mental health and addiction services. Most of these initiatives acknowledge the fragmentation of current mental health, substance abuse, and social services and explicitly encourage better integration of these services. However, none has given serious consideration to the role of social factors in the etiology, prevention, or treatment of behavioral health disorders. Rather, emerging policies focus almost exclusively on behavioral health disorders as barriers to economic self-sufficiency.[4]

At the same time, international concern about the public health consequences of violence, particularly violence against women and children, continues to grow. Campaigns are being waged against genital mutilation, international child prostitution, and war-related sexual crimes. Interventions are being designed for victims of torture and political oppression. The world stands riveted as the anguish and mental health consequences of decades of politically inspired violence are aired at "tribunals" in South Africa and Bosnia. Surely we understand, as a society, that there are serious public health consequences to this "epidemic" of violence.[5] So why is it so difficult to apply these principles to mental health delivery systems in America?

The chapters in this book suggest at least three contributing factors: the patriarchal structure of mental health and substance abuse delivery systems; our conceptual inability to integrate the consequences of environmental events with genetic and biological vulnerabilities into a true public health model; and the fragmentation of health and social services into discrete sectors, leading, for example, to the same behavior being attributed to "illness" in the mental health system, to "bad behavior" in jails or prisons, or just to "old age" in nursing homes and long-term facilities.

This chapter will examine current deficiencies in the organization of women's mental health services and will briefly summarize the major epidemiologic studies of women's mental disorders in community settings. The chapter will conclude with suggestions for reconceptualizing current mental health delivery systems within a public health framework.

STRUCTURAL BARRIERS

Over 20 years ago, feminist scholars made a convincing argument that the mental health system was structured on an essentially patriarchal model[6] and that the most basic tool of mental health professionals, psychotherapy, was inherently sexist.[7] Since that time, there have been substantial efforts on the part of many professional associations and women's organizations to promote nonsexist forms of treatment and to develop and support a consciously feminist approach to therapy.[8] Although these efforts have reduced the level of overtly sexist practice, key elements of feminism remain largely ignored in the practice of psychotherapy and the treatment of individuals with mental disorders and substance abuse. Factors such as the role of context and power imbalances in relationships are still infrequently addressed as part of the healing process, and as a result, women may not be receiving help in recognizing oppressive conditions and working to overcome them.[8]

Despite 20 years of research, there is scant evidence that "women's issues" are adequately addressed in mental health systems today,[9] and some therapists argue that there is little room within the profession for a truly female idiom of practice.[10] The failure of mental health systems to make structural adaptations to women's work patterns or to enlist women fully into leadership positions contributes to this situation.[11]

LACK OF AN INTEGRATED
PUBLIC HEALTH MODEL

Despite considerable rhetoric about the interaction of biology and the environment, there is little to suggest that the mental health professions have moved much beyond a simplistic either/or dichotomy with reference to the etiology of severe mental illnesses. Increasingly, these conditions are referred to as "brain disorders," "biologically based illnesses," or "neurobiological dysfunctions," clearly implying a single, biological cause despite substantial evidence that attending to environmental and contextual factors is critical to the recovery of people diagnosed with severe mental illnesses.[12]

A recent article by Coursey and colleagues attempts to create a more complex picture, postulating a shift from a pathology-based model of serious mental illness to a competence paradigm based on a broadened concept of causality.[13] Their proposed model includes environmental factors interacting with genetic predispositions, leading to physical brain abnormalities and deficits in cognition and attention, and ultimately to both positive and negative symptoms. The model also acknowledges that environmental factors such as stress, drug abuse, and homelessness can affect the nature and course of the illness. However, the only causal environmental factor specifically cited is "viral infection," and nowhere in the article is interpersonal violence mentioned. This absence is particularly glaring in light of growing knowledge about the interaction of biological and social factors in the manifestation of post-traumatic stress disorders.[14,15]

It is important to recognize that adopting an integrated public health or "biopsychosocial" model such as that proposed by Coursey and colleagues implies variability in causation, not a wholesale rejection of the "medical model." Symptoms of severe mental illness may result from extreme or chronic stress (including physical or sexual abuse as well as more chronic conditions like homelessness), biological malfunctioning (genetically predisposed or unexplained chemical imbalances), environmental conditions or assaults (allergic and toxic reactions or nutritional deficits), developmental blocks, or physical trauma (neurological diseases, drug abuse, or head injuries). Widening the scope of our interventions to address the psychosocial aspects of behavioral health disorders will ultimately improve the organization, financing, and delivery of mental health and substance abuse services.

It is no coincidence that recognition of the importance of gender differences among people diagnosed with severe, long-term mental illnesses was slow to develop. Despite being brought to the attention of the mental health community by Test and Berlin in 1981,[16] little attention has been paid to explaining the gender differences that have consistently been found in both diagnosis and service utilization patterns within this population.[17] For example, in an entire special section devoted to innovative approaches to the treatment of serious mental illness in a recent national mental health publication, there is not a single reference to gender differences.[18] The medical model, which is so dominant in the treatment of serious mental illness, has apparently blinded us to the relationship between the conditions of women's lives and their manifestations of severe emotional turmoil.[19]

FRAGMENTATION OF CARE

The large gap between epidemiologic estimates of the rates of behavioral health disorders and the actual number of women receiving treatment over the course of a lifetime leads to the inevitable conclusion that many women handle their problems without professional help, or receive assistance through other health and social service systems, including the primary health care, welfare, correctional, or long-term care systems. In fact, research has shown that from 5 to 40 percent of all welfare recipients have substance abuse problems and treatment needs. Among women receiving Aid to Families With Dependent Children (AFDC), twice as many individuals abuse substances as their non-AFDC counterparts (27 percent vs. 12 percent), and over 15 percent need substance abuse treatment services.[4] Similarly, nearly 20 percent of female jail detainees have significant psychiatric disorders that require treatment.[20]

The current fragmentation of health, behavioral health, and social services makes it difficult to take a holistic approach to the etiology or treatment of alcohol, drug abuse, and mental disorders. This problem is compounded by the fact that people who use mental health and social services are devalued by our society and are stereotyped accordingly. Once people are labeled (e.g., as a mental patient, a criminal, or a welfare recipient), they are assumed to be more alike than they are different. Similarly, the nature of their problem or problems is assumed to be reflected by the institution within which they were served.[21] Thus, a woman with a severe behavioral health disorder will probably be treated for a behavioral (but possibly not physical) illness if she enters a mental health facility, punished for her behaviors if she goes to jail or prison, and deemed an unfit mother and lose custody of her children if she applies for welfare. Because each service system focuses exclusively on one aspect of her life, it is difficult to discern the underlying roots of her problems. This situation is compounded if comorbid disorders exist. Thus, the causal role of social factors such as interpersonal violence or poverty goes undetected and/or untreated.

Labeling and stereotyping have an immediate impact on the individuals involved as well as on societal attitudes and institutional responses. Although research fails to support the hypothesis that labeling determines chronicity, there is substantial evidence that the causal attributions people make regarding their own problems (as well as their beliefs about the attributions that others are making) can have a significant impact on their personal identity and emotional state.[22]

In one study of "illness identity work," Estroff found that many informants defined mental health as the ability to balance and control their emotions. Furthermore, they believed that anger or psychological trauma could accumulate over time, eventually resulting in symptoms of mental illness. As one informant stated, "It's almost as though I have a deep depression coming from things I've kept inside all these years." Similarly, another informant reflected: "Anger is natural. What makes it an illness is when it gets too heavy at one end. It needs balance."[22]

Both race and gender appear to affect illness attributions and identity work. Regardless of race, men are more likely than women to attribute their mental illness to social/situational factors (e.g., lack of housing or a job) or to believe that they have "no problem." White men are substantially more likely than any other race or gender to accept a mental illness label, while white women alone compose 58 percent of those whose illness explanations were coded as emotional/developmental.[22] It seems quite possible that these differences could reflect actual differences in people's lives, and in the etiology of their emotional disorders. Unfortunately, the epidemiology of mental illness has been based on standard diagnostic categories, and we have no comparable scientific epidemiology of interpersonal violence.

PUBLIC HEALTH AND EPIDEMIOLOGY

Improving the overall health of Americans is the fundamental objective of federal, state, and local public health agencies. Historically, epidemiologic research has been used to determine the frequency, distribution, and etiology of disease in specified populations. However, until recently, research on women's health services has been focused primarily on the reproductive health of women, while epidemiologic and health services research specific to women's issues (including mental health services research) has been generally neglected.

Over the past ten years, a renewed national focus on women's health has emerged, emphasizing increased funding for health services research, inclusion of women in clinical trials, and training and educational opportunities for women pursuing research, clinical, administrative, and other health care professions. In addition, the Office of Women's Health was established in the early 1990s within the Public Health Service to coordinate the various women's health initiatives within the U.S. Department of Health and Human Services.[23]

The National Center for Health Statistics highlighted recent trends in women's health services. Findings presented in the resource volume included the following:[24]

- Women have a higher risk (vis-à-vis men) of nonfatal chronic conditions, including arthritis, osteoporosis, depressive disorders, and anxiety disorders.
- Heart disease, cancer, and stroke were the leading causes of death for women in the United States.
- Women were nearly seven times as likely as men to experience violent crimes by an intimate (spouse, former spouse, or partner) or relative.
- Poor women 25-64 years of age were more than three times as likely not to have health care coverage vis-à-vis nonpoor women.
- Between 1965 and 1990, cigarette smoking declined more among men than among women.
- Age-adjusted prevalence of a sedentary lifestyle among persons 25 years of age and older was greater for women compared with men.

Despite the willingness of women to seek somatic health services (women 15-64 years of age had 66 percent more than the average number of physician visits made by men[24]), mental disorders in women have been largely unrecognized and untreated, and if they are treated, it is most likely by a primary care provider. Explanations for this absence of treatment have included unequal insurance coverage for mental health and substance abuse services compared with physical (or somatic) health services, the continued social stigma of mental disorders, the lack of access to mental health specialty providers (particularly within managed health care), and the problems of seeking care for women who work, care for their families, and have additional responsibilities.

In response to the President's Commission on Mental Health chaired by Rosalynn Carter, the Epidemiologic Catchment Area (ECA) study[25] was established by the National Institute of Mental Health (NIMH) to identify baseline rates of mental disorders within treated and untreated populations in the United States. This comprehensive study sampled 18,000 community residents and 2,290 institutional residents in five sites of at least 200,000 residents: New Haven, Baltimore, St. Louis, Durham, and Los Angeles. The ECA study incorporated an interview design comprised of two basic parts: the Diagnostic Interview Schedule (DIS) and a health services questionnaire examining the use of somatic health and mental health services.

Overall, results of the study indicated comparable rates of mental disorder for women and for men. Approximately 20 percent of the women and men interviewed in this study had a mental disorder within the past 12 months of the study. The lifetime prevalence of mental disorders was also nearly equivalent for women and for men. The median age of onset was 16 years, while 90 percent of the sample experienced initial symptoms by age 38. The disorders with the highest lifetime prevalence rates were phobia (14 percent) and alcohol abuse (9 percent).

Results of the ECA study also underscored important gender differences in the rates of specific mental disorders. Women had higher rates of affective disorders and anxiety disorders, while men had significantly higher rates of alcohol abuse/dependence, drug abuse/dependence, and antisocial personality disorders. The ECA study found equivalent prevalence rates for women and men for schizophrenia, obsessive-compulsive disorder, and bipolar disorder.

More recently, the National Comorbidity Study (NCS)[26] of more than 8,000 people was designed to improve on the ECA study by incorporating *DSM-III-R* nomenclature, more extensively examining risk factors that affect particular mental disorders, and conducting the study on a national sample of noninstitutionalized individuals 15 to 54 years old. Results from the NCS revealed that approximately 52 million people (29.5 percent) between the ages of 15 and 54 had a diagnosable alcohol, drug abuse, or mental disorder. About 5 percent of the people experienced both a mental disorder and substance abuse/dependence within the past year, while approximately 14 percent of the population had both disorders in their lifetime. The most prevalent behavioral disorders within the previous 12 month period were anxiety disorders, affective disorders, or substance abuse/dependence.

The NCS revealed differences in prevalence of specific mental disorders according to age (see Chapter 18 in this volume), race/ethnicity (see Chapter 3 in this volume), and gender (see Chapters 2 and 3 in this volume). While men were more likely than women to have alcohol and drug abuse/dependence and antisocial personality disorder, approximately 7 percent of women between the ages of 15 to 54 abused alcohol and/or other drugs in the past year. Women were more likely to have affective disorders (approximately 21 percent of women in the United States, compared with about 13 percent of men, suffer from major depression during their lifetime) and anxiety disorders (approximately 30 percent of women, compared with about 19 percent of men, suffer from anxiety disorders during their lifetime). Women were also found to have higher prevalence rates (compared with men) of lifetime comorbidity of three or more disorders.[26]

A growing body of evidence suggests that specific mental disorders may affect women at particular stages of life: certain eating disorders often affect young women;[27] women are at increased risk for major depression during the postpartum period of their life;[28] and there is increasing evidence of relationships between mental health, maltreatment, and elderly women.[29] In addition, women of color and of lower socioeconomic status have higher rates of depression than the general population.[30]

SERVICE BARRIERS AND USE

The use of mental health services may differ by gender, based, in part, on factors that create barriers to seeking and using these services. Data collected from both the ECA[31] study and the NCS[26] confirmed that the majority (approximately 60 percent) of people with diagnosable mental disorders did not receive treatment, and of those who did seek treatment, even fewer received treatment in the mental health specialty sector (approximately 25 percent) or in a substance abuse facility (approximately 8 percent). This underuse of mental health services relative to need appears greater for members of ethnic minority groups (see Chapter 3 of this volume) and has been attributed to a number of factors. These factors include the current organization and structure of mental health services in America (including the lack of insurance coverage of mental disorders), poverty, problems of accessibility to mental health services (including time constraints and parenting responsibilities), the lack of coordination between mental health delivery systems within a given community as well as the lack of coordination between health organizations and mental health organizations in a community, sociocultural factors (including language barriers), knowledge (including attitudes and beliefs) of available mental health services, willingness to use mental health services, existence of alternative mental health services, fear of stigma attached to using mental health services, and employment discrimination.[32] In addition, women who have been victims of trauma (by intimates or others) or women who have experienced retraumatization (particularly within mental health facilities) are at risk of developing mental illness (see Chapters 11 through 16 in this volume).

Most women (and men) who have a diagnosable mental disorder do not seek treatment in either the formal somatic or mental health delivery systems. Nevertheless, women are more likely to use ambulatory mental health services compared with men (for further discussion, see Chapter 2 in this volume), while men are more likely to use hospital care compared with women. However, socioeconomic status, diagnosis, and other variables are important correlates of mental health utilization rates for women. Glied and Kofman[32] provide a recent summary and discussion of gender differences in the use of mental health services. In addition, further discussion of service use appears in Chapters 2, 3, 9, and 18 in this volume.

In addition to gender differences in mental health service use, little research has been conducted regarding gender differences in the efficacy of treatment for mental disorders. Ridgely and van den Berg[33] suggest that outcome studies have not analyzed the impact of gender differences on treatment for mental health services. Glied and Kofman[32] suggest that outcome studies have not addressed the impact of managed mental health services on outcomes in women.

IMPLICATIONS FOR WOMEN'S
MENTAL HEALTH SERVICES

Recent epidemiological research suggests that women may be at higher risk for mental illness than men. This pattern appears to hold across ethnicity and culture in the United States as well as cross-culturally.[34] Moreover, research evidence overwhelmingly supports the conclusion that violence, including domestic violence, is an important factor affecting women's mental health.[34] Violence may also have serious physical health consequences, which are often not recognized as stress related or trauma-related. The financial costs of ignoring these problems are enormous, conservatively calculated at billions of dollars annually.[35]

This edited volume presents a public health perspective on women's mental health services. Adopting a public health policy framework would require that we attempt to "control the agents" causing mental health problems in women; "strengthen the host" to improve resistance to the agents; provide an "environment" more responsive to women's mental health issues, and design and fund treatments and delivery systems that reflect an accurate picture of causation. A mental health system that truly responds to women's needs would help women to connect with each other, and to stay connected to their children and families, rather than isolating and separating them. It would also pay serious attention to the role of social context in the etiology of health and mental health problems and would recognize and support women's strengths and capacities.[19]

It is imperative that we consider the public health aspects of women's mental health at this point in time. Although particular models and technologies of managed care may come and go, the underlying need to control the costs of health and mental health care is likely to remain unchanged for several decades and will increase as the baby boom generation ages. Experience to date suggests that managed care organizations do not serve the poor or uninsured, although they increasingly draw revenue-generating Medicaid patients from the public sector.[36] In addition, managed care companies often restrict access to mental health services to people diagnosed with serious mental illness (usually defined diagnostically, and presumed to be "biologically based") and often require that treatment be focused on functional disabilities related to these diagnostic categories.[37] As a result, women (and men) with trauma-related health and mental health problems may either be denied services or be forced to accept a diagnosis that ignores the role of trauma, thereby reenacting the "silencing" that so many trauma victims have experienced. Moreover, any treatment they do receive will likely focus on specific symptoms, rather than addressing more global concerns or undertaking the sometimes lengthy process of healing from trauma.

Finally, "specialty approaches" of all types are at risk in managed care systems.[38] Managed care, like all normative approaches to health care, seeks to increase predictability and reduce variability. Without corrective pressure, "outliers" will be ignored or excluded. As behavioral health care is increasingly subsumed within generic health care (i.e., medical model) delivery systems, a focus on the unique aspects of "mental health," including the conjunction of social and biological concerns, is likely to be lost. Those whose disorders do not respond to strictly biological interventions may find themselves unwelcome and remain untreated. Unfortunately, the only safety net left for those individuals may be homeless shelters, jails or prisons, and long-term facilities.

REFERENCES

1. U.S. Department of Health and Human Services: *Table 31, National Health Care/Trends.* http://www.hcfa.gov/stats/hstats96/blustat2.html. Washington, DC: Office of the Actuary, Health Care Financing Administration, 1996.
2. *Recommendation for the FY 1998 Appropriations for the National Institute of Mental Health, National Institute on Drug Abuse, National Institute on Alcohol Abuse and Alcoholism, and Center for Mental Health Services.* Washington, DC: Mental Health Liaison Group, 1997.
3. *Prevalence and Cost of Uncured Disease in the United States.* http://www.phrma.org/facts/industry/profile97/figures97/1-7.html. Washington, DC: Pharmaceutical Research and Manufacturers of America, 1997.
4. Center for Substance Abuse Treatment: *Substance Abuse Treatment and Welfare Reform.* Working draft. July 16, 1997.
5. Bloom SL: The Germ Theory of Trauma: The Impossibility of Ethical Neutrality. In: Stamm BH (Ed.): *Secondary Traumatic Stress: Self-Care Issues for Clinicians, Researchers and Educators.* Lutherville, MD; Sidran, 1995, pp. 257-276.
6. Chesler P: *Women and Madness.* New York: Doubleday, 1972.

7. Broverman I, Broverman D, Clarkson F, et al.: Sex role stereotypes and clinical judgment of mental health. *Journal of Consulting Psychology* 1970; 24:1-7.
8. Mowbray CT: Nonsexist therapy: Is it? *Women and Therapy* 1995; 16(4):9-30.
9. Subotsky F: Issues for women in the development of mental health services. *British Journal of Psychiatry* 1991; 158(10):17-21.
10. Wooley SC: The female therapist as outlaw. In: Falloon P, Katzman MA, Wooley SC (Eds.): *Feminist Perspectives on Eating Disorders.* New York: Guilford, 1994, pp. 318-338.
11. Blanch AK, Feiden-Warsh C: Women's mental health services: The need for women in mental health leadership. *Journal of Mental Health Administration* 1994; 21(4):332-337.
12. Anthony WA, Blanch AK: Community support programs: What have we learned? *Psychosocial Rehabilitation Journal* 1989; 12(3):55-81.
13. Coursey RD, Alford J, Satarjan B: Significant advances in understanding and treating serious mental illness. *Professional Psychology: Research and Practice* 1997; 28(3):205-216.
14. van der Kolk BA: The trauma spectrum: The interaction of biological and social events in the genesis of the trauma response. *Journal of Traumatic Stress* 1988; 1:273-290.
15. van der Kolk BA, Fisler RE: The biological basis of post-traumatic stress. In: Elliott BA, Halverson KC, Hendricks-Matthews M (Eds.): *Primary Care Clinics of North America* (Special Issue: Family Violence and Abusive Relationships) 1993; 20(2):417-432.
16. Test MA, Berlin SB: Issues of special concern to chronically mentally ill women. *Professional Psychology* 1981; 12:136-145.
17. Mowbray CT, Herman SE, Hazel KL: Gender and serious mental illness: A feminist perspective. *Psychology of Women Quarterly* 1992; 16:107-126.
18. Coursey RD, Sullivan M, Brow RA (Eds.): Special section: Servicing the seriously mentally ill. *Professional Psychology: Research and Practice* 1997; 28(3):205-245.
19. Stefan S: Reforming the provision of mental health treatment. In: Moss KL (Ed.): *Man-Made Medicine: Women's Health, Public Policy, and Reform.* Durham, NC: Duke University Press, 1996, pp. 195-218.
20. GAINS Center: *1996-1997 Annual Report.* Delmar, NY: Policy Research, 1997.
21. Blanch AK: Issue paper: Stigma and discrimination in mental health. *Community Support Network News* 1990; 6(4):12-13,15.
22. Estroff SE, Lachicotte WS, Illingworth LC, et al.: Everybody's got a little mental illness: Accounts of illness and self among people with severe, persistent mental illnesses. *Medical Anthropology Quarterly* 1991; 5:331-369.
23. Office of Women's Health: *PHS Action Plan on Women's Health.* Washington, DC: U.S. Department of Health and Human Services, 1991.
24. National Center for Health Statistics: *Health, United States, 1995.* Hyattsville, MD: Public Health Service, 1996.
25. Robins LN, Regier DA (Eds.): *Psychiatric Disorders in America: The Epidemiologic Catchment Area Study.* New York: Free Press, 1991.
26. Kessler RC, McGonagle KA, Zhao S, et al.: Lifetime and 12-month prevalence of DSM-III-R psychiatric disorders in the United States: Results from the national comorbidity survey. *Archives of General Psychiatry* 1994; 51:8-19.
27. Munoz RF, Hollon SO, McGrath E, et al.: On the AHCPR depression in primary care guidelines. *American Psychologist* 1994; 49:42-61.
28. Gitlin MJ, Pasnau RO: Psychiatric syndromes linked to reproductive function in women: A review of current knowledge. *American Journal of Psychiatry* 1989; 146:1413-1421.

29. Nadien M: Aging women: Issues of mental health and maltreatment. In: Sechzer JA, Pfafflin SM, Denmark FL, et al. (Eds.): *Women and Mental Health*. New York: New York Academy of Sciences, 1996, pp. 129-145.
30. Weissman MM, Klerman JK: Sex differences and the epidemiology of depression. *Archives of General Psychiatry* 1977; 34:98-111.
31. Shapiro S, Skinner EA, Kessler LG, et al.: Utilization of health and mental health services: Three Epidemiological Catchment Area sites. *Archives of General Psychiatry* 1984; 41:971-978.
32. Glied S, Kofman S: *Women and Mental Health: Issues for Health Reform*. New York: Commonwealth Fund Commission on Women's Health, Columbia University, 1995.
33. Ridgely MS, van den Berg P: *Women & Coercion in Mental Health Treatment: Commitment, Involuntary Medication, Seclusion & Restraint*. Tampa: Louis de la Parte Florida Mental Health Institute, University of South Florida, 1997.
34. WHO says women at higher risk of mental illness. *Mental Health Weekly* 1996; 6(43):7.
35. Reilly MA: A question of illness, injustice, or both? In: Harris M (Ed.): *Sexual Abuse in the Lives of Women Diagnosed With Serious Mental Illness*. Amsterdam: Harwood, 1997, pp. 235-258.
36. APHA president warns of health care inequities. *The Medicaid Letter* 1996; July.
37. Staton D: Psychiatry's future: Facing reality. *Psychiatric Quarterly* 1991; 62:165-175.
38. Schreter RD: Ten trends in managed care and their impact on the biopsychosocial model. *Hospital and Community Psychiatry* 1993; 44:325-327.

2

Gender Differences in the Use of Outpatient Mental Health Services

Anne Rhodes, R.N., M.Sc.
Paula Goering, R.N., Ph.D.

Current economic constraints necessitate careful planning and evaluation of outpatient mental health services. Epidemiologic studies are a valuable source of information to assist with these tasks. This chapter will examine gender differences in need for outpatient mental health services and the type of service use. Issues of concern for women will be the main focus. Hypotheses about gender differences in need and use of outpatient mental health services will be discussed as will implications for planning and evaluation. Mental health services are defined as "any and all services provided for the purpose of identification, diagnosis and treatment of mental health problems" (p. 306).[1] Outpatient mental health services are "provided in a clinic or office to ambulatory clients. Outpatient care typically lasts for less than three hours per session and can be provided on either an individual or group basis" (p. 306).[1]

NOTE: This chapter appeared as an article in the *Journal of Mental Health Administration,* 1994, Vol. 21, No. 4, pp. 338-346.

GENDER DIFFERENCES IN THE NEED
FOR MENTAL HEALTH SERVICES

Need has been conceptualized in various ways, for example, distress, psychiatric symptoms, number and type of psychiatric diagnoses, and number of disability days.[2-4] Most of the scientific literature focuses on distress, symptoms, or psychiatric diagnoses. Recent studies have indicated that there is only a small amount of overlap between indicators of diagnosis, distress, and disability.[5,6] Thus, the importance of considering several dimensions is underscored. Recently, more attention has been given to disability, comorbid physical disorders, subsyndromes, and severe symptoms, for example, suicidal behaviors, as indicators of need for mental health services. Although persons with these conditions may not meet criteria for a psychiatric diagnosis, high prevalence rates are common and the impact on society is considerable. These conditions may be the residual effects of past disorder or precursors of the onset of a disorder. Identification and treatment of them is critical.[4,5,7-9]

Historically, women were thought to have more mental health needs than men. Treatment rates were often equated with prevalence of mental disorder and women sought treatment more frequently. In addition, early population-based surveys relied on measures of distress to define need, and women consistently reported more distress than men. Measures of substance abuse/dependence were seldom considered in such surveys.[10,11] Given these findings, some concluded that women were differentially exposed to social stressors that contributed to mental health problems.[12,13]

Specific diagnostic criteria and reliable techniques for diagnosing mental disorders were not available until the mid-1970s.[10,14] After their development, however, a population-based study of the prevalence of mental disorders was initiated. The Diagnostic Interview Schedule (DIS) was developed based on the *Diagnostic and Statistical Manual of Mental Disorders*, third edition (*DSM-III*),[15] system of classification. In 1980, five large surveys, known as the Epidemiologic Catchment Area (ECA) studies, were conducted in the United States, using the DIS.[16] Bland et al.[17] conducted a similar survey in Edmonton, Alberta. Prevalence and incidence rates for specific *DSM-III* mental disorders are now available for the United States as are prevalence rates for Edmonton, Alberta.[18-20]

From these studies, three issues particularly relevant to women's health needs emerged. First, there is little evidence of an excess of mental disorders among women compared with men, although type of mental disorders differs between the sexes. Second, it appears that elderly persons, a group composed predominantly of women, have less mental disorders than younger or middle-aged groups. Third, drinking problems appear to be increasing in young women. When interpreting these findings, it is important to recognize the strengths and limitations of the study design and examine findings from other research. Each of these three issues will be discussed in more detail.

One of the main strengths of the ECA studies was the detailed information provided regarding psychiatric diagnoses. More men than women met criteria for a psychiatric diagnosis in their lifetime (36 percent vs. 30 percent); however, men and women did not differ in active symptoms in the past year (20 percent).[20] In terms of types of mental disorders, men were more likely to suffer from substance abuse or dependence (largely alcohol), regardless of the length of time examined. A lifetime diagnosis of alcoholism was over five times more likely in males than females.[21] For varying periods of time, prevalence rates for anxiety disorders and affective disorders remained higher for women. Women were approximately two times more likely to suffer from affective disorders in their life.[22] Lacking in the ECA studies, though, was comprehensive information regarding other need indicators such as disability or suicidality.

Because of gender differences across types of mental disorders, women may experience more disability than men. Depressive symptoms and disorders are associated with increased disability days, and time lost from work.[4,9,23] Depression may be as disabling or more disabling than eight chronic medical conditions in terms of social functioning, role functioning, physical functioning, and days spent in bed.[24] Since the effects of having a chronic medical condition and depressive symptoms appear to be additive,[7] those with physical illness and depression are at particular high risk for disability. Depressed women account for a large proportion of need for mental health services when disability is used as an indicator.

Even within substance abuse/dependence disorders, women may experience more disability than men. In the ECA surveys, the chance of having a comorbid psychiatric diagnosis is higher among alcohol dependent women (65 percent) than men (44 percent). Among women, comorbid diagnoses were usually depressive or anxiety disorders and depression usually preceded the alcoholism. Among men, the secondary diagnoses are most often other types of substance abuse or dependence and antisocial personality disorder.[21] In a Canadian survey, women problem drinkers reported more psychiatric symptoms and more disability at home, work, and school than male problem drinkers.[25]

Based on disability, it might be concluded that women have more need than men; however, other need indicators give a different picture. Men are known to have premature mortality due to accidents and suicide,[26] and suicide rates are consistently higher for males compared with females.[27-30] The change in the use of alcohol over time is highly correlated with changes in suicide rates over time,[29] and alcoholism has been estimated to contribute to 25 percent of suicides.[31] It is more reasonable to conclude that need is a multidimensional construct and specific dimensions differ by gender. A variety of need indicators, in addition to diagnosis, should be assessed.[32]

The second significant issue raised by recent epidemiological studies concerns the mental health needs of elderly women. In the ECA studies, elderly persons had the lowest prevalence rates for all mental disorders (except for cognitive impairment, which increased with age.) The lifetime prevalence for those over 65 years of age was 21 percent, with 13 percent active in the past year.[16] When birth cohorts are examined, it appears that increasing rates of depression in younger age groups account for the relatively lower prevalence rates among elderly persons.[14,33]

The concern is that those who plan and develop mental health services may not consider other indicators of need and accept these findings without questioning their validity. For instance, these findings could be hastily used to justify a diversion of funds from mental health services for elderly persons to younger age groups. The consequences would have particular relevance for women, since this rapidly expanding demographic group is composed of more women than men. It is important, then, to examine these findings more closely.

From a social causation framework, the ECA findings do not fit with the losses and declining health and income that elderly persons face.

Nor do these findings concur with high suicide rates or psychotropic drug use in the elderly population.[34,35] Unfortunately, prevalence rates from other studies do not clarify the picture. Some find higher rates in elderly persons, some find lower rates. These differences may be due, in part, to variation in case identification, samples, and types of disorder examined. In particular, higher prevalence rates of disorder or symptoms are found when organic mental disorder is included.[36]

With respect to the design of the ECA studies, it is possible that the true prevalence of mental disorder in elderly persons is underestimated because results are presented for the community-based sample. Persons who might have had a mental illness in the time frame studied die or are institutionalized prior to sample selection. Simon and VonKorff[37] examined the ECA data further and concluded that it is unlikely the decreased prevalence rates in elderly persons could be explained solely by selective mortality or institutionalization. Deterioration of memory, though, may be an important factor. Tweed et al.[34] hypothesized that elderly persons would have more difficulty remembering past states as opposed to more recent ones. When the DIS algorithm for depression is modified to rely on current recall of symptoms, more elderly persons meet criteria for depression and fewer younger persons do. Until such methodological issues are resolved and a broader range of need indicators are examined, the findings regarding elderly persons should be interpreted with caution.

The third issue of concern for women is alcoholism in younger age groups. While alcoholism predominates in males, younger age groups, particularly women, have been affected by increased trends in alcohol consumption over time. The male to female ratios of alcoholism in the past month, past 6 months and lifetime are smallest among those aged 18-29 years.[21] A related trend may be suicide attempts in women. Although more data are needed, trends for suicide attempts appear to follow trends for suicide, and therefore, alcohol use. Women appear to have higher rates of suicide attempts. Those who attempt suicide are at greater risk for later completing suicide.[28,29] Further information about these women and their service needs is desirable.

Longitudinal research is necessary to sort out age-, period-, and cohort-effects with gender over time in the rates of mental disorder. In particular, attention should be given to age-specific differences in mental health needs. It is clear, though, that women are at an elevated risk for depressive disorders and their associated disabilities throughout the life span.

Due to longevity, elderly women are more susceptible to the mental health problems associated with physical and social changes. The increase of alcoholism and suicidal behaviors among young women is alarming and warrants further study.

GENDER DIFFERENCES IN THE USE OF OUTPATIENT MENTAL HEALTH SERVICES

Before discussing gender differences, some background information about studies of use of outpatient mental health services is necessary. It should be noted that the majority of studies of use do not achieve the detailed definition of outpatient mental health service use described at the beginning of this chapter. Use is typically determined by:

1. A visit made for mental health problems (self- or proxy report) to specific providers/settings, or
2. Visits connected to a psychiatric diagnosis/mental health procedure/ psychotropic drug prescription (medical records or insurance claim forms).

Given variations in sample selection and availability of mental health resources in each study setting, it is difficult to generalize across these studies. It is compelling, though, that in the majority of studies, women are consistently more likely to use outpatient mental health services than men. This difference remains even when a variety of predisposing, enabling, and need indicators are controlled[38-42] including free care.[43-45] Why this difference persists is not well understood. We will return to this question in a subsequent section.

Higher overall rates of service use by women do not ensure better care or care appropriate to level of need. For example, it is unclear whether specific age groups are receiving care in proportion to need because the effect of age and gender have not been examined together. In most studies, the young (under 24) and the old (65 or more) are less likely to use outpatient mental health services. If these findings apply to both sexes, then two important groups, young women and elderly women, may be less likely to have their needs met.

In addition to asking who is getting services, it is important to determine what type of care is received and whether it is appropriate to need. Types of outpatient mental health services have been conceptualized as two sectors: primary and specialty care. Again definitions vary from study to study, but primary care usually incorporates nonpsychiatrist physicians, who are for the most part general practitioners or family doctors. Specialty care tends to include visits to psychiatrists, psychologists, psychiatric social workers, and other trained mental health professionals, along with visits to specific mental health or alcohol/drug treatment settings.

With respect to the type of services used, the principal concern is that women may not be receiving care appropriate to level of need. Studies suggest that the gender differences lie largely within the primary sector.[3,24,41,46] The actual magnitude of gender differences in use of primary care settings for mental health problems is difficult to estimate because of the problems faced in detecting and/or defining "cases" in primary care settings.[47-50] There may be considerable underreporting of cases and undetected need for outpatient mental health services in primary care settings.[6]

Women who use the primary care sector for much or all of their health needs may not have their mental health problems detected or adequately treated. Studies that describe mental health care in primary care settings illustrate the risks. The National Ambulatory Medical Care Study found that nonpsychiatrist physicians performed more procedures, prescribed more psychotropic drugs, and spent less time with their patients than psychiatrists did. This study implies that primary care practitioners over-rely on drug therapy.[51] Since women receive anxiolytics and antidepressants more than men,[52] they were most vulnerable. The RAND studies reveal that nonpsychiatrist physicians are insensitive to changes in the level of distress their patients experienced. In contrast, specialty providers increased the number of visits in response to increased levels of patient distress in patient.[53] Persons who use the primary care sector are seen less often than those who are seen in the specialty sector.[54] It is feared that this form of treatment will be an attractive alternative to specialty care because of the decreased cost.[55]

Although questions have been raised about the quality and quantity of mental health care given in primary care settings, it is not realistic for all mental health problems to be referred and treated in the specialty care sector. It is likely that some mental health problems can be treated in the primary care sector at reduced costs (human and monetary). The boundaries between the two sectors, though, are far from clear. Although some studies suggest a filtering process where persons treated in the specialty care sector have more severe symptoms or syndromes,[56,57] others find that need indicators do not differ.[58] Clearly, more research about patterns of use over time is needed. With a more comprehensive definition of need, selection factors or barriers to care can be better understood.

EXPLAINING GENDER DIFFERENCES IN THE NEED AND THE USE OF OUTPATIENT MENTAL HEALTH SERVICES

Further study of social roles and behaviors may help to explain gender differences in need and use of outpatient mental health services.

One indicator of need is distress. It is puzzling that women, who often cite more social resources than men, consistently report more distress than men. Given that changes in social relationships can be beneficial or harmful[59-61] and that the timing of such effects are not known, it is plausible that at a cross section in time, both processes are operating.[62-64] Because women report more persons as important in their social networks, they are affected more by stressful events occurring to others. This hypothesis has been called the "cost of caring."[65,66] This hypothesis is alluring because women spend more time and effort in providing health care to their family and in the larger community, and this burden may increase given an aging society.[67] The term "sandwich generation" has been used to describe the dual responsibility of raising children and caring for elderly parents.[68]

In addition to affecting need, social roles and behaviors may also affect the process of help seeking. Kessler et al.[69] examined gender differences in terms of service use for mental and emotional problems in four large surveys conducted in the United States. In all four samples, women reported higher levels of distress than men and were more likely to perceive having an emotional problem than men who had a similar level of symptoms. Once men recognized they had a problem, they were not less likely to use mental health services. These findings may reflect gender differences in orientation toward health.[70]

Gourash[71] hypothesized that mental health problems mobilize social relationships. Once mobilized, these social relationships either increase or decrease service use depending on the information, attitudes, and beliefs conveyed to the person in need. In the New Haven ECA site, Leaf and Bruce[46] examined gender differences more closely in use of outpatient mental health services in the primary care sector. They found that a three-way interaction between the presence of a psychiatric diagnosis, attitudes toward mental health services, and gender predicted use of services. In men, poor attitudes about mental health services were important, whereas favorable attitudes were important for women. These results did not seem to be affected by type of psychiatric diagnosis or previous treatment. Leaf and Bruce conjectured that men may resist referral to specialty services more than women. This study highlights the importance of examining gender differences in primary and specialty care sector use and the social processes that may affect attitudes and behavior.

In summary, further study of social roles and behaviors over time may explain why men and women differ in type of need. Studies have begun to explore how perceptions of health and attitudes toward services influence the use of outpatient mental health services differently for men and women.

IMPLICATIONS FOR PLANNING OUTPATIENT MENTAL HEALTH SERVICES

Information from community surveys is useful for assessing needs, evaluating existing services, and identifying prevention strategies. It supplements knowledge gained from studies of treated populations, which cannot tell us about unmet needs for services or changes in patterns of illness in the general population. In particular, the findings with regard to gender differences that have been summarized suggest directions for better planning, organizing, and delivering services to meet the special needs of women.

Those who plan services must be aware of the various ways of measuring need and should take care not to rely on any one indicator of need for mental health services. Indicators of need for men and women should include disability and dysfunction. The prevalence of depression is high among women, and it is often a chronic disabling illness. Fewer women have a diagnosis of substance abuse, but when they do, they are more likely to be disabled than are men. Elderly women may appear to have less diagnosable disorders, but measurement problems contribute to this finding, and other indicators of need, particularly the coexistence of physical illness, suggest that their needs are considerable. The subgroup of women with psychotic disorders are not adequately represented in community household surveys because prevalence rates are relatively low and they may be in institutions or on the streets. Still, they are heavy users of a service system that is woefully inadequate for their needs.[72]

Most outpatient mental health care services are provided to anxious and depressed women in the primary care sector. There are many reasons to question whether they receive appropriate care. Over-reliance on drugs, insufficient attention to psychosocial factors, and insensitive and unresponsive treatment and referral practices have been described. Such conditions disadvantage the women who are the recipients of care in this sector. A wider range of treatment options, better training of general practitioners, and better coordination of primary and specialty care are required. In addition to elderly persons, the increasingly visible group of young women with drinking problems and suicidal behaviors may also be better served by such changes.

The influence of social relationships on women's need for and use of mental health services has implications for primary and secondary prevention. Strategies to alleviate the cost of caring are needed. As service systems increasingly shift away from institutional to community care, it is women who are at increased risk as primary caregivers for family members and friends. Adequate supports must be put into place to prevent stress that can lead to illness. The critical role, for women, of informal resources in the detection of mental health problems and facilitation of help seeking should be recognized. Building and educating social support networks can encourage early and appropriate use of formal services by those who are in need.

In summary, there are several implications for managers and planners. Needs surveys should expand on measurement of symptoms and diagnosis and include measures of functioning. Information systems (e.g., case mix groupings and management information systems) that do not include measures of disability may not represent women's special needs. Those who plan and administer health services for elderly persons should be alerted that physical and social problems may be indirect indicators of mental health needs that should not be overlooked. Interventions must be multifaceted, and the coordination of mental health, social, and medical services is particularly necessary. Women treated in the primary care sector will be better served when psychosocial interventions replace an over-reliance on drug therapy. In medical school and continuing medical education courses, physicians need to be educated about the range of health problems and treatment options for women of all ages. Social agencies can be involved in educating and coordinating the efforts of primary care practitioners and key personnel in school, work, or other settings. Strategies to reduce the stress associated with the cost of caring range from improved working conditions (e.g., more day care, flexible work hours, and increased availability of employee assistance programs) to the creation and support of informal social networks and self-help groups. Both early recognition and referral, and less reliance on formal treatment services, could be expected from such primary prevention efforts.

REFERENCES

1. George LK: Definition, classification, and measurement of mental health services. In: Taube C, Mechanic D, Hohmann AA (Eds.): *The Future of Mental Health Services Research*. DHHS Pub. No. (ADM) 89-1600. Washington, DC: Superintendent of Documents, U.S. Government Printing Office, 1989, pp. 303-319.
2. Shapiro S, Skinner EA, Kramer M, et al.: Measuring need from mental health services in the general population. *Medical Care* 1985; 23(9):1033-1043.
3. Leaf PJ, Bruce ML, Tischler GL, et al.: Factors affecting the utilization of specialty and general mental health services. *Medical Care* 1988; 26(1):9-26.
4. Johnson J, Weissman MM, Klerman GL: Service utilization and social morbidity associated with depressive symptoms in the community. *Journal of the American Medical Association* 1992; 267(11):1478-1483.

5. Ciarlo JA, Shern DL, Tweed DL, et al.: The Colorado Social Health Survey of Mental Health Service Needs: Sampling, instrumentation and major findings. *Evaluation and Program Planning* 1992; 15(2):133-148.

6. Cleary PD: The need and demand for mental health services. In: Taube C, Mechanic D, Hohmann AA (Eds.): *The Future of Mental Health Services Research*. DHHS Pub. No. (ADM) 89-1600. Washington, DC: Superintendent of Documents, U.S. Government Printing Office, 1989, pp. 161-184.

7. Wells KB, Stewart A, Hays RD, et al.: The functioning and well-being of depressed patients: Results from the Medical Outcomes Study. *Journal of the American Medical Association* 1989; 262(7):914-919.

8. Regier DA, Farmer ME, Rae DS, et al.: One-month prevalence of mental disorders in the United States and sociodemographic characteristics: The Epidemiologic Catchment Area study. *Acta Psychiatrica Scandinavica* 1993; 88:35-47.

9. Broadhead WE, Blazer DG, George LK, et al.: Depression, disability days, and days lost from work in a prospective epidemiologic survey. *Journal of the American Medical Association* 1990; 264(19):2524-2528.

10. Dowhrenwend BP, Dowhrenwend BS: Sex differences and psychiatric disorders. *American Journal of Sociology* 1976; 81(6):1447-1454.

11. Kessler RC, Reuter JA, Greenley JR: Sex differences in the use of outpatient facilities. *Social Forces* 1979; 58(2):557-571.

12. Gove W: The relationship between sex roles, mental illness and marital status. *Social Forces* 1972; 51:34-44.

13. Gove W, Swafford M: Sex differences in the propensity to seek psychiatric treatment: Prevailing folk beliefs and misused log-linear analysis—Comment on Kessler et al. *Social Forces* 1981; 59(4):1281-1296.

14. Weissman MM, Klerman GL: Depression: Current understanding and changing trends. *Annual Review of Public Health* 1992; 13:319-339.

15. American Psychiatric Association: *Diagnostic and Statistical Manual of Mental Disorders*. 3rd ed. Washington, DC: American Psychiatric Association, 1980.

16. Robins LN, Regier DA (Eds.): *Psychiatric Disorders in America: The Epidemiologic Catchment Area Study*. New York: Free Press, 1991.

17. Bland RC, Newman SC, Orn H: Epidemiology of psychiatric disorders in Edmonton. *Acta Psychiatrica Scandinavica* 1988; 77(338):7-80.

18. Regier DA, Narrow WE, Rae DS, et al.: The de facto U.S. mental and addictive disorders service system: Epidemiologic Catchment Area prospective 1-year prevalence rates of disorders and services. *Archives of General Psychiatry* 1993; 50:85-94.

19. Eaton WW, Kramer M, Anthony JC, et al.: The incidence of specific DIS/DSM-III mental disorders: Data from the NIMH Epidemiologic Catchment Area program. *Acta Psychiatrica Scandinavica* 1989; 79:163-178.

20. Robins LN, Locke BZ, Regier DA: An overview of psychiatric disorders in America. In: Robins LN, Regier DA (Eds.): *Psychiatric Disorders in North America*. Toronto: Collier Macmillan, 1991, pp. 328-366.

21. Helzer JE, Burnam A, McEvoy LT: Alcohol abuse and dependence. In: Robins LN, Regier DA (Eds.): *Psychiatric Disorders in North America*. Toronto: Collier Macmillan, 1991.

22. Weissman MM, Bruce ML, Leaf PJ, et al.: Affective disorders. In: Robins LN, Regier DA (Eds.): *Psychiatric Disorders in North America*. Toronto: Collier Macmillan, 1991, pp. 53-80.

23. Klerman GL, Weissman MM: The course, morbidity and costs of depression. *Archives of General Psychiatry* 1992; 49(10):831-834.

24. Wells KB, Manning WG Jr, Duan N, et al.: Cost-sharing and the use of general medical physicians for outpatient mental health care. *Health Services Research* 1987; 22(1):1-17.

25. Cochrane J, Goering P, Lancee W: Gender differences in the manifestations of problem drinking in a community sample. *Journal of Substance Abuse* 1992; 4:247-254.

26. Wilkins K, Mark E: Potential years life lost, Canada, 1990. *Chronic Diseases in Canada* 1992; 13(6):111-115.

27. Monk M: Epidemiology of suicide. *Epidemiologic Reviews* 1987; 9:51-69.

28. National Health & Welfare: *Suicide in Canada: Report of the National Task Force on Suicide in Canada*, 1987.

29. Diekstra RFW: Suicidal behaviour and depressive disorder in adolescents and young adults. *Neuropsychobiology* 1989; 22:194-207.

30. Leenars AA, Lester D: Suicide in adolescents: A comparison of Canada and the United States. *Psychological Reports* 1990; 67:867-873.

31. Murphy GE, Wetzel RD: The lifetime risk of suicide in alcoholism. *Archives of General Psychiatry* 1990; 47:383-392.

32. Lin E, Goering PN: *Psychiatric Disability: Multiple Domains and Multiple Perspectives.* Paper presented at the Ontario Psychiatric Association meeting, Toronto, 1991.

33. Wickramaratne PJ, Weissman MM, Leaf PJ, et al.: Age, period and cohort effects on the risk of major depression: Results from five United States communities. *Journal of Clinical Epidemiology* 1989; 42(4):333-343.

34. Tweed DL, Blazer DG, Ciarlo JA: Psychiatric epidemiology in elderly populations. In: Wallace RB, Woolson RF (Eds.): *The Epidemiologic Study of the Elderly.* New York: Oxford University Press, 1992, pp. 213-233.

35. Koenig HG, Blazer DG: Epidemiology of geriatric affective disorders. *Clinics in Geriatric Affective Disorders* 1992; 8(2):235-251.

36. George L, Blazer DG, Winfield-Laird I, et al.: Psychiatric disorders and mental health service use in later life: Evidence from the Epidemiologic Catchment Area program. In: Brody JA, Maddox GL (Eds.): *Epidemiology and Aging: An International Perspective.* New York: Springer, 1988, pp. 189-219.

37. Simon GE, VonKorff M: Reevaluation of secular trends in depression rates. *American Journal of Epidemiology* 1992; 135(12):1411-1422.

38. Kessler LG, Burns B, Shapiro S, et al.: Psychiatric diagnoses of medical service users: Evidence from the Epidemiologic Catchment Area program. *American Journal of Public Health* 1987; 77:18-24.

39. Shapiro S, Skinner EA, Kessler LG, et al.: Utilization of health and mental health services: Three Epidemiologic Catchment Area sites. *Archives of General Psychiatry* 1984; 41:971-978.

40. Leaf PJ, Livingston MM, Tischler GL, et al.: Contact with health professionals for the treatment of psychiatric and emotional problems. *Medical Care* 1985; 23(12):1322-1337.

41. Horgan CM: Specialty and general ambulatory mental health services. Comparison of utilization and expenditures. *Archives of General Psychiatry* 1985; 42(6):565-572.

42. Greenley JR, Mechanic D, Cleary PD: Seeking help for psychologic problems. A replication and extension. *Medical Care* 1987; 25:1113-1128.

43. Bland RC, Newman SC, Orn H: Health care utilization for emotional problems: Results from a community survey. *Canadian Journal of Psychiatry* 1990; 35:397-400.

44. D'Arcy C, Schmitz JA: Sex differences in the utilization of health services for psychiatric problems in Saskatchewan. *Canadian Journal of Psychiatry* 1979; 24(1):19-27.

45. Wells KB, Manning WG Jr, Duan N, et al.: Sociodemographic factors and the use of outpatient mental health services. *Medical Care* 1986; 24(1):75-85.
46. Leaf PJ, Bruce ML: Gender differences in the use of outpatient mental health-related services: A re-examination. *Journal of Health and Social Behaviour* 1987; 28:171-183.
47. Jencks SF: Recognition of mental illness and diagnosis of mental disorder in primary care. *Journal of the American Medical Association* 1985; 253:1903-1097.
48. Morlock LL: Recognition and treatment of mental health problems in the general health care sector. In: Taube C, Mechanic D, Hohmann AA (Eds.): *The Future of Mental Health Services Research.* DHHS Pub. No. (ADM) 89-1600. Washington, DC: Superintendent of Documents, U.S. Government Printing Office, 1989, pp. 39-61.
49. Schulberg HC: Mental disorders in the primary care setting: Research priorities for the 1990s. *General Hospital Psychiatry* 1991; 13:156-164.
50. Jones LR, Badger LW, Ficken RP, et al.: Inside the hidden mental health network. Examining mental health care delivery of primary care physicians. *General Hospital Psychiatry* 1987; 9:287-293.
51. Schurman RA, Kramer PD, Mitchell JB: The hidden mental health network. Treatment of mental illness by nonpsychiatrist physicians. *Archives of General Psychiatry* 1985; 42:89-94.
52. Hohman AA: Gender bias in psychotropic drug prescribing in primary care. *Medical Care* 1989; 27(5):478-490.
53. Ware JE Jr, Manning WG Jr, Duan N, et al.: Health status and the use of outpatient mental health services. *American Psychologist* 1984; 39(10):1090-1100.
54. Narrow WE, Regier DA, Rae DS, et al.: Use of services by persons with mental and addictive disorders. Findings from the National Institute of Mental Health Epidemiologic Catchment Area program. *Archives of General Psychiatry* 50:95-107.
55. Mechanic D: Treating mental illness: Generalist vs. specialist. *Health Affairs* 1990; 9(4):61-75.
56. Goldberg D, Huxley P: *Mental Illness in the Community: The Pathway to Psychiatric Care.* London and New York: Tavistock, 1980.
57. Anthony JC, Romanoski AJ, Nestadt G, et al.: Psychiatric syndromes among persons in contact with general medical and psychiatric services in eastern Baltimore. In: Cooper B, Eastwood R (Eds.): *Primary Health Care and Psychiatric Epidemiology.* London & New York: Tavistock/Routledge, 1992, pp. 319-339.
58. Frank RG, Kamlet MS: Determining provider choice for the treatment of mental disorder: The role of health and mental status. *Health Services Research* 1989; 24(1):83-103.
59. Turner RJ: Direct, indirect and moderating effects of social support on psychologic distress and associated conditions. In: Kaplan HB (Ed.): *Psychosocial Stress.* New York: Academic Press, 1983, pp. 105-155.
60. House JS, Umberson D, Landis KR: Structures and processes of social support. *Annual Review of Sociology* 1988; 14:293-318.
61. Schuster TL, Kessler RC, Aseltine, RH Jr: Supportive interactions, negative interactions, and depressed mood. *American Journal of Community Psychology* 1990; 18:423-438.
62. Pearlin LI, Lieberman MA, Menaghan EG, et al.: The stress process. *Journal of Health and Social Behaviour* 1981; 22(12):337-356.
63. Pearlin LI: The sociological study of stress. *Journal of Health and Social Behaviour* 1989; 30:241-256.
64. Gore S, Colton ME: Gender, stress, and distress. In: Eckenrode J (Ed.): *The Social Context of Coping.* New York: Plenum, 1991, pp. 139-161.

65. Kessler RC, McLeod JD: Sex differences in vulnerability to undesirable life events. *American Sociological Review* 1984; 49:620-631.

66. Turner RJ, Avison W: Gender and depression: Assessing exposure and vulnerability to life events in a chronically strained population. *Journal of Nervous and Mental Disease* 1989; 177(8):443-485.

67. Dowler JM, Jordan-Simpson DA, Adams O: Gender inequalities in caregiving in Canada. *Health Reports* 1992; 4(2):125-136.

68. Shumaker SA, Hill DR: Gender differences in social support and physical health. *Health Psychology* 1991; 10(2):102-111.

69. Kessler RC, Brown RL, Broman CL: Sex differences in psychiatric help-seeking: Evidence from four large-scale surveys. *Journal of Health and Social Behaviour* 1981; 22:49-64.

70. Hibbard JH, Pope CR: Gender roles, illness orientation and use of medical services. *Social Science and Medicine* 1983; 17:129-137.

71. Gourash N: Help-seeking: A review of the literature. *American Journal of Community Psychology* 1978; 6(5):413-423.

72. Bachrach LL, Nadelson C (Eds.): *Treating Chronically Mentally Ill Women*. Washington, DC: American Psychiatric Press, 1988.

3

Women and Outpatient Mental Health Services

Use by Black, Hispanic, and White Women in a National Insured Population

Deborah K. Padgett, Ph.D.
Cathleen Patrick Harman, Ph.D.
Barbara J. Burns, Ph.D.
Herbert J. Schlesinger, Ph.D.

Empirical studies of the use of mental health services by ethnic minority women are rare despite the recent growth of research on the mental health needs of subpopulations such as women and ethnic minorities. Specific attention to the needs of ethnic minority women was given by the Special Populations Subpanel on Women of the President's Commission on Mental Health report of 1978, which highlighted potential barriers arising from discrimination because of gender, ethnicity, and social class.[1] Soon after this report was issued, Olmedo and Parron noted the absence of reliable, systematic national data on the epidemiology of mental disorders among ethnic minority women and on their use or nonuse of mental health services.[2] Data that are pre-

NOTE: This research was supported by NIMH Grant MH-46005. This chapter appeared as an article in the *Journal of Mental Health Administration*, 1994, Vol. 21, No. 4, pp. 347-360.

sented are broken down either by ethnic group *or* by gender—the interaction of the two is seldom explored.[2]

Subsequent research in the 1980s, including the National Institute of Mental Health-sponsored Epidemiologic Catchment Area (ECA) surveys,[3-6] has produced a wealth of important national data, but has done little to close this information gap. Thus far, several publications using the ECA data have reported prevalence rates of mental disorders or use of mental health services comparing Hispanics to non-Hispanic Whites,[7,8] Blacks to Whites,[9] and men to women.[10]

Several articles have addressed the special mental health needs of ethnic minority women in general[2,11] as well as the needs of Black women,[12,13] Hispanic women,[14,15] and Asian women[16] in particular. A number of issues have been raised in these articles with respect to socioeconomic and cultural barriers to use of mental health services as well as the need to consider special circumstances of each group of women including English-language acquisition, immigration history, social isolation, family and gender role-related burdens, and cultural beliefs and values that may stigmatize women who seek formal mental health treatment.

The absence of empirical data severely limits understanding of help-seeking behavior of ethnic minority women and how, if at all, it differs from the behavior of their White non-minority counterparts. There is a particular gap in understanding how women who are members of ethnic minority groups use outpatient mental health services in both the public and private sectors. A few key questions underlie this study: Do women from various ethnic groups differ in their use of outpatient mental health services? If the effects of lower socioeconomic status, insurance coverage, and other sociodemographic factors are controlled, will ethnic differences among women persist or disappear?

From the existing literature, a few generalizations about ethnic and gender differences in use of outpatient mental health services can be offered. As mentioned earlier, studies typically focus on either ethnicity or gender as the basis for comparison. First, while all ethnic/racial groups (including Whites) underuse mental health services relative to need as indicated by the general prevalence of mental disorders revealed by the ECA studies,[5] the gap between need and use is greatest for members of ethnic minority groups. Using data from the Los Angeles site of the ECA studies, Hough et al.[7] and Wells et al.[8] found that

Mexican Americans had significantly lower rates of use of outpatient specialty mental health care when compared with non-Hispanic Whites. Similar patterns of lower use relative to Whites have been shown for Blacks.[9]

Second, while ethnic differences in the amount of mental health services used have also been noted, findings are inconsistent. While Blacks, Asian Americans, and Hispanics generally use fewer outpatient visits than Whites,[8,17-20] O'Sullivan et al.[21] found few ethnic differences among these groups. Wells et al.[8] also report no significant differences between Mexican Americans and non-Hispanic Whites in level of use, given any use.

Third, it has been shown that women have lower lifetime rates of mental disorder than men[3] and that Black, Hispanic, and White men are more likely than their female counterparts to be hospitalized for a severe mental illness.[22-25] However, Black, Hispanic, and White women are more likely to seek outpatient psychiatric treatment than are men from these ethnic groups.[3,10,23,25-27]

Fourth, greater use of outpatient mental health services by women does not negate the ethnic differential—Black and Hispanic men and women alike still use fewer services than White men and women.[24,25,27,28] Some researchers have noted that ethnic differences in mental health services use are the result of differences in age, education, and income levels and are minimized when these factors are controlled.[8,29,30] However, in a study of Medicaid enrollees in upstate New York, Temkin-Greener and Clark[28] found that Whites had twice the rate of mental health use as non-Whites (Blacks and Hispanics were combined)—12.4 percent compared with 6.0 percent. Ethnicity by gender interactions revealed that White women used significantly more mental health visits in 1984 ($p < .001$) followed by Black and then Hispanic women. Thus, there is evidence that ethnic differences in use of services occur in a poor Medicaid population of women.

A question arises at this point: Does this ethnic differential hold for women who are generously insured? This study examined an insured, non-poor population of Black, Hispanic, and White women to assess differences in service use and to assess the effects of an array of predisposing, enabling, and need factors[31] as they predict outpatient mental health service use. Based on previous research, it is hypothesized that White women will be more likely to use outpatient mental health services than Black or Hispanic women even after controlling for the effects of socioeconomic status and other predisposing, enabling, and need variables. It is further hypothesized that White women who use mental health services will make more visits than their Black or Hispanic counterparts after controlling for the effects of socioeconomic status and other potentially intervening variables.

With regard to the predictive power of predisposing, enabling, and need factors, the absence of previous research on women in which these factors are measured and analyzed led to the decision to engage in analyses of these variables driven by research questions rather than hypotheses. Which of these factors are the strongest predictors of the probability of use of outpatient mental health services? Which most strongly predict the number of visits among those who have entered treatment?

This study's database of over 1.2 million federal employees and their family members insured by Blue Cross/Blue Shield in 1983 offers a rare opportunity to examine and compare service use by White, Black, and Hispanic women in a national insured population. Advantages of this database include: (1) population-based rather than facility-based data on use, thus allowing the calculation of per capita rates, and (2) inclusion of visits to mental health specialists in private office-based practice, data that are rarely available on a national basis.

If ethnic differences are found even in this well-insured population, this would lend support to the notion that Black, Hispanic, and White women respond differently to mental symptoms and manifest distinct patterns of help seeking that are related to cultural and attitudinal factors seldom considered in studies of mental health services use. This study's focus on women is intended to highlight their cross-ethnic diversity and thus contribute to the field of women's mental health.

METHOD

Description of the Federal Employees' Blue Cross/ Blue Shield Insurance Claims Database

This study used insurance claims and related enrollment data from federal employees and their family members who were insured by the Blue Cross and Blue Shield (BC/BS) Association's Federal Employees

Plan (FEP) in 1983. Family members who were insured elsewhere and/or who were not BC/BS claimants during 1983 were not available for inclusion in the study. (A claimant is a person who filed at least one claim in the year for any type of medical service.)

Information obtained from the Office of Personnel Management employee files included education, salary, and ethnic designation (Black, White, or Hispanic) of the insured federal employee. There were insufficient numbers of Asian Americans and American Indians for analysis, and ethnic subgroups of Hispanics, Blacks, and Whites were not identified in the database. The Bureau of Health Professions Area Resource File (ARF) was obtained to provide county-level data on the availability of psychiatric services and on the ethnic composition of the county.

For outpatient mental health care, the high option plan co-payment was 30 percent with a $200 deductible and a 50-visit maximum, and the low option plan co-payment was 25 percent with a deductible of $250 and a 25-visit maximum. The most significant difference between the two plans appears to be in the higher cap on visits allowed in the high option plan. It is likely that use below the deductible is included in these data since BC/BS encouraged enrollees to file claims even when they did not exceed the deductible limit.

The study sample was composed of all Black, Hispanic, and White women over age 18 who had at least one outpatient mental health visit in 1983 and random samples of nonoutpatient women in each group (n = 2,440 for Blacks, n = 2,046 for Hispanics, and n = 2,187 for Whites). The preexisting structure of the database required that the sample was aggregated in this way. In subsequent analyses, these samples were weighted to estimate the total number of women who did not have outpatient mental health treatment in each year. In 1983, there were 67,795 Black female claimants, 13,063 Hispanic female claimants, and 362,494 White female claimants.

The structure of the FEP database placed two restrictions on the study that should be noted. First, since ethnic designation was available only for federal employees, the ethnic group membership of women who were spouses of federal employees was considered the same as that of their husbands. While the FEP database did not allow ascertaining the extent of mixed-ethnic marriages (or the ethnicity of women who were spouses), U.S. Census Bureau data reveal that the rate for

Black/White couples versus all married couples in 1980 was extremely low—335 per 100,000. (There were no data for Hispanic/non-Hispanic marriages.) It was considered reasonable under these circumstances to assign the ethnic designation of federal employee husbands to their spouses. Second, only long-term enrollee families were included; this study examined use in 1983 for women in families enrolled for at least five years. An advantage of this restriction is that it minimizes the risk of bias due to "adverse selection" whereby families with individuals in greater need are likely to choose (or reject) plans on that basis.

Predictors of Probability and Amount of Use of Outpatient Mental Health Services

Following the Andersen and Newman model of factors explaining health service use,[31] three sets of independent variables were developed. Predisposing factors included sociodemographic characteristics of age, number of years of education of the employee, family size, and percentage of the county that was Black, Hispanic, or White. The latter was a continuous variable used as a measure of the level of ethnic congruity in the surrounding community. Tweed et al.[32] found that persons residing in areas characterized by numerical dominance of own-group members manifested lower levels of psychological distress when compared with persons living in racially mixed, or "dissonant," areas. It was reasoned that the level of ethnic congruence in the woman's geographic area might also influence her decision to seek mental health care.

Enabling factors included region of the country (with the three-state Washington, D.C./Virginia/Maryland area contrasted against the other four regions—Northeast, North central, West, and South), salary of the employee, and high versus low option plan. Region of country was considered enabling since the availability of mental health services and of providers varies considerably across these areas.[33] For analyses predicting amount of use, that is, number of visits, the setting of the first visit (hospital clinic vs. office) and the type of provider (physician, psychologist, or mental health worker) were included. (As classified in the claims data, mental health workers included clinical social workers and psychiatric nurses.) Two enabling variables were available from the ARF to provide countywide measures of the relative availability of outpatient mental health services: (1) percentage urban, and (2) ratio of the number of psychiatrists to the number of physicians.

Because of the nature of these insurance claims, no direct measures of need factors such as specific mental diagnoses were available; however, several variables were useful as indexes of risk factors of the need for mental health treatment. These included the individual woman's total annual medical expenses, the rest of her family's total annual medical expenses, whether anyone else in the family received inpatient psychiatric treatment during the year, and the sum of the number of outpatient mental health visits made by all other family members. For the amount of use analyses, whether the woman also had inpatient mental health treatment was included. In the analyses and tables presenting results, "index person" refers to the individual woman and is used to contrast her medical expenses or use of inpatient psychiatric treatment from that of other members of her family.

Dependent Variables: Probability and Amount of Use of Outpatient Mental Health Treatment

Probability of use and amount of use constituted the two dependent variables in the study. The first dependent variable was coded "1" if the woman had an outpatient visit claim coded "nervous and mental" during the year and "0" otherwise. The second dependent variable was the number of mental health visits she had during the year. Only women who used outpatient mental health services were included in analyses of this variable. This approach—restricting analyses of amount of service use to service users only—follows the well-established precedent of previous research on mental health use.[34-36] Given that a very small proportion of women in the general population use specialty mental health services, analyses of number of visits that included all persons in the study population would risk providing misleading findings due to this maldistribution.

Data Analysis

Weighted logistic regression models were developed separately for each group using the logit procedure of Systat[37] to predict the probability of at least one mental health visit using odds ratios (ORs). The Systat procedure allows the use of random samples for one or both of the dichotomous groups and provides a weighting procedure for properly analyzing these samples. For predicting the amount of use, ordinary least squares (OLS) regression was used. Variables were entered into the regression equation following hierarchical procedures recommended by Cohen and Cohen[38] and were ordered according to the Andersen-Newman model: the predisposing variables first, followed by the enabling variables, and then the need variables. Within each set, variables were entered hierarchically according to presumed causal priority. In cases where no causal priority could be inferred, all such variables were entered into the regression equation at the same time.

To test the two study hypotheses, logistic and linear regression models were run with all three groups simultaneously to assess if White women had higher rates and amounts of services use after controlling for predisposing, enabling, and need factors.

RESULTS

As shown in Table 3.1, White women in the population were somewhat older than their Black and Hispanic counterparts with an average age of 51 years compared with 48 years and 49 years, respectively. Regional geographic distribution differs across the three groups: While Black women were disproportionately concentrated in the Washington, D.C., area, Hispanic women were overwhelmingly concentrated in the southern and western states, and White women were more evenly distributed geographically.

Black and Hispanic women were equally and far more likely to be enrolled in the high option plan—79 percent compared with 61 percent of White women.

The remaining variables in Table 3.1 report the educational level and salary of the federal employee/subscriber who may or may not be female and therefore the unit of analysis of this study. As mentioned earlier, data on education and salary were available only for the federal employee, spouses, and dependents. As shown in Table 3.1, White

TABLE 3.1 Sociodemographic Characteristics of Women in Blue Cross/Blue
Shield Federal Employees Plan, by Ethnic Group

Characteristic	Blacks (n = 67,795)	Hispanics (n = 13,063)	Whites (n = 362,494)
Age (in percentages)			
18-29	13.0	11.8	9.7
30-49	35.3	32.2	28.2
50 or more	51.7	56.0	62.1
Average age (in years)	47.9	48.8	51.3
Region (in percentages)			
Washington, D.C., area	43.0	4.2	22.8
Northeast	9.6	2.7	16.5
North central	20.7	3.5	18.6
West	6.2	34.4	12.8
South	20.4	55.2	29.3
High versus low option (in percentages)			
Low option	21.3	21.3	39.2
High option	78.7	78.7	60.8
Years of education of employee (in percentages)			
< 12 years	28.2	39.0	12.2
High school graduate	50.1	41.9	52.8
Some college	12.4	9.4	10.0
College graduate	9.3	9.8	25.1
Average years of education of employee (in years)	11.8	11.2	13.1
Average salary of employee	$21,512	$23,086	$27,759

NOTE: n refers to the total number of claimants in 1983. Column percentages within each demographic group sum to 100%.

employees averaged more education and salary than their Black and
Hispanic counterparts.

Rates of Outpatient Use

Table 3.2 shows the percentage of women who made at least one
outpatient mental health visit during 1983 and results of statistical significance tests of ethnic differences in rates of use ($p < .05$). Overall, Black
women had the lowest rate (2.64 percent), Hispanic women were
slightly higher (3.31 percent), and White women had the highest rate
(4.35 percent), a statistically significant difference. Breakdowns of rates
by age, region, option, and education resulted in similar patterns in

almost all cases. Black versus White differences in rates were statistically significant for the following subgroup categories: women 30-49 years old and 50 or more years old, women residing in the Washington, D.C., area, women enrolled in the high option, and women with some college education. No differences between Hispanic rates and Black or White rates were significant.

A few noteworthy findings can be seen in Table 3.2. For White and Hispanic women, the highest rate of use was in the Washington, D.C., area, while for Black women, the highest rate of use was in the western states. While those with high option enrollment had significantly higher rates of use than low option enrollees, the discrepancy between high versus low option rates was greater for Whites. For all three groups, rates of use increased as the level of education of the federal employee/subscriber increased.

Mean Number of Outpatient Mental Health Visits

As shown in Table 3.2, Hispanic women averaged the fewest visits, followed by Black women, and then White women. Differences between Whites and Blacks and between Whites and Hispanics were statistically significant. Older women in outpatient treatment in all three groups averaged fewer visits than women under age 49. Those living in the Washington, D.C., area and in the northeastern states averaged the most visits while those living in the South averaged the fewest visits. High option enrollees averaged between four and five more visits during the year than low option enrollees. In general, those with more education made more visits.

Results of pairwise tests of group differences in average number of visits (Table 3.2) reveal significant findings for almost all subgroup categories. There is consistently greater use of outpatient mental health services by White women when compared with Black and Hispanic women across various age strata, geographic regions, plan options, and educational levels.

Tests of Study Hypotheses

Results of the logistic and linear regression analyses showed that White women had a greater likelihood of using outpatient mental

TABLE 3.2 Women Who Made an Outpatient Mental Health Visit in 1983 (in percentages) and Mean Total Visits During the Year for Those With a Visit

Characteristic	Blacks (n = 67,795)			Hispanics (n = 13,063)			Whites (n = 362,494)			A	B
	n	%	Mean Visits	n	%	Mean Visits	n	%	Mean Visits		
Overall	1,787	2.64	10.0	432	3.31	8.7	15,773	4.35	13.0	a	ab
Age											
18-29	198	2.24	11.6	37	2.41	9.8	1,458	4.14	15.2	a	a
30-49	958	4.01	11.1	190	4.51	12.0	7,076	6.92	16.5	a	ab
50 or more	631	1.80	7.8	205	2.80	5.4	7,239	3.22	9.1		abc
Region											
Washington, D.C., area	779	2.67	12.5	31	5.71	21.4	4,638	5.60	18.2	a	ac
Northeast	149	2.28	11.6	12	3.35	14.7	2,696	4.51	13.6		a
North central	350	2.49	8.5	18	3.95	7.5	2,468	3.67	10.5		b
West	144	3.41	9.4	148	3.29	8.0	2,071	4.46	11.9		a
South	365	2.64	5.6	223	3.09	7.1	3,900	3.6	8.6		
Option											
Low option	356	2.47	7.0	68	2.45	5.0	4,434	3.12	8.9	a	ab
High option	1,431	2.68	10.8	364	3.54	9.4	11,339	5.14	14.6		ab
Years of education of employee											
<12 years	329	1.94	7.7	125	2.66	5.2	1,272	3.21	7.1		c
High school graduate	829	2.75	9.5	155	3.07	8.4	6,075	3.53	10.9		ab
Some college	207	2.78	11.2	47	4.14	10.1	1,727	5.29	12.4	a	
College graduate	222	3.98	14.2	57	4.83	14.4	5,201	6.36	17.5		a

NOTE: The sums of those who had outpatient treatment across education groups are 1,578, 384, and 14,275 for blacks, Hispanics, and whites, respectively, because not all persons were able to be matched to the Office of Personnel Management database. Column A indicates significant differences in percentage with an outpatient visit; Column B indicates significant differences in number of outpatient visits. For both columns, alpha was specified as .05.
a. Whites and Blacks were significantly different.
b. Whites and Hispanics were significantly different.
c. Hispanics and Blacks were significantly different.

health services ($p < .001$) and had more outpatient psychotherapy visits ($p < .001$) even after controlling for all predisposing, enabling, and need factors. Thus, both hypotheses were affirmed by the data in this study.

Predicting the Odds of Making a Mental Health Visit

Significant predictors ($p < .05$) for all three groups of women (see Table 3.3) include younger age (ORs = 2.3 for Blacks, 1.6 for Hispanics, and 2.2 for Whites); medical dollars of the index person (ORs = 1.1 for Blacks, 1.2 for Hispanics, and 1.3 for Whites), and outpatient mental health visits by other family members (ORs = 2.5 for Blacks, 2.5 for Hispanics, and 1.7 for Whites). Family factors appear to be associated with help-seeking in this population. For every increment of ten outpatient mental health visits by other family members, the likelihood of seeking outpatient mental health treatment increased 1.7 times for White women and 2.5 times for Black and Hispanic women.

Although no other variables were significant for Black or Hispanic women, additional significant predictors for White women included employee education; several regions of residence in contrast to Washington, D.C.; percentage urban of the county; high option enrollment; the psychiatrist to physician ratio in the county; and inpatient mental health treatment of other family members. The strongest of these odds ratios was associated with the latter variable. Thus, White women whose families included at least one member who had inpatient psychiatric treatment were almost 3 times more likely to seek outpatient mental health treatment as their White female counterparts without a family member in inpatient care. Comparable odds ratios for Black and Hispanic women with versus without a family member in inpatient psychiatric care were 1.7 and 2.5, respectively (see Table 3.3).

Predicting the Number of Mental Health Visits

As shown in Table 3.4, most of the variables in the OLS regression models were statistically significant. Only one variable was not statistically significant for White women: salary of the employee. While many of the significant variables—younger age, higher educational level, high option plan, and region of residence—are predictably asso-

TABLE 3.3 Logistic Regression Results Showing Odds of Making at Least One Outpatient Psychotherapy Visit by Women in Blue Cross/Blue Shield Federal Employees Plan

	Blacks		Hispanics		Whites	
Characteristic	Odds Ratio	Signifi-cance	Odds Ratio	Signifi-cance	Odds Ratio	Signifi-cance
Predisposing factors						
(1) Age 30-49 versus 18-29	1.82	.059	1.92	.120	1.72	.000
(1) Age 30-49 versus 50+	2.28	.000	1.64	.036	2.24	.000
(2) Education, employee	1.06	.155	1.05	.226	1.09	.000
(3) Family size	1.02	.894	1.05	.727	0.95	.235
(4) Ethnic % in county	1.00	.340	1.00	.410	1.00	.124
Enabling factors						
(5) Northeast vs. Washington, D.C.	0.94	.876	0.56	.470	0.93	.550
(5) North central vs. Washington, D.C.	0.97	.909	0.65	.547	0.75	.015
(5) West vs. Washington, D.C.	1.30	.517	0.62	.354	0.86	.215
(5) South vs. Washington, D.C.	1.01	.965	0.63	.410	0.73	.003
(5) % Urban in county	1.00	.832	1.01	.340	1.00	.005
(6) Salary ($10,000)	1.00	.995	0.91	.511	1.01	.705
(7) High option? (yes = 1)	1.27	.328	1.61	.131	2.04	.000
(8) Psychiatrist to physician ratio (.1)	1.11	.765	0.74	.517	1.27	.020
Need factors						
(9) Medical $, index person ($5,000)	1.14	.030	1.16	.013	1.27	.000
(10) Medical $, others ($5,000)	0.99	.945	1.04	.707	1.03	.482
(11) Outpatient mental health visits, others	2.49	.000	2.52	.001	1.69	.000
(12) Inpatient mental health, others? (yes = 1)	1.72	.408	2.54	.148	2.89	.000

NOTE: Odds ratios were calculated for (1) salary in units of $10,000, (2) psychiatrist to physician ratio in units of .1, (3) total medical charges for the index person and for the rest of the family in units of $5,000, and (4) outpatient mental health visits for others in the family in units of ten visits.

ciated with higher levels of use, others are lesser known. For example, ethnic congruence is significant in predicting the number of visits for all three groups, though not in the same direction. For Black women, ethnic congruence is positively associated with number of outpatient psychiatric visits, but it is negatively associated for Hispanic and White women. Provider type and setting are also significant, with more visits associated with visiting an office, as opposed to an outpatient hospital mental health clinic, and with visiting a psychologist as opposed to a physician for all three groups.

TABLE 3.4 Ordinary Least Squares Regression Results Predicting Number of Outpatient Psychotherapy Visits for Women With at Least One Visit

Characteristic	Blacks (n = 1,787)		Hispanics (n = 432)		Whites (n = 15,773)	
	B	SE	B	SE	B	SE
Predisposing factors						
(1) Age (range 18 to 99)	-0.15 [b]	0.02	-0.24 [b]	0.05	-0.27 [b]	0.01
(2) Education, employee	0.63 [b]	0.13	-0.80 [b]	0.18	1.01 [b]	0.04
(3) Family size	-0.15	0.42	-0.92	0.71	-0.35 [b]	0.13
(4) Ethnic % in county	0.03 [a]	0.01	-0.08 [b]	0.03	-0.03 [b]	0.00
Enabling factors						
(5) Northeast versus Washington, D.C.	-1.07	1.15	-10.37 [b]	3.84	-3.23 [b]	0.33
(5) North central versus Washington, D.C.	-3.91 [b]	0.87	-15.23 [b]	3.32	-6.12 [b]	0.34
(5) West versus Washington, D.C.	-3.14 [b]	1.22	-11.67 [b]	2.40	-5.24 [b]	0.36
(5) South versus Washington, D.C.	-6.99 [b]	0.81	-11.34 [b]	2.65	-7.72 [b]	0.30
(5) % Urban in county	0.02 [a]	0.01	0.11 [b]	0.03	0.04 [b]	0.00
(6) Salary [c]	0.76 [a]	0.37	-0.18	0.67	0.01	0.09
(7) High option? (yes = 1)	4.29 [b]	0.73	3.65 [a]	1.46	6.86 [b]	0.23
(8) Psychiatrist to physician ratio [c]	2.45 [a]	1.06	3.80	2.50	2.71 [b]	0.29
(9) Office versus hospital	6.75 [b]	0.61	3.63 [b]	1.36	5.80 [b]	0.32
(9) Physician versus psychologist	-2.25 [b]	0.43	-3.14 [b]	0.76	-1.67 [b]	0.13
(9) Physician/psychologist versus other	-1.15	0.75	1.57	1.68	-1.34 [b]	0.24
Need factors						
(10) Medical $, index person [c]	-0.43 [a]	0.20	-0.60	0.34	-0.37 [b]	0.07
(11) Medical $, others [c]	-0.21	0.25	-0.64	0.58	-0.25 [b]	0.09
(12) Outpatient mental health visits, others [c]	2.39 [b]	0.37	2.43 [b]	0.42	2.18 [b]	0.09
(13) Inpatient mental health, others? (yes = 1)	-0.37	1.82	-3.59	2.68	-3.19 [b]	0.72
(14) Index have inpatient mental health?	0.75	0.72	1.27	1.30	1.84 [b]	0.30

a. Statistically significant at the .05 level of alpha.
b. Statistically significant at the .01 level of alpha.
c. Regression weights were calculated for (1) salary in units of $10,000, (2) psychiatrist to physician ratio in units of .1, (3) total medical charges for the index person and for the rest of the family in units of $5,000, and (4) outpatient visits for others in the family in units of ten visits.

DISCUSSION

As demonstrated by this study of a national population of Black, Hispanic, and White women, ethnic differences in use of outpatient mental health services persist even after a number of potentially confounding factors are controlled. As hypothesized, White women were consistently higher users of these services. Although Black women were least likely to receive treatment during the year, Hispanic women averaged the lowest number of visits among users of outpatient mental health treatment. The pattern of higher use by White women held true for a number of sociodemographic subgroups defined by age, geographic region, plan option, and education.

It is particularly noteworthy that differences in salary and educational level were not responsible for higher use by White women. For example, it could be argued that the higher average salary of Whites in the sample explained higher use levels since they could more likely afford the deductible and co-payment requirements of the insurance plan. Yet the analyses found that White women were both more likely to use mental health services and made more visits than their Black and Hispanic counterparts even after controlling for the effects of these and other differences in enabling factors.

Analyses of individual characteristics that predict the probability of service use revealed that regardless of ethnicity, younger women, women with higher medical costs, and women whose family members were in outpatient mental health treatment were more likely to make a mental health visit. These findings might be seen as indicating the influence of stress within the woman's family and related to her own physical health.

Among significant predictors of amount of use given any use, it is notable that significantly higher levels of use were associated for all three groups with visiting an office-based practitioner and with visiting a psychologist. This effect of visiting a psychologist was also reported by Taube et al.[36] It is intriguing that White and Hispanic women in counties with lower proportions of residents of their own ethnic group averaged more mental health visits. This finding fits with the ethnic congruence approach[32] since levels of distress are predicted to be higher among persons residing in counties with fewer residents from their own ethnic group. Of course, higher levels of distress need not necessarily lead to more treatment visits. By contrast, for Black women, a higher percentage of Blacks in the county was significantly associated with more mental health visits—a finding that conflicts with the ethnic congruence approach. In the absence of data necessary to fully test this hypothesis, these findings are only suggestive. They could as well reflect local practice patterns or obscure underlying socioeconomic indicators reflecting greater need for mental health treatment.

As noted earlier, lower use of mental health services by Black and Hispanic women relative to White women was found in a Medicaid-enrolled population.[28] What is noteworthy from this study is that this phenomenon is discernible in a non-poor population of women where presumably even fewer socioeconomic and system barriers are present to inhibit use. It is also worth noting that the influence of differential acculturation is minimized since these women, who are either federal employees or their spouses, are less likely to be unacculturated and/or non-English speaking.

The absence of diagnostic data in the FEP database limited understanding of the nature and severity of the mental problem. While the measures used in this study allowed some approximation of need for mental health services, the findings were possibly affected by this limitation. Future studies would be enhanced by inclusion of measures of mental health status that are reliable and validated for use in diverse ethnic populations. Some researchers have underscored this problem by arguing that the diagnostic data used in cross-ethnic comparisons are suspect since symptom scales may convey different meanings to members of different ethnic groups.[39] In this context, it can be argued that insurance claims data have an advantage over self-report data in studies of ethnic groups where underreporting of embarrassing or socially stigmatizing events such as visiting a mental health specialist is not uncommon.[39]

A second limitation of the FEP database (and of many, if not most other, large empirical databases) is the lack of information on intra-group diversity within the broadly defined ethnic categories. For example, Hispanic groups include Puerto Ricans, Mexican Americans, and Cuban Americans, among many others—all groups that could not be identified for separate analysis in this study. It is an unfortunate necessity in many studies that the "ethnic group" under study typically refers to an array of culturally heterogeneous groups.

Third, the FEP database did not afford analysis of potentially important factors such as marital status and number of children of women in the study. Similarly, sociocultural factors such as gender role burdens and attitudes and beliefs about mental illness and its treatment were not captured by these claims data. Finally, the latest year in the FEP data was 1983 and questions may be raised regarding the relevance of this study's findings given the changes in mental health services delivery that took place in the latter 1980s and early 1990s. It should be noted that the national representativeness of this database would almost definitely have been reduced in the later 1980s as several alternative insurance plans were introduced to provide greater choice. BC/BS's prominence as the major insurer of federal employees virtually disappeared as the proportion of enrollees who opted for BC/BS dropped considerably. In the following section, it is argued that these data have direct relevance to discussions of changes in health and mental health benefits under a national plan for health care.

IMPLICATIONS FOR MENTAL
HEALTH SERVICES DELIVERY

Two key issues arise from previous research and from the present study that have relevance for mental health policies and services delivery: (1) Unmet need for mental health treatment appears greater among Black and Hispanic women compared with White women, and (2) even generously insured Black and Hispanic women are less likely to use outpatient mental health services and make fewer visits after entry into treatment when compared with White women. The types of changes in services delivery required to reduce unmet need among ethnic minority women are not fully understood and require critical attention. This study's finding that socioeconomic factors cannot explain ethnic differences in use points to a need to go beyond conventional wisdom that liberalizing health benefits will be sufficient to address the health and mental health needs of ethnic minority groups. Thus, changes in health policies designed to reduce economic barriers to care

are necessary but not sufficient to close the gap in unmet need for these groups.

It is highly unlikely that lower use of outpatient mental health services by Black and Hispanic women is attributable to a lack of need for these services. It is more plausible to reason that even generously insured ethnic women encounter system delivery barriers or have attitudes and beliefs that inhibit use of psychotherapeutic services.

Many researchers have suggested that cultural or attitudinal factors play a role in lower use by Blacks and Hispanics.[7,8,28] Such factors can take many forms, from reluctance to use a mental health delivery system dominated by English-speaking Whites to a preference for alternative healers or clergy more attuned to the culture of the individual. The presence of female traditional healers in many cultures further enhances the likelihood that a woman in distress may feel more comfortable with seeking help from a familiar source.

It is recommended that mental health providers improve their understanding of ethnic women's perceptions of barriers as well as their use of alternative sources of help. A more balanced and complete picture would also include attention to protective factors and coping resources related to ethnic identity,[40,41] rather than exclusively focusing on individual psychopathology. Older ethnic minority women in particular have been identified as having strengths as "psychological survivors"[11]—self-reliant strategists with coping skills honed by years of adversity.[40] At the same time, it would be misleading to imply that these women do not suffer from stress or experience mental illness and therefore do not have unmet needs.

In addition to cultural and attitudinal barriers, aspects of the services delivery system play a role in lower use of outpatient mental health services by ethnic women. The absence of ethnic providers is one of the most conspicuous barriers. Also, the intersection of lower-social-class status, ethnicity, and residential segregation leads to inequities in services delivery that disproportionately affect Blacks and Hispanics. An inner-city resident who has insurance coverage will still have more difficulty finding a clinic or provider than a resident of an affluent neighborhood.

An ignorance of more subtle aspects of cultural, social-class, and gender differences may contribute to an appearance of insensitivity, which may be unintended, but is nevertheless powerful in its impact.

For ethnic minority women, fears of discrimination due to ethnicity and gender cannot be easily dismissed. Furthermore, treatment programs that rely on psychotherapeutic modalities requiring intimate self-disclosure may be seen as inappropriate or irrelevant in addressing the problems faced by ethnic minority women. These problems may arise from poverty and discrimination and from familial and social responsibilities and whose resolution lies in a more holistic approach to treatment.

Qualitative studies are needed to examine the process of mutual estrangement that can result from cultural and gender-based misunderstandings between therapist and client. In the meantime, mental health program planners and administrators can enhance use of services by employing more culturally sensitive outreach and referral programs.

Taking a broader perspective, it can be argued that this study's findings have applicability to planning mental health services for women in the United States as the 21st century approaches. While information on all forms of mental health services use by various subpopulations is critical to establishing sound policies in financing and services delivery, empirical studies of women's mental health use are particularly needed since so little attention has been given to women's health and mental health needs.

Clearly, Black and Hispanic women in the FEP population are not fully representative of their uninsured counterparts in the general U.S. population where the prevalence of severe mental disorders is reported to be higher.[3] Although differences may be expected due to greater need associated with the lower socioeconomic status of ethnic minorities, this study's primary finding is that White women use more mental health services even in an insured population. Increasing equity and access, although certainly worthy goals, will not necessarily close the "ethnic gap" in women's use of mental health services. Further research is needed to establish the extent to which this gap is due to lower availability of services, lower acceptability of services, or both. Mental health policies and programs designed to meet the needs of ethnic minority women will be more effective if they address barriers arising from the intersection of gender and ethnic differences.

REFERENCES

1. President's Commission on Mental Health: *Volume 2: Task Panel Reports: The Nature and Scope of the Problem*. Washington, DC: U.S. Government Printing Office, 1978.
2. Olmedo EL, Parron DL: Mental health of minority women: Some special issues. *Professional Psychology* 1981; 12:103-111.
3. Robins LN, Regier DA (Eds.): *Psychiatric Disorders in America: The Epidemiologic Catchment Area Study*. New York: Free Press, 1991.
4. Shapiro S, Skinner EA, Kessler LG, et al.: Utilization of health and mental services: Three Epidemiologic Catchment Area sites. *Archives of General Psychiatry* 1984; 41:971-978.
5. Shapiro S, Skinner EA, Kramer M, et al.: Measuring need for mental health services in a general population. *Medical Care* 1985; 23:1033-1043.
6. Regier DA, Narrow WE, Rae DS, et al.: The de facto U.S. mental and addictive disorders service system. *Archives of General Psychiatry* 1993; 50:85-94.
7. Hough RL, Landsverk JA, Karno M, et al.: Utilization of health and mental health services by Los Angeles Mexican Americans and non-Hispanic Whites. *Archives of General Psychiatry* 1978; 44:702-709.
8. Wells KB, Golding JM, Hough RL, et al.: Factors affecting the probability of use of general and medical health and social/community services for Mexican Americans and non-Hispanic Whites. *Medical Care* 1988; 26:441-452.
9. Sussman LK, Robins LN, Earls F: Treatment-seeking for depression by Black and White Americans. *Social Science and Medicine* 1987; 24:187-196.
10. Leaf PJ, Bruce ML: Gender differences in the use of mental health-related services: A re-examination. *Journal of Health and Social Behavior* 1987; 28:171-183.
11. Rodeheaver D, Datan N: The challenge of double jeopardy: Toward a mental health agenda for aging women. *American Psychologist* 1988; 43:648-654.
12. Mays VM: Black women and stress: Utilization of self-help groups for stress reduction. *Women and Therapy* 1986; 4:67-79.
13. Penn NE, Levy VL, Penn BP: Professional services preferred by urban elderly women. *American Journal of Social Psychiatry* 1986; 4:129-130.
14. Palacios M, Franco JN: Counseling Mexican-American women. *Journal of Multicultural Counseling and Development* 1986; 14:124-131.
15. Amaro H, Russo NF: Hispanic women and mental health: An overview of contemporary issues in research and practice. *Psychology of Women Quarterly* 1987; 17:393-407.
16. True RH: Psychotherapeutic issues with Asian American women. *Sex Roles* 1990; 22:477-486.
17. Yamamoto J, Silva JA: Do Hispanics underutilize mental health services? In: Gaviria M, Arana JD (Eds.): *Health and Behavior: Research Agenda for Hispanics*. Chicago: Simon Bolivar Hispanic American Psychiatric Research and Training Center, 1987, pp. 88-99.
18. Sue S: Community mental health services to minority groups. *American Psychologist* 1977; 32:616-624.
19. Armstrong HE, Ishiki P, Heiman J, et al.: Service utilization by Black and White clientele in an urban community mental health center: Revised assessment of an old problem. *Community Mental Health Journal* 1984; 20:269-280.
20. Scheffler RM, Miller AG: Demand analysis of mental health service use among ethnic subpopulations. *Inquiry* 1989; 26:202-215.

21. O'Sullivan MJ, Peterson PD, Cox GB, et al.: Ethnic populations and community mental health services ten years later. *American Journal of Community Psychology* 1989; 47:17-30.

22. Rosenfield S: Race differences in involuntary hospitalization: Psychiatric versus labeling perspectives. *Journal of Health and Social Behavior* 1984; 25:14-23.

23. Russo NF, Sobel SB: Sex differences in the utilization of mental health facilities. *Professional Psychology* 1981; 12:7-19.

24. Russo NF, Amaro H, Winter M: The use of inpatient mental health services by Hispanic women. *Psychology of Women Quarterly* 1987; 11:427-441.

25. Rosenstein MJ: *Hispanic Americans and Mental Health Services: A Comparison of Hispanic, Black, and White Admissions to Selected Mental Health Facilities, 1975.* Washington, DC: U.S. Government Printing Office, 1980.

26. Wells KB, Manning WG, Duan N, et al.: Sociodemographic factors and the use of outpatient mental health services. *Medical Care* 1986; 24:75-85.

27. Neighbors HW, Howard CS: Sex differences in professional help-seeking among adult Black Americans. *American Journal of Community Psychology* 1987; 15:403-417.

28. Temkin-Greener H, Clark KT: Ethnicity, gender, and utilization of mental health services in a Medicaid population. *Social Science and Medicine* 1988; 26:989-996.

29. Broman CL: Race differences in professional help seeking. *American Journal of Community Psychology* 1987; 15:473-480.

30. Lopez S: Mexican-American usage of mental health facilities: Under-utilization considered. In: Baron A (Ed.): *Explorations in Chicano Psychology.* New York: Praeger, 1981, pp. 139-148.

31. Andersen R, Newman JF: Societal and individual determinants of medical care utilization in the United States. *Milbank Memorial Fund Quarterly: Health and Society* 1973; 51:95-124.

32. Tweed DL, Goldsmith HF, Jackson DJ, et al.: Racial congruity as a contextual correlate of mental disorder. *American Journal of Orthopsychiatry* 1990; 60:392-400.

33. Knesper DJ, Wheeler JR, Pagnucco DJ: Mental health services providers' distribution across counties in the United States. *American Psychologist* 1984; 39:1424-1434.

34. Wells K, Manning W, Duan J, et al.: *Cost Sharing and the Demand for Ambulatory Mental Health Services.* Santa Monica, CA: RAND, 1982.

35. Horgan CM: The demand for ambulatory mental health services from specialty providers. *Health Services Research* 1986; 21:291-298.

36. Taube CA, Kessler LG, Burns BJ: Estimating the probability and level of ambulatory mental health services use. *Health Services Research* 1986; 21:321-327.

37. Steinberg D, Colla P: *Logit: A Supplementary Module for Systat.* Evanston, IL: Systat, 1991.

38. Cohen J, Cohen P: *Applied Multiple Regression/Correlation for the Behavioral Sciences.* Hillsdale, NJ: Lawrence Erlbaum, 1983.

39. Vernon SW, Roberts RE: Prevalence of treated and untreated psychiatric disorders in three ethnic groups. *Social Science and Medicine* 1982; 16:1575-1582.

40. Padgett DK: Aging minority women: Issues in research and health policy. *Women and Health* 1989; 14:213-225.

41. Vega WA, Rumbaut RG: Ethnic minorities and health. *Annual Review of Sociology* 1991; 17:351-383.

4

Great Expectations

Challenges for Women as Mental Health Administrators

Susan D. Scheidt, Psy.D.

Women are developing a higher profile in many areas of leadership as the year 2000 approaches. Concerns about women's ability to be competent, effective leaders are increasingly challenged. However, barriers to women achieving power remain. Despite recent additions of women to the U.S. Senate, women are still profoundly underrepresented in politics.[1] Corporate business is still dominated by men.[2] Women leaders are glaringly absent in academia. In 1990, 16.9 percent of U.S. physicians were women, and that number is predicted to increase to 30 percent by the year 2010. And yet, while 20 percent of full-time medical school faculty are women, as of 1991 there were no women deans in any of the 126 medical schools. Although the percentage of female residents in psychiatry grew from 36.2 percent to 42.9 percent between 1980 and 1990, as of 1990, there were only two women chairs of academic psychiatry departments in the United States.[3]

Hurdles to women's leadership have been explored and challenged by several women at the University of California, San Francisco, in the San Francisco General Hospital Department of Psychiatry. Together we have developed an inpatient team focused on serving women who have serious mental illness. There have been challenges in creating treatment

NOTE: This chapter appeared as an article in the *Journal of Mental Health Administration,* 1994, Vol. 21, No. 4, pp. 419-429.

opportunities for this underserved population, struggles related to an all-female leadership group establishing authority, and internal soul-searching as each of us comes to terms with our own expectations and stereotypes of powerful women. There have also been numerous rewards, from the responses of patients and trainees who participate on the Women's Focus Team to the mutual support of working with other women. This chapter addresses both the challenges and the rewards. It describes the inpatient program and presents case examples of the manifestations of women's leadership in a psychiatric setting. The chapter concludes by describing the implications for mental health administration and offers suggestions for promoting women's leadership.

San Francisco General Hospital's Specialized Inpatient Programs

The Department of Psychiatry at San Francisco General Hospital (SFGH), a major teaching site for the University of California (UCSF), is unique in many ways. A prominent feature of the department, and that for which it has gained the most recognition, is the commitment to culturally competent inpatient treatment for ethnic and gender minorities. Each of the five locked psychiatric inpatient units is organized with a specific focus. The units have treatment programs geared toward African Americans, Asians, Latinos, women, gay and lesbian patients, and HIV/AIDS and forensic issues. Each unit attempts to recruit staff who are interested in the unique needs of that population and are willing to learn and participate in the appropriate treatment interventions. Neither the staff nor the patients on a unit are exclusively from the "focus" group; ethnic and gender diversity within units is common.

Each of the units has the capacity to treat approximately 20 patients, with the exception of the forensic ward, which has a capacity of 12. Ninety-five percent of the patients are admitted on involuntary commitments, and the average length of stay is 11 days. All of the units treat general psychiatric problems, particularly major psychotic and affective disorders, serious personality disorders, and coexisting psychiatric and substance abuse disorders. SFGH is the only public hospital in San

Francisco; consequently, many of the patients are uninsured or are undocumented immigrants.

The Women's Focus Program

The Women's Focus Team began on Unit 7A in 1984. The need for a specific women's focus arose from the observation that a number of women being admitted to the department had particular problems related to childbearing. Most prominent were women who presented as pregnant and psychotic. The unique needs of these women were often overlooked, and neither behavioral nor psychopharmacological interventions were differentiated from those for the general psychiatric population. The women were rarely thought to be sexually active, and detailed gynecological histories were not consistently obtained. Attention was seldom paid to these women's children, who had often been placed in foster care at birth, but whose existence was still significant to the patients. Treatment strategies that were developed by the team to address these issues are documented elsewhere.[4]

Over time, other needs specific to women with serious mental illness became prominent. Most dramatic was the incidence of sexual trauma in the lives of the women admitted for inpatient treatment. Consistent with the literature linking sexual trauma to severe psychiatric disorders,[5-12] histories of childhood sexual and physical abuse are common in the women admitted to the team. A simple yes/no question ("Have you ever been sexually abused?") revealed a 43 percent endorsement in 93 women admitted over a period of one year.[13] Often just asking the question helps the patient to feel less isolated. There are also specific women's groups held on the unit to discuss these issues, and attempts are made to link the patients with treatment and self-help groups in the community to continue with recovery after hospitalization. However, the degree of psychological disintegration is often profound, and some of the women are unable to tolerate direct discussion of the trauma in their lives. Other modes of expression, particularly nonverbal art and creative projects in occupational therapy, are incorporated into treatment, with symbolic representations of abuse acknowledged by the staff and interpreted when appropriate.

While not an explicit goal of the team, a benefit has been the development of women as leaders. Female staff at all levels serve as role models for women patients and trainees. Most of the staff on the Women's Focus Team are women. The executive leadership group on the inpatient ward (which includes the Latino Focus Team) are four women: the unit chief psychologist, the unit chief psychiatrist, and two master's-level nurses, all of whom hold faculty appointments with UCSF. The Women's Team is led by a female attending psychiatrist, and other women hold the positions of social worker, occupational therapist, registered nurses, and licensed psychiatric technicians. Although there are a few male nursing staff on the team, other male staff on the unit working with the Latino Focus Team, and male patients on the ward, the women admitted to the Women's Focus Team are primarily treated by other women.

CHALLENGES FOR WOMEN LEADERS

Classic ideas about femininity are not associated with power. As Cantor and Bernay write in their 1992 book *Women in Power: The Secrets of Leadership,*[1]

> The old-fashioned spectrum of femininity typically encompasses attributes such as affectionate, sympathetic, sensitive to the needs of others, understanding, compassionate, warm, tender, fond of children, gentle, yielding, cheerful, shy, responsive to flattery, loyal, soft-spoken, gullible, or even childlike. There is no room in the traditional female stereotype for powerful. Femininity doesn't imply tough, strong, or decisive. (p. 35)

Stereotypes of gender roles are mirrored in traditional attitudes toward child rearing. Many girls are still socialized to be good, kind, and virtuous rather than adventurous and risk taking. They are also often taught that being accepted is a higher aim than being powerful and competent. The little girl who has been raised traditionally to see herself as wife and mother is seldom supported in the same way to be an independent, self-reliant leader. Indeed, the priority placed on relationships may seem antithetical to the independence associated with a career. Although society rewards power, a woman who seeks it may still lose acceptance.

In our work as a group of four women who lead the complex inpatient unit housing a women's treatment team described above, we have found that we need to acknowledge and address stereotypes that may interfere with women's leadership in relation to several groups. These include our own stereotypes about ourselves and each other as female leaders, the expectations and biases of the staff and trainees we supervise, the projections of our patients onto us as leaders, and our relationship to the executive administration within our department. Each of these areas is discussed below.

Addressing Our Own Stereotypes
of Women as Leaders

Women in leadership positions must confront their own negative images about women's competence. Each of us in this setting has had to accept her own desire for power and have confidence in her ability to effectively exert it. Self-doubt sometimes arises; the beauty of working with other competent women is that we can do a "reality check" with each other. When one of us is uncertain about a perception or decision, she can ask the others for feedback, trusting that her self-reflection will not be misconstrued as weakness as it might be by men. There is also enough safety within the group that we can point out times when one of us is distorting or overreacting to a situation, and this constructive advice is usually well received.

However, there are times that our own negative images of women leaders may interfere with the way we work with each other. Luise Eichenbaum and Susie Orbach wrote about some of these more difficult issues in their 1988 book *Between Women*.[14] Originally published in Great Britain under the title *Bittersweet*, the book discusses "love, envy and competition in women's friendships." They acknowledge the positive, supportive, and cooperative aspects of women's relationships with each other, stressing the joy and pleasure that can emerge from such collaborations. However, women sometimes have such a need to idealize these relationships that the more negative aspects of the interaction may be repressed. Feelings of hurt and anger, envy and competition, and even guilt and sorrow are not uncommon between women. Some of the feelings are in response to particular conflicts; others come from

the disappointment of admitting there are any conflicts or any differences at all, thereby losing the idealized object.

Eichenbaum and Orbach discuss the prohibitions that women place
on being able to talk about these very real phenomena with each other.
They write,

> There is a post-feminist self-imposed censorship on certain feelings that
> women consider unacceptable. Feelings, for example, of competition
> and envy are rampant. No woman today escapes them, but every
> women feels conflicted by them. There is a new privatization of
> women's experience, but this isolation is not identical to the old isola-
> tion. It is similar in that just as before women are experiencing self-
> doubt, self-blame, feelings of inadequacy, envy of other women. But this
> time around the conflicts are more complex.
> There are stronger forces at odds. (pp. 31-32)

The need for connection sometimes makes it painful to confront each
other directly. For instance, the two clinical nurse specialists, who are
also close personal friends, were forced to make a decision about which
of them would take a less desirable work assignment. Although neither
of them wanted the job, they had difficulty being direct with each other,
for fear it would threaten their friendship. When there are conflicts such
as these, it is often painful and inconsistent with our self-perception of
working as a cooperative group. Subtleties of competition may emerge
without being addressed. The challenge for us as female leaders, then,
is to be able to acknowledge what are common phenomena in women's
relationships with each other and not feel threatened should the idyllic
merger not be flawless, to take the risk of saying, "I'm angry" or "I'm
envious" and trusting the relationship to survive.

Stereotypes of Staff/Trainees
of Women in Leadership

The inpatient environment is often a very intense milieu with a culture and life of its own. Working with psychotic patients promotes an
atmosphere where primary process is the norm, and staff often become
desensitized to expressions of rage, sexuality, threatening, and even
murderous impulses. While people who work in this setting may become somewhat accustomed to the patients' distortions and projec-

tions, staff are often vulnerable to their own primary processes becoming activated.

Staff members in such an intense and stressful work environment often look to their leaders, male or female, to direct, to advocate for them, and to provide nurturance. However, simultaneously the leaders' authority is often met with resistance. These expectations and ambivalence seem to be heightened toward women leaders.

The pervasive cultural view that women should be powerless, nurturing, and submissive coexists with, and is perhaps a response to, the fantasy that women are potentially more powerful and dangerous than men. Femininity has been characterized as artistic and mystical representations of "Mother" throughout the ages: The Good Mother is portrayed as nurturing, loving, and caretaking; the Terrible Mother is aggressive, engulfing, devouring, ensnaring; the Great Mother encompasses all of these features.[15]

These ancient archetypes become powerful projections when associated with women leaders. Women are approached with both fascination and fear. In current society, however, the Good Mother image is often considered to be the most desirable and acceptable. As described earlier, girls are traditionally raised to be sweet, loving, nurturing, receptive; aggressive impulses are discouraged, and expressions of anger or even discontent are not acceptable. The first projection onto a woman leader can be a desire for limitless nurturance and care along with fear that she is too weak to protect the group. There is often bitter disappointment when the leader is inevitably unable to gratify all the needs of the individuals or the unit. The staff can become resentful, angry, and act out over the frustration of not being given enough. The leader may be devalued as weak, ineffective, and rendered powerless by those she is attempting to lead.

The Terrible Mother archetype gets expressed as the "Nurse Ratched" image in psychiatric hospitals. This is the projection of a powerful, destructive, castrating woman, a "bitch on wheels" who wields her power in particularly evil ways. She is feared and hated. Women leaders who appropriately set limits and exert their authority are often devalued with this sort of stereotype.

Sometimes when there is a group of women working together, the women get split from each other in staff perception. For example, we have noticed in the Unit 7A executive leadership group of four women that we are often split into "two and two" by the staff. The two clinical nurse specialists, who by definition are direct supervisors and evaluators of the nursing staff, receive projections consistent with the Terrible Mother, that is, powerful, and not nurturing enough. The psychiatrist and psychologist, largely because we do not give direct evaluations to the nursing staff, are often seen as accepting and responsive. This sometimes leads to us responding to the projections of the Good Mother and trying to take on tasks in unrealistic ways to fulfill all the expectations of the unit staff. As a group of four leaders, we need to recognize the potential for this split and support one another. It is sometimes tempting for those of us being portrayed as the Good Mother to play into the split; it feels more tolerable than being devalued. What we need to recognize, however, is that we are all ultimately rendered ineffective as leaders when we foster unrealistic expectations and allow ourselves to become polarized.

The combination of a Latino team and a women's team on the same unit makes for interesting similarities and contrasts. Both teams have developed considerable expertise in treating post-traumatic stress disorder. The Latino team sees many Central Americans who have witnessed civil war and have been exposed to torture, and the women's team has specialized in addressing issues of childhood and adult sexual trauma in women. Both teams also place a high value on family issues and children. However, projections of the Good Mother are prominent in Latino culture, as exemplified by the concept of the Madonna, selfless and devoted to her children. And though machismo is a misunderstood concept that unfairly stereotypes Latino men as controlling or even abusive, the protective authority assumed by males in many traditional Latino households leaves little room for recognizing female leadership.

This has implications for the mixed groups of staff on Unit 7A, which includes both men and women from Caucasian, Latino, African American, and Asian backgrounds. Various cultural norms may contribute to both men and women viewing women's leadership with ambivalence. Frustration is sometimes expressed by staff in terms of "not knowing who is in charge," yet when women's authority is asserted, resistance is often seen in the form of the staff ignoring or protesting directives from the leaders. When two new psychiatrists started on the unit at the same time, one a Caucasian woman and the other a Latino man, the woman was subject to much more staff criticism than the man. Critique often centered on her not being nurturing enough and not seeking enough staff input into decisions, even though the man and woman did not seem to differ dramatically in their approaches.

Another unit debate centers on who is able to help in situations in which a patient is highly agitated and may require extra staff to calm him or her down. In some cases, this may require physically restraining the patient. While all staff are trained in both the psychological and physical interventions to help calm or contain a patient, there are often heated debates whether or not female staff should be involved, particularly with physical restraint. The majority of women on the unit feel capable of such intervention and are offended when it is suggested that only men are equipped to handle such crises. It seems to most frequently be the male staff who mention feeling safer with other men helping in these situations. Overall, it is important to acknowledge that both genders are trained and competent in these interventions and to make clinical decisions on the basis of the combination of staff to which an individual patient is most likely to respond.

There are trainees from all disciplines on the unit: psychiatry residents; psychology fellows; and nursing, social work, and occupational therapy students. The majority of trainees who work on the women's team are women. They typically report positive experiences, mostly regarding the impact of seeing strong, effective women in leadership positions. The psychiatry residents in particular, who come from the male-dominated field of medicine, express an appreciation for the more egalitarian style of leadership demonstrated on the Women's Focus Team. However, there are sometimes complaints about the diffused nature of our decision making. Needing to coordinate with several staff members around treatment decisions as opposed to giving and receiving direct orders is often a formidable challenge for trainees who are already bombarded with learning new information.

Not all of the trainees or staff on the inpatient unit are women. The men who work on the unit are sensitive to women's issues and are involved in our discussions of gender-related issues. They have sometimes expressed the discomfort of being a minority on the unit, and they have talked about wanting more seminars on men's issues to balance the emphasis on women's treatment. Overall, the men and women who work on Unit 7A know that the leadership is composed of women and are interested enough in the concept to choose to work in this environment.

Patients' Reactions to Women Leaders

Most often the reactions of women patients to having women-focused treatment, a female peer group, and competent women treaters as role models are positive. They state that they feel more comfortable with women when discussing issues such as sexual abuse by men or gynecological problems. Yet our patients are subject to maintaining the same negative stereotypes as others in society, sometimes even more so. Those patients who have been raised in chronically dysfunctional systems have often developed rigid gender stereotypes, perhaps in an attempt to order their chaotic worlds. We have seen this as a devaluation of women as effective professionals. One woman patient with rigid sex role stereotypes said to the female psychiatrist treating her, "Woman's place is at home in service to her husband. You have no business being here. And proper ladies always wear dresses!" Other patients with histories of maternal abuse or neglect may have difficulty accepting the compassion shown to them by the treatment team. They may defend against being disillusioned again by becoming hostile, devaluing, or increasingly paranoid. Some women patients with borderline features feel especially threatened by the potential loss of boundaries and psychological merger they fear with women caregivers. It is not uncommon for them to engage in a struggle with the clinician in what might be understood as a need to maintain their separateness and sense of self.

Women patients are sometimes particularly intrusive with women leaders. They want to know if we are married, have children, or where we live. Comments on the leaders' clothing is quite common. The female leaders on Unit 7A are reasonably comfortable engaging our patients on such issues. While we do not answer all of their questions, we conceptualize them as the patient's attempt to identify with a positive woman role model, and respond accordingly.

Male patients also exhibit a range of reactions to women leaders. It seems that in many instances, men are less likely to be threatening or assaultive toward a female than male, and a woman can often soothe or "talk down" an agitated male quite effectively. However, we also see patients who turn to ethnic or gender slurs when angry, and the female staff are frequently subject to verbal abuse, such as being called a "bitch." Some non-Latino males have expressed resentment at being on a unit with a women's focus and Latino focus, and worry that their specific needs will not be addressed.

Resolving power issues within genders as well as across genders is a challenge on a locked inpatient unit where 95 percent of the patients are involuntarily admitted. We have attempted to address these issues by integrating principles from psychiatric rehabilitation literature.[16] This involves making patients more active participants in treatment and giving them choices wherever possible. For instance, patients may make choices as simple as which chair they prefer when meeting with the therapist to more complex decisions such as medication preferences. While it is therapeutic for all staff to apply these principles, one could argue that it is a style that comes more naturally to women, who tend to focus more on relationship and less on power.

Women's Leadership and Department Administration

There is much evidence that the administration in the Department of Psychiatry at SFGH supports women in this setting. While the chief and assistant chief of the department at SFGH are men, 7 of the 12 members of the departmental Executive Committee are women, as are half of the six unit chiefs. The director of residency training at this site is female, and the Ethnic Minorities and Gender Committee (EMGIC), an influential group within the department, is also led by a woman. In terms of our inpatient unit, the development of a women's team and the support of an all-female leadership group and the dual-leadership model of two women as "co-chiefs" speaks to administration's commitment to women's treatment as well as to the career development of female staff.

One dynamic our department has begun to acknowledge is that though we have extolled the virtues of our diversity programs and congratulated ourselves for our ingenuity and openness in developing them, there exists a shadow side to these accomplishments. We too can be vulnerable to our own subtle or not-so-subtle racism and sexism. When we cling too tightly to our self-perceptions of being "above all that," we miss opportunities to evaluate our own vulnerabilities and grow.

This is illustrated in the difficulty the department administration sometimes has in understanding our unit's model of collaborative leadership. We really have conceptualized our leadership style as collaborative, with the group of four in our leadership group sharing the responsibilities of managing a diverse and complex staff of about 35 people. While our roles and tasks are well defined and we each hold specific areas of responsibility, we do share the major decision making on the unit with one another. If all of us are not available in a crisis, any one or any combination of us is likely to make the decision and process it with the group later. Understandably, this is a break from the usual hierarchical structure, and one that others may not fully endorse. We are often asked by both male and female members of the department administration, "But who's really in charge?" "*We* are," is one answer we sometimes give, or we ask, "In charge of what specific tasks?" This does require more explaining and more effort on the part of others to understand how we function. And yet overall we have found this to be an effective way of managing our ward, one that is rich in its complexities and one that models cooperation and shared responsibility to our staff and our trainees.

Each of the other four inpatient units in our department has one designated unit chief, a psychiatrist. Our ward's co-unit chief model, shared by two women, a psychiatrist and a psychologist, is unique in its leadership structure. The question, "Who's really in charge?" sometimes arises in this context as well, though over time our colleagues have learned to see us as a team. The psychiatrist clearly has responsibility for supervising all medical aspects of care, which are numerous in this urban setting. The psychologist has more responsibility for developing and managing the program on the ward. We are both outspoken and affectively expressive women, and we find that this combination is quite dynamic. As two women leading the inpatient unit (with our nursing colleagues), the main drawback of our combined persona tends to be that we are sometimes seen as "overly emotional" or "having too much affect." While we are comfortable with our level of expression, we are sometimes perceived as having more problems managing our ward than others simply because we express the issues openly. Incidentally, this has also been a stigmatization that has plagued the African American focused unit, the only other ward headed by a woman. Over time, with continued demonstration of our competence, our leadership skills are being recognized and acknowledged.

In the harsh economic realities of the current health care market, it is not enough to say that it simply "feels good" to work with other women. We must be able to demonstrate the value of a women's focus team and show that our leadership model is effective. These are not easy effects to measure, but our unit has kept pace with the other wards in the department in terms of numbers of patients admitted and discharged and maintaining the department's target level of acuity for reimbursement purposes.

We want to be able to demonstrate that our style of leadership can contribute to moving the field ahead to new areas, beyond simply maintaining current standards and practices. Stereotypes of female passivity may lead others to misinterpret our cooperative approach as not active or aggressive enough to make needed changes. This is not our concern. Fighting against the status quo is a familiar arena for strong, professional women even if the "fight" is not in the context of male war metaphors such as "going to battle" or being "in the trenches."

It is important to be aware of possible vulnerabilities our style may bring to our work. Recently, we have reflected on some of the difficulties our unit has had in moving toward a more acute treatment model with less time for the psychological interventions we value. This is clearly not just a women's issue; it is one with which everyone in our department must come to terms. Our hope is that the process-oriented tone we have set on the unit as women leaders will help our staff cope with the inevitable changes in the health care arena.

Qualities of Female Leadership: The Value of a Woman's Perspective

We believe many of the features of our leadership style to be a function of having an all-women executive group as opposed to all-men or a mixed-gender management team. Admitting our vulnerabilities to one another seems to come easier than it does in mixed groups; we often integrate examples from our personal lives to make a point when meeting with only women that we do not share as easily when men are present, for fear of appearing "nonprofessional."

Gilligan[17] has introduced a concept she terms "the strategy of the web" to describe a particularly female paradigm of leading; it is further developed in Helgesen's book *The Female Advantage: Women's Ways of Leadership.*[2]

The concept is one of a nonhierarchical organizational structure: The leader is in the center of the web, reaching out, instead of at the top of a pyramid reaching down. The priority is inclusion, and the figurehead is the *heart* rather than the *head*. Therefore, a woman leader is the heart of an organization; her authority comes from connection to the people around her rather than from obedience from those below. As is seen in the Unit 7A executive leadership group, there is less emphasis on rank. Yet although the lines of authority may seem more diffuse, the women in these organizations are very much the leaders, taking final responsibility for decisions.

The "strategy" of the web is that of weaving. It is, as Helgesen describes, "guided by opportunity, proceeds by the use of intuition, and is characterized by a patience that comes of waiting to see what comes next," "a recognition and acceptance of destiny as the interweave of past and future, of chance and work."[2] This is not a passive stance; successful women need to be actively involved in shaping their destiny. Yet the awareness and acceptance that one ultimately cannot control the universe is key to this philosophy, trusting that opportunities for growth will continually present themselves. The web structure promotes interaction, the acknowledgment of individuals, and direction from the heart of the organization, which can lead to a more humane workplace.

Another feature of women's leadership is that women tend to have a more holistic approach to health care. The women's treatment team at SFGH has found that many of the women we treat have multiple, complex variables affecting their lives that are not adequately addressed within the prevailing medical model. We have to broaden our perspective and view the woman as a whole being. This requires paying attention to sociocultural factors such as poverty, violence in the home and on the streets, lack of education, and the effects of substance abuse on families and individuals. We gather detailed reproductive histories for our women patients, including discussions of abortions as well as children they may have relinquished. Some issues that may appear to be "nonpsychiatric" but that need to be addressed include attention to child care needs, housing, gynecological health maintenance such as birth control and safe sex education, and referrals to women's programs treating substance abuse and sexual trauma. With staff, more flexible work hours may be established for child care needs or attending important family functions, recognizing that work is only one part of people's lives. This sort of approach, as long as it operates within clear guidelines and is fair to all staff, can create greater job satisfaction and effectiveness.

We believe that women tend to be less linear in decision making than men and that we are able to synthesize conflicting, sometimes contradictory, pieces of information to produce creative treatment plans. While men certainly have the capacity to think holistically, it seems to us that it comes to women somewhat more easily. The early developmental task whereby boys need to separate from mother to establish a sense of self[18] may contribute to men's view of the world as separate pieces that are rationally linked together. The woman's experience of connectedness and relationship allows her to see the interdependence of people and the universe.

IMPLICATIONS FOR MENTAL HEALTH ADMINISTRATION

Some men and women deny that there are any hurdles to women in leadership positions, claiming that with the recent "Year of the Woman" phenomenon, women may actually have an advantage. Other women so embrace the concept of being disadvantaged that they sabotage their own opportunities, isolating themselves from the mainstream or becoming so angry about the challenges that they are not able to network with male colleagues. Our experience in leadership, particularly in a clinical/academic setting, requires a perspective somewhere between these two. One cannot deny the difficulties that women face based on gender; neither can one wallow in a victim stance. Following are some suggestions for establishing oneself as a female leader based on the experiences described above.

1. *Acknowledge gender differences.* Early literature on women's leadership encouraged women to "become like a man" to succeed.[19] While

this thinking is outdated, some women still approach organizations pretending that there are no gender differences. A first step to excelling as a woman leader is to acknowledge that differences between men's and women's work styles, problem-solving approaches, and communication styles do exist.[20] These things are important for women to recognize and admit to themselves, allowing them to become more aware in their interactions with both male and female colleagues. These phenomena can also be conveyed to others to help break cycles of discrimination. As leaders in a mental health setting, we encourage our colleagues to look at these issues and discuss them more openly than might be acceptable in corporate settings.

2. *Seize opportunities for leadership.* Women need to begin to see themselves as leaders, fighting their own self-imposed sexism. When women are asked to take on leadership positions, the first response is sometimes a self-defeating fear, such as, "I could never handle all of that responsibility." Those who see themselves as clinicians may feel comfortable in a helping role, but hesitate to move into leadership positions. In mental health settings, as in others, becoming an administrator can have overtones of "selling out," of joining the patriarchal system instead of resisting it. Yet the way to change the system is to become involved. One cannot always wait to be asked to assume more leadership; women are encouraged to be active in stepping forward to take on more authority.

One note of caution, however: Women may also be more vulnerable than men to taking on too many tasks in an effort to be recognized. Women are often tempted to volunteer for numerous committees, unable to refuse when asked, feeling like they must do everything to be successful. In our hospital setting, we often find ourselves becoming social directors as well as administrators, organizing potlucks or bringing food in for the staff. It is important to set limits and prioritize what is the best use of one's time. Otherwise, women can become so fragmented that it inhibits their careers rather than enhancing them.

3. *Connect with other women.* While many organizations may not be willing to develop a specific women's focus, it remains useful for the women who work together in predominantly male settings to connect with each other, acknowledging their commonalities as well as differences. They should also seek out women in other organizations for for-

mal or informal supports. For example, in addition to supporting each other on the unit, the Women's Focus Team at SFGH has established links with other women as well as other women's treatment programs in San Francisco: the Rape Treatment Center, women's outpatient programs, and women representatives on the local Mental Health Board and the SFGH Community Advisory Board. We have also nurtured our national contacts, particularly in the areas of sexual trauma, women with serious illness, and women in academia.

4. *Seek female role models/become a mentor.* The limited number of female mentors has been widely discussed.[21,22] However, as more women do become successful leaders, increasing numbers of mentors are available to become positive role models and help the women who will come after them. As women recognize the value of mentoring in mental health settings, a new generation of women leaders will emerge.

5. *Learn to promote one's self.* Related to lack of confidence in leadership skills, women often have a difficult time with self-promotion. Boys' games involve much more boasting and one-upmanship than girls' cooperative play; it is often uncomfortable for women to declare their successes publicly. Yet this is required to be recognized and make gains in most organizations. This writer began in the Department of Psychiatry at SFGH over ten years ago as a psychology intern. At that time the only faculty positions for psychologists in the department were for those who were trained researchers, which I was not. It was largely through seeking out new opportunities and convincing the male administrators that I was capable of fulfilling these positions that I became an inpatient team leader and eventually unit chief. Both positions had formerly been held only by physicians. It took a combination of skill, confidence, self-promotion, and willingness to take risks for me to develop these roles as a psychologist.

6. *Promote each other to persons in authority.* Equally important as self-promotion is women learning to promote one another in mixed-gender meetings, as men often do. A woman can show her respect for another woman's work as well as validate it as worthy of recognition by using this strategy in treatment planning meetings, clinical conferences, and administrative meetings. Specific identification of a female peer's suc-

cess to male leaders can also promote women's accomplishments, both publicly and in memos or other written formats. As women support each other in this way, it improves the image of all the women in the organization by demonstrating frequent examples of female competence.

7. *Develop ties with male leaders.* Having female support, role models, and mentors is important for women aspiring to leadership positions; developing ties with male colleagues and leaders is also essential. Although there are important gender differences in leadership style, there are also many general principles of administration to learn. Men who have held these positions and have diverse experiences as leaders have much to offer. The key for women is to accept this information and adapt it so that it works for them instead of trying to emulate men identically.

The support of male leaders and connections they provide are also valuable to successful women. While we may eschew the concept of an "old boys' network" and the nepotism it suggests, it is a fact that it is difficult to rise in an organization without the leaders knowing one's work and believing it supports the group's mission. Many women mistakenly segregate themselves from men in an organization, and then feel wronged when these same men do not welcome them into leadership positions. Women need to create opportunities to establish credibility and to foster mutual trust with male colleagues. While my confidence, self-promotion, and encouragement from female peers were necessary to establish the role of an attending psychologist in our department, I would not have had the opportunity to prove myself without the direct support of my male colleagues as well. They had seen my competence in our prior work together, and my efforts to maintain respectful, warm, professional relationships gave them the confidence that I would be a reasonable leader. Although I was not consciously aware of these strategies at the time, the links I established in our department contributed to my promotions as well as my job satisfaction.

Conclusion

Mental health administrators face multiple challenges, often managing complex clinical systems and large groups of staff with little formal administrative training. Women who aspire to these leadership positions also confront societal ambivalence about powerful women. This chapter asserts that it is possible for women to carve out ways of leadership that capitalize on their unique perspectives. One hopes that in the future men and women will be able to share ways of leading that draw from one another's strengths.

REFERENCES

1. Cantor DW, Bernay T: *Women in Power: The Secrets of Leadership.* New York: Houghton Mifflin, 1992.
2. Helgesen S: *The Female Advantage: Women's Ways of Leadership.* New York: Doubleday/Currency, 1990.
3. Kopriva P (Ed.): *Women in Medicine in America.* Chicago: American Medical Association, 1991.
4. Spielvogel A, Wile J: Treatment of the psychotic pregnant patient. *Psychosomatics* 1986; 27:487-492.
5. Briere J, Zaidi LV: Sexual abuse histories and sequelae in female psychiatric emergency room patients. *American Journal of Psychiatry* 1989; 146:1602-1606.
6. Bryer JB, Nelson BA, Miller JB, et al.: Childhood sexual and physical abuse as a factor in adult psychiatric illness. *American Journal of Psychiatry* 1987; 144:1426-1430.
7. Craine LS, Henson CE, Colliver JA, et al.: Prevalence of a history of sexual abuse among psychiatric patients in a state hospital system. *Hospital and Community Psychiatry* 1988; 29:300-304.
8. Goodwin JM, Cheeves K, Connell V: Borderline and other severe symptoms in adult survivors of incestuous abuse. *Psychiatric Annals* 1990; 20:22-32.
9. Jacobsen A, Herald C: The relevance of childhood sexual abuse to adult psychiatric inpatient care. *Hospital and Community Psychiatry* 1990; 41:154-158.
10. Kluft R (Ed.): *Incest-Related Syndromes of Adult Psychopathology.* Washington, DC: American Psychiatric Press, 1990.
11. Pribor EF, Dinwiddie SH: Psychiatric correlates of incest in childhood. *American Journal of Psychiatry* 1992; 149:52-56.
12. Whitwell D: The significance of childhood sexual abuse for adult psychiatry. *British Journal of Hospital Medicine* 1990; 43:346-352.
13. Scheidt SD, Thomas TJ, Thomas B: *A Survey of Patient Data.* San Francisco: University of California, July 1990.
14. Eichenbaum L, Orbach S: *Between Women: Love, Envy and Competition in Women's Friendships.* New York: Penguin, 1987.
15. Bayes M, Newton PM: *Women in Authority; A Sociological Analysis.* New York: Penguin, 1987.
16. Anthony W, Cohen M, Farkas M: *Psychiatric Rehabilitation.* Boston: Center for Psychiatric Rehabilitation, 1990.
17. Gilligan C: *In a Different Voice.* Cambridge, MA: Harvard University Press, 1982.

18. Chodorow N: *The Reproduction of Mothering: Psychoanalysis and the Sociology of Gender.* Berkeley: University of California Press, 1978.
19. Hennig M, Jardim A: *The Managerial Woman.* New York: Pocket, 1976.
20. Tannen D: *You Just Don't Understand: Women and Men in Conversation.* New York: Ballantine, 1990.
21. Folger Jacobs K, Wolman CS: Strategies of women academics. In: Frank H (Ed.): *Women in the Organization.* Pittsburgh: University of Pennsylvania Press, 1977, pp. 256-262.
22. Barnett RC, Baruch GK: *The Competent Woman: Perspectives on Development.* New York: Irvington, 1978.

5

Disparities in Data Collection on Women's Issues in the Mental Health and Substance Abuse Communities

Sandra L. Forquer, Ph.D.
Pamela McDonnell, M.P.A.

When collecting and organizing data about any subject, which data are collected (or not collected) as well as later presentation, organization, and analysis can greatly influence our perception of the subject. The most popular presentation of this idea is the tale of the blind people investigating and then describing an elephant. Each blind person's perception of what the elephant "is," is based on his or her own limited set of data (i.e., which part of the elephant he or she touched).

In some cases partial data are adequate for our purposes, perhaps because we are interested only in describing the elephant's trunk or its leg. In fact, the specialization that we are all so familiar with often leads us as researchers to adopt a very myopic view of our subject and present our findings in excruciating detail to our peers. However, in some cases we need to present a full picture of the elephant to provide a context in which to place more detailed work.

The Substance Abuse and Mental Health Services Administration (SAMHSA) is the agency with congressionally chartered responsibility for the prevention and treatment of addictive and mental health problems and disorders. Within SAMHSA, the Office for Women's Services (OWS) is charged with addressing women's issues in the prevention and treatment of these disorders. The establishing legislation mandates that the OWS perform the following data collection tasks:

- Review data currently collected by SAMHSA to determine uniformity and applicability;
- Develop data standards for all programs funded by SAMHSA so that data are to the extent practical, collected, and reported using common reporting formats, linkages, and definitions; and
- Report to the administrator a plan for incorporating the standards developed into all SAMHSA programs and a plan to assure that the data collected are accessible to health professionals, providers, researchers, and the public.

In response to this mandate from Congress, the OWS, in early 1994, initiated a baseline assessment of data collection within SAMHSA pertaining to women's mental health and substance abuse (MH/SA) issues. The study was organized to support the first task above and to lay the groundwork for the second and third tasks. This study, then, is not so much about interpreting data related to women's MH/SA issues but rather focuses on gathering and interpreting data about existing data. The type of data that describe other data are frequently referred to as "meta-data."

The study first attempted to define all possible types of data that might be gathered about women's issues as they relate to MH/SA. Second, a review of a selected set of databases developed by SAMHSA and other agencies was conducted to determine what data were actually being collected and to present those data in a comprehensive format. Third, the study attempted to define standards for future data collection efforts.

The OWS at SAMHSA established a coordinating committee shortly following its inception. The OWS Internal Coordinating Committee (composed of SAMHSA's directors or their designees) was charged with identifying priority issues for OWS. These priority areas were used to compile the data elements against which the databases would be scanned to determine what data were currently being collected.

Selected issue areas include (1) physical/sexual abuse of women; (2) women as mothers and caretakers; (3) women with mental and addictive disorders; (4) women with HIV, AIDS, and/or other sexually transmitted diseases (STDs), with or without tuberculosis (TB); (5) older women; and (6) women involved in the criminal justice system.

The OWS also has established an external Advisory Committee for Women's Services to provide advice to the associate administrator for Women's Services and to SAMHSA's administrator regarding appropriate activities to be undertaken by SAMHSA with respect to women's MH/SA services. The Advisory Committee was composed of ten nonfederal physicians, practitioners, treatment providers, and other health professionals, whose clinical practice, specialization, or professional expertise includes a significant focus on women's MH/SA problems.

To avoid the "elephant is like a tree" danger of searching the databases for data unrelated to the issue areas, a considerable effort was expended early on in the study to define the data elements that would be used to determine the presence or absence of relevant information.

A candidate data element list representing the six issue areas was produced by the OWS staff and project consultants. This list was reviewed by professionals both inside and outside SAMHSA until consensus on a valid list was achieved.

This chapter is organized into four sections. The first section focuses on the study objectives, methodology, and design. Key findings are highlighted in the second section. Implications of the findings for the MH/SA fields are discussed in the third section. The fourth section concludes with a focus on the future of data collection and women's initiatives at SAMHSA.

STUDY OBJECTIVES, METHODOLOGY, AND DESIGN

The study had three broad objectives:

- To define a data set that would represent an encompassing set of quantitative measures and qualitative descriptors of issues related to women's MH/SA treatments. These measures and descriptors, referred to as global variables, could be used as a template against which the inclusiveness of SAMHSA and other data collection efforts on women's mental health care and/or alcohol or substance abuse treatment issues could be measured;

- To produce a single-source reference document in which the data collected by SAMHSA and other selected agencies relevant to women's MH/SA treatments would be described and tabulated for easy reference; and

- To cross-reference the data using the global variables defined in the first objective as linkages to determine:

  a. Whether information on each global variable related to the priority issue areas has been or is being collected; and

  b. Whether a measure of uniformity for similarly defined data could be identified across multiple databases (e.g., is age defined as age in years or by date of birth, or represented only by a range of ages?).

A cursory examination of the databases revealed that databases referenced to individuals such as the Hispanic Health and Nutrition Examination Survey[1] differed to some extent from databases referenced to institutions such as the National Nursing Home Survey.[2] In general, aggregate facility-based data are useful to study the types of services provided, but are of limited applicability in studying the use of these services by women. In addition, in those databases in which service use by women is broken out, there is almost no information on the characteristics of the women using the services. For these reasons, the facility-based and individual-based databases were treated separately when developing the global variables.

The definition process began by defining classes of variables as well as the global variables themselves, along with an indication of their relevance to individual- or facility-oriented databases. This list was circulated among SAMHSA professional personnel to generate consensually validated sets of variable classes. This process was continued for several iteration/revision cycles. Tables 5.1 and 5.2 reflect the final consensus on the global variables actually used in the study. As Table 5.1 indicates, four classes of variables were identified and consensually validated. These four classes represent demographic, medical, service-related, and payment variables. The global variables against which each SAMHSA or other national database was scanned appear under each variable class. Table 5.2 identifies each of the global variables to be

TABLE 5.1 Summary Information to Be Collected for Individual-Level Databases: Global Variable Definitions

Demographic variables
Age, dependent children, education, employment, entitlements, family income, gender, individual income, marital status, other caretaking responsibilities, race/ethnicity, region, urban/rural

Medical variables
Alcohol/drug current, alcohol/drug diagnosis, alcohol/drug history, alcohol severity measure, drug severity measure, medical diagnosis, medical history, mental health severity measure, current medication, HIV/AIDS status, other hospitalizations, other STDs, physical abuse, pregnancy history/abortions, pregnancy status, previous treatment, sexual abuse, TB status

Services received variables
Alcohol/drug testing, child care, collateral sessions, comprehensive assessment/ diagnosis, drug testing, family therapy/counseling, general health assessment, group therapy/counseling, HIV risk education, individual therapy/counseling, individual treatment plan, prescription medications, self-help groups, aftercare/follow-up, community support programs, crisis intervention, employment/vocational/educational counseling, family/parenting assessment, family planning, financial counseling, HIV screening or treatment, housing assistance, medical care, other preventive services, other services, other STD screening or treatment, prenatal care, psychosocial rehabilitation, TB screening or treatment

Payment variables
Cost/charges/expenditures, HMO/managed care, primary payment source

TABLE 5.2 Summary Information to Be Collected for Facility-Level Databases: Global Variable Definitions

Facility variables
Actual active clients, client capacity, costs/charges/expenditures, linkage agreements with special providers, sources of funds, staff trained in programs for women, substance abuse services provided, type of fee charged, types of third-party payment accepted

mapped against each facility-level database; facility-level databases were also analyzed against the individual-level data elements listed in Table 5.1.

In addition to the definition of the global variables to be used in this study, SAMHSA also provided a list of databases to be analyzed. The selected databases were chosen to provide a broad representation of the types of data being collected by SAMHSA and those most heavily relied on by the research community. In addition, the list of selected databases was validated by the External Advisory Committee of the OWS. Hundreds (perhaps thousands) of reports have been based on the data in these databases; one publication alone lists nearly 200 reports based primarily on a few of the databases included in the study.[3] In turn, the MH/SA policymakers relied on these reports as the basis for setting MH/SA policy, requesting funding for new or refined collection instruments and providing critical information in securing funding for treatment initiatives, especially in the six priority areas targeted to address MH/SA issues.

The sample size of the databases examined ranged from relatively modest, such as the Inventory of Local Jail Mental Health Services,[4] to very large, such as the Medicaid Statistical Information System.[5] The scope or focus of the databases examined ranged from very narrow, such as the Pregnancy Risk Assessment Monitoring System,[6] to very broad, such as the National Health and Nutrition Examination Survey.[7]

Descriptive information on each database was provided by the agencies responsible for generating and maintaining the database. The most common form of information was a document containing the actual data collection forms along with instructions for the interviewer and/or participant. Both the Inventory of Local Jail Mental Health Services[4] and the Medicaid Statistical Information System[5] are typical of the descriptive information used.

A number of tables were designed to capture the information contained in the database descriptions (full copies of the report can be obtained from SAMHSA/OWS). Descriptions of each of the databases analyzed in the study are available in *The Inventory of Public Health Data Projects and Systems, Fiscal Years 1993-1995, Developed by the Public Health Service Task Force on State and Community Data*.[8] Tables 5.3 and 5.4 are lists of databases reviewed for this project, listed in alphabetical order for convenience. Table 5.3 lists mental health databases, and Table 5.4 lists substance abuse databases. Twenty-one mental health and 29 substance abuse databases were analyzed in this study.

Summary tables (Tables 5.5 to 5.7) were produced to allow "at a glance" comparisons of the content of the various databases. In Table

TABLE 5.3 Summary of Textual Descriptions of Mental Health Databases

Database Acronym	Database Name
BRFSS	Behavioral Risk Factor Surveillance System
CPSS	Client Patient Sample Survey
CSSOP	Client Sample Survey of Outpatient Programs
DIS	Diagnostic Interview Schedule
ECAS	Epidemiologic Catchment Area Survey
HHANES	Hispanic Health and Nutrition Examination Survey
ILJMHS	Inventory of Local Jail Mental Health Services
IMHO&GHMHS	Inventory of Mental Health Organizations and General Hospital Mental Health Services
IMHSSACF	Inventory of Mental Health Services in State Adult Correctional Facilities
LPDSMHIS	Longitudinal Patient Data for State Mental Hospital Inpatient Services
MSIS	Medicaid Statistical Information System
M&CHSBGP	Maternal & Child Health Services Block Grant Program
NHANES III	National Health and Nutrition Examination Survey
NHDS	National Hospital Discharge Survey
NHIS	National Health Interview Survey
NMFS	National Mortality Followback Survey
NMIHS	National Maternal and Infant Health Survey
NNHS	National Nursing Home Survey
NSFG	National Survey on Family Growth
PRAMS	Pregnancy Risk Assessment Monitoring System
SCMHIS	State and County Mental Hospital Inpatient Services

5.5, each row in the table identifies a database and each column identifies a global variable. An "X" indicates the global variable is represented in the corresponding database by at least one datum. A single page from the mental health database analysis is included for reference purposes.

Table 5.6 allows the reader to peruse the content of a single database in extensive detail. This table represents mental health databases, and Table 5.7 represents substance abuse databases. A single page from the mental health databases is included here for reference purposes. Each row in the table identifies one value of one data element in one database and maps that data element into a global variable. The examples displayed in Table 5.6 demonstrate the different values associated with age, education, and employment. Additionally, it is possible to observe:

TABLE 5.7 Detail of Global Variables Across Substance Abuse Databases

Database Acronym	Full Name	Form or Questionnaire ID	Variable Category	Global Variable	Local Question No.	Answer or Description
CDS	Client Data System		Demographics	Age	Age	Date of birth
DAWN	Drug Abuse Warning Network		Demographics	Age	Age in years	Age
DSRS	Drug Services Research Survey		Demographics	Age	On 3/30/90 how many clients under 15 were undergoing: Alcohol treatment all modalities and environments	Number
DSRS	Drug Services Research Survey		Demographics	Age	On 3/30/90 how many clients under 15 were undergoing: Hospital inpatient drug detoxification	Number
DSRS	Drug Services Research Survey		Demographics	Age	On 3/30/90 how many clients under 15 were undergoing: Hospital inpatient drug maintenance	Number
DSRS	Drug Services Research Survey		Demographics	Age	On 3/30/90 how many clients under 15 were undergoing: Hospital inpatient drug-free	Number
DSRS	Drug Services Research Survey		Demographics	Age	On 3/30/90 how many clients under 15 were undergoing: Outpatient drug detoxification	Number
DSRS	Drug Services Research Survey		Demographics	Age	On 3/30/90 how many clients under 15 were undergoing: Outpatient drug maintenance	Number
DSRS	Drug Services Research Survey		Demographics	Age	On 3/30/90 how many clients under 15 were undergoing: Outpatient drug-free	Number

DSRS	Drug Services Research Survey	Demographics	Age	On 3/30/90 how many clients under 15 were undergoing: Residential drug detoxification	Number
DSRS	Drug Services Research Survey	Demographics	Age	On 3/30/90 how many clients under 15 were undergoing: Residential drug maintenance	Number
DSRS	Drug Services Research Survey	Demographics	Age	On 3/30/90 how many clients under 15 were undergoing: Residential drug-free	Number
DSRS	Drug Services Research Survey	Demographics	Age	On 3/30/90 how many clients 15-17 were undergoing: Alcohol treatment all modalities and environments	Number
DSRS	Drug Services Research Survey	Demographics	Age	On 3/30/90 how many clients 15-17 were undergoing: Hospital inpatient drug detoxification	Number
DSRS	Drug Services Research Survey	Demographics	Age	On 3/30/90 how many clients 15-17 were undergoing: Hospital inpatient drug maintenance	Number
DSRS	Drug Services Research Survey	Demographics	Age	On 3/30/90 how many clients 15-17 were undergoing: Hospital inpatient drug-free	Number
DSRS	Drug Services Research Survey	Demographics	Age	On 3/30/90 how many clients 15-17 were undergoing: Outpatient drug detoxification	Number

89

TABLE 5.8 Summary of Missing Variables for Mental Health Databases

Variable Category	Missing Variable	Total Variable Count in Category	Variables Collected by 2 or Fewer Databases	Variables Not Collected
Demographics	Dependent children		1	1
	Other caretaking responsibilities		1	1
	Total	**13**	**2**	
Medical	Alcohol drug current		1	
	Current medication		1	
	HIV/AIDS status		1	
	Medical diagnosis		1	1
	Medical history		1	
	Mental health severity measure		1	
	Other hospitalizations		1	
	Physical abuse		1	
	Previous treatment		1	
	Sexual abuse		1	
	TB status		1	1
	Total	**23**	**11**	**2**
Services	Alcohol/drug testing		1	1
	Child care		1	1
	Collateral sessions		1	1
	Community support programs		1	
	Crisis intervention		1	
	Drug testing		1	
	Family planning		1	
	Financial counseling		1	1
	General health assessment		1	1
	HIV risk education		1	1

Category	Element			
	Housing assistance		1	
	Medical care		1	
	Individual treatment plan		1	1
	Psychosocial rehabilitation		1	
	TB screening or treatment		1	1
	Total	**29**	**15**	**10**
Payment	Cost/charges/expenditures		1	1
	HMO/managed care		1	1
	State psychiatric hospital/IMD*		1	1
	Total	**4**	**3**	**3**
Outcomes	Abstinence		1	1
	Functioning status		1	1
	Health status		1	1
	Other measures of outcome		1	1
	Quality of life		1	
	Total	**5**	**5**	**4**
Facility	Client capacity		1	
	Cost/charges/expenditures		1	
	Provider ownership		1	1
	Provider site location		1	
	Sources of funds		1	
	Staff trained in programs for women		1	1
	Substance abuse services provided		1	1
	Type of fee charged		1	1
	Types of third-party payment accepted		1	1
	Total	**11**	**9**	**5**
	Total	**85**	**44**	**25**

*IMD = Institutions for Mental Disorders

TABLE 5.9 Summary of Missing Variables for Substance Abuse Databases

Variable Category	Missing Variable	Total Variable Count in Category	Variables Collected by 2 or Fewer Databases	Variables Not Collected
Demographics	Gender		1	1
	Total	**13**	**1**	**1**
Medical	Alcohol severity measure		1	
	Drug severity measure		1	
	Mental health severity measure		1	
	Other STDs		1	
	Physical abuse		1	
	Pregnancy history/abortions		1	
	Primary diagnosis		1	
	Sexual abuse		1	
	TB status		1	
	Total	**23**	**9**	**0**
Services	Collateral sessions		1	1
	Community support programs		1	1
	Comprehensive assessment/diagnosis		1	1
	Diagnosis		1	1
	Drug testing		1	1
	Family parenting assessment		1	

Category	Item			
	General health assessment		1	
	Other preventive services		1	
	Psychosocial rehabilitation		1	
	Total	29	9	5
Payment	State psychiatric hospital/IMD*		1	
	Total	4	1	0
Outcomes	Abstinence		1	
	Quality of life		1	
	Total	5	2	0
Facility	Actual active clients		1	
	Client capacity		1	
	Cost/charges/expenditures		1	1
	Provider ownership		1	
	Provider site location		1	
	Source of funds		1	1
	Substance abuse services provided		1	
	Type of fee charged		1	1
	Type of third-party payment accepted		1	
	Total	11	9	3
Total		85	31	9

*IMD = Institutions for Mental Disorders

comes, and facility), 90 percent of the databases collect less than 10 percent of the variables.

Within the substance abuse databases, in five of the six variable categories, more than 80 percent of the databases each collect more than 15 percent of the data elements defined as part of each category. In the facility category, however, almost 90 percent of the databases collect less than 10 percent of the variables. Overall, in the substance abuse databases, about one tenth of the variables are not included by any database.

Included in these variables were data elements deemed necessary for addressing the six issue areas identified as priorities by the OWS. The analysis of the 21 mental health databases and 29 substance abuse databases reviewed for this study established that, in large part, the desired data are not being collected. Within the mental health databases, issue areas identified as priority areas for the OWS in which data collection efforts were minimal (e.g., addressed only by two or fewer databases) or nonexistent included:

- Physical abuse
- Sexual abuse
- Women with HIV infection or AIDS
- Other STDs
- TB status
- Women as mothers or caretakers

Within the substance abuse databases, they included:

- Physical abuse
- Sexual abuse
- STDs
- TB status

Task 1 has provided SAMHSA with ample material to make recommendations on improving its database collection activities and to enable it to move ahead with Task 2, developing data standards for SAMHSA-funded programs.

IMPLICATIONS FOR MENTAL
HEALTH SERVICES DELIVERY

Clearly, the most important issue emerging from the study is the absence or minimal availability of critical data elements necessary to provide information on the six high-priority policy areas identified by SAMHSA as the focus of their OWS. Issues such as sexual and/or physical abuse are still not routinely assessed in many clinical settings, nor is their role in establishing a differential diagnosis between post-traumatic stress disorder and schizophrenia delineated in the fourth edition of the *Diagnostic and Statistical Manual of Mental Disorders (DSM-IV).*[9]

Senior policy advisers and administrators understand the critical links between data and information to support funding for services research and treatment interventions. These decision makers are increasingly wary of investing dollars where a clear need has not been demonstrated. Data, particularly collected across different population samples and broad geographic areas, are essential in building a convincing picture of need. While the priority areas for women's issues have been the focus of national conferences, and small studies have demonstrated the value of investing dollars and the value of improved outcomes, our field must be able to use data from large, national databases. As currently constructed, these national databases, in particular the mental health databases, do not provide critical data elements necessary to justify need for research and intervention dollars in the priority areas. This lack of data creates serious policy issues for women's services. The scarcity of data could have a negative impact in supporting the need for intervention in these areas: No single or combined set of national surveys could be identified that could provide the type of information necessary to convince Congress or the Office of Management and Budget to fund large-scale studies or intervention programs focused on women's MH/SA issues.

Without a formal study of how data collection decisions are derived, one can only speculate as to why such important areas have been neglected. It seems reasonable to assume that the reasons would include the following. First, it takes time for a controversial issue such as sexual abuse and/or physical abuse to become socially acceptable for study. In light of the debates on how best to reform welfare and medical assis-

tance, even issues such as "caregiving responsibilities" and "dependent children" can be viewed as controversial.

Second, after the acknowledgment of the issue, there is a period of time before the issue and its defining parameters coalesce to allow for its inclusion in a data collection instrument. Third, once general agreement has been reached that a study is in order and operational definitions determined, normal bureaucratic delays exist before the changes are incorporated into a national survey. Last, changes in data collection strategies and definitions in large-scale national surveys can take years to implement.

The relative neglect of these data elements may also result from a specific focus on the part of policy communities who fund and charter these data collection efforts and the researchers who design and carry them out. The policy communities generally are asking either:

- What can be done about issue "X"?

or

- Is what we are doing about issue "X" producing any results?

In general, researchers are looking to increase their depth of knowledge rather than their breadth. We are a nation of specialists. Unfortunately, this bias tends to perpetuate existing lines of inquiry rather than stimulate new ones.

This study provides a number of useful tools for researchers. A consensually validated set of MH/SA variables deemed necessary to address six priority issue areas concerning women's MH/SA status has been identified. In addition, a cross-sectional view of many national data collection efforts offers researchers a tool to use in defining their own data collection efforts and in comparing those efforts to others. The tables on operational definitions provide researchers with a definitional database that should foster increased uniformity in how basic data elements are defined. The MH/SA communities are encouraged to use these tools in defining their own future data collection efforts. Finally and perhaps most important, this study has clearly identified a lack of data in several areas considered important by the MH/SA policy-making communities.

FUTURE EFFORTS

When collecting and organizing data about any subject, determining which data are collected, as well as their presentation, organization, and analysis can greatly influence our perception of the subject. Data collection is an expensive, resource-intensive activity.

The congressional mandate to "develop data standards for all programs funded by SAMHSA so that data are to the extent practical, collected, and reported using common reporting formats, linkages and definitions" (Public Law 102-321) must become a priority. Accomplishing this, however, will require a standardization effort on several levels:

- An agreed-on set of standard definitions of global variables. Even a cursory study of the tables produced in this study indicates that an acceptable definition of many, perhaps most, of the global variables could be easily achieved. This is particularly true of the naturally quantitative variables (i.e., when measuring alcoholism severity, should we measure episodes per week or episodes per month?) and many of the qualitative variables. Most of the qualitative variables such as "severity of mental illness" have been objectified if not quantified already (e.g., *DSM* codes, facility admission dates and discharge dates, and frequency of admissions);

- An agreed-on set of minimum information to be gathered independent of the particular focus of the study, including basic demographic information. This information could be used as the minimum set of comparison variables when attempting to relate data collected in multiple studies; and

- The use of automation (i.e., the development of a formal data dictionary), which would further enhance the utility of standardized data elements.

Finally, based on the minimal information related to women's issues in the national databases reviewed in this study, current data collection instruments should be updated to include physical and sexual abuse, HIV/AIDS and other STDs, information on caregiver responsibilities, issues facing aging women, and women in the criminal justice system.

REFERENCES

1. Russell-Briefel R, Dresser C, Ezzati TM, et al.: National Center for Health Statistics: Plan and Operation of the Hispanic Health and Nutrition Examination Survey, 1982-84. In: *Vital and Health Statistics*, Series 1, Number 19. DHHS Pub. No. (PHS) 85-1321. Public Health Service. Washington, DC: U.S. Government Printing Office, September, 1985.
2. *Plan and Operation: National Nursing Home Survey Follow-Up 1987, 1988, 1990.* PHS 93-1306. Washington, DC: U.S. Government Printing Office, 1993.
3. *Catalog of Publications 1990-1993.* Washington, DC: U.S. Department of Health and Human Services, Public Health Service, Centers for Disease Control and Prevention.
4. *Inventory of Local Jail Mental Health Services.* OMB Number 0930-162. Washington, DC: Department of Health and Human Services, Public Health Service, Substance Abuse and Mental Health Services.
5. *Medicaid Statistical Information System, Tape Specifications and Data Dictionary.* Washington, DC: Health Care Financing Administration, Bureau of Data Management and Strategy, Office of Programs Systems, Division of Medicaid Statistics. Version 2.6, January 26, 1994.
6. *Pregnancy Risk Assessment Monitoring System* (Questionnaire). Washington, DC: U.S. Department of Health and Human Services, Public Health Service.
7. Plan and operation of the third National Health and Nutrition Examination Survey, 1988-1994. In: *Vital Health and Statistics*, Volume 1, Number 32. Washington, DC: National Center for Health Statistics, 1994.
8. *The Inventory of Public Health Data Projects and Systems, Fiscal Years 1993-1995, Developed by the Public Health Service Task Force on State and Community Data.* Washington, DC: U.S. Government Printing Office, 1996.
9. American Psychiatric Association: *Diagnostic and Statistical Manual of Mental Disorders.* 4th ed. Washington, DC: American Psychiatric Association, 1994.

6

Independent Community Living Among Women With Severe Mental Illness

A Comparison With Outcomes Among Men

Judith A. Cook, Ph.D.

The field of mental health services research has become increasingly concerned with the lives of women who have severe psychiatric disorders.[1] One area of interest is that of independent living, and one related question is the extent to which men and women experience differential outcomes following residential rehabilitation. This chapter investigates whether or not women and men display differen-

NOTE: The contents of this publication were developed under a grant from the National Institute on Disability and Rehabilitation Research, U.S. Department of Education cooperative agreement number H133B00011, and the Center for Mental Health Services, Substance Abuse and Mental Health Services Administration. This publication does not necessarily reflect the views of either agency and does not imply endorsement by the U.S. government. Earlier versions of this chapter were presented at the University of Chicago, School of Social Service Administration Conference, Mental Health Research: Critical Issues for the 90's and Beyond, May 3-4, 1991, Chicago, and the American Sociological Association annual meetings, Pittsburgh, PA, 1992. The author gratefully acknowledges the assistance of Lisa Razzano, Madison Straiton, Mark Gervain, Mardi Solomon, Sitha Pugh, Helen Rosenberg, Stephanie Lazarus, and the members and staff of Thresholds. This chapter appeared as an article in the *Journal of Mental Health Administration,* 1994, Vol. 21, No. 4, pp. 361-373.

tial ability to live on their own in commercial housing following psychiatric rehabilitation.

REVIEW OF THE LITERATURE

A review of the literature on women with severe psychiatric disorders suggests that gender influences the experiences of mental illness because of women's status, role expectations, and differential illness course. As discussed below, some of these influences may promote women's attempts to live independently in the community while others may act as barriers.

One gender difference that may favor residential independence is a later onset of mental illness among women than men. While women are typically hospitalized for the first time during middle age, onset of mental illness among men tends to occur earlier, during their twenties and thirties.[2,3] A later age at onset may enable women greater opportunities to learn domestic skills and establish competencies such as budgeting, money management, housekeeping, cooking, and shopping before becoming ill. Residential rehabilitation for women may, thus, involve relearning independent living skills acquired before the illness while for men it involves first-time skill acquisition, which is, presumably, more difficult.

Related to later onset is the frequent finding of better premorbid functioning among women than men.[4,5] Women with severe mental illness are more likely than men to have married and borne children[6-8] and to have attained higher levels of education[9] before becoming ill. Most important, women were more likely to have lived on their own before the onset of illness in at least three studies.[4,9,10] Thus, women may bring to the independent living effort a greater repertoire of related experiences that help promote greater success.

Another gender difference favoring women's community living is the differential pattern of inpatient admissions among men and women. In several studies, women remained in the community significantly longer between hospitalizations[11,12] and had lower readmission rates following discharge.[13,14] Women's longer community tenure means that they have longer periods of time to pursue residential goals. This is relevant in an area such as obtaining public housing, given that people with mental illness have trouble competing for available housing and have difficulty using subsidy or voucher programs.[15] The long waiting lists and application process for public housing might favor those clients with longer periods of community tenure, thereby enhancing women's chances of obtaining and maintaining commercial housing.

Another potential advantage is the finding that women with psychiatric disabilities have wider community support networks than their more isolated male counterparts. One study of 971 persons receiving Community Support Program services[16] found that women were more likely than men to be engaged with others in activities outside their homes. Women's higher rates of marriage and child rearing suggest that they have a greater number of social relationships that may support independence.[1]

While the foregoing factors may promote residential independence, there are several additional factors that may be negative influences. First, women in North American society are socialized into passive, dependent roles in comparison to men.[17] These dependent positions may be inadvertently encouraged by service provision models emphasizing comprehensive, wrap-around services.[9] For example, one study found that homeless women, many with mental illness, received encouragement from shelter providers for passive behavior.[18] In other studies of independent living skills training, programs tacitly accepted lower levels of independence for women clients than for men.[19,20]

Also supporting dependency may be the attitudes and behaviors of family members, especially parents, toward their ill daughters. There is evidence that parents of ill daughters are more protective of them because they see them as more vulnerable than sons.[21] Seeman[10] found that families lowered their expectations for their ill daughters while continuing to hold pre-illness achievement expectations for ill sons. Several studies have reported that parents feel higher caregiver burden for daughters than sons.[22-24] Expectations that they will be dependent may create barriers for those women who wish to live on their own.

Women's more limited financial resources and economic vulnerability[6,25] may be a barrier to obtaining commercial housing. Disabled women's poorer work histories mean that they receive less generous benefits from programs such as disability insurance, supplemental security income, and workers' compensation.[26] Along with this, disabled women's lower employment rate[27] means that they bring fewer financial resources to the effort to obtain residential independence. Women with disabilities also may have lower financial resources for other reasons such as child care[28] or the need to care for elderly parents.[29]

The close connection between poverty and residence means that many women with mental illness live in unsafe housing in unsafe neighborhoods.[9] This is one reason that women with severe mental illness, especially those who are homeless, are targets of crime and violence. Partly as a result, disproportionately more women with mental illness report physical and sexual assault in adulthood than men.[30] Moreover, homeless women, many of whom are mentally ill,[18] may be more vulnerable to exclusion from shelters, creating greater risks of victimization as targets of violent crime[31] or untreated incarceration.[32]

Prior Outcome Studies in Residential Rehabilitation

Outcome research in the area of residential rehabilitation offers some clues as to the effects of gender on independent living. Interestingly, these studies suggest that women have superior residential outcomes in comparison to men. In a study of 187 aftercare patients following release from an urban state psychiatric hospital,[33] women were significantly more likely to be in stable housing and less likely to be homeless than men. A study of 122 young adults with schizophrenia and schizophrenia-related disorders[3] found that women spent significantly more time than men residing in apartments and houses while men spent more time than women living in rooming houses. A review of 320 records of patients in seven psychiatric hospitals[1] found that women were more likely to live independently (but also more likely to live in nursing homes) while men were more likely to live in group or foster homes, in jail, or with family.

Level of Functional Impairment

Level of functional impairment appears to be an additional client-level influence on residential outcomes. In one study of board and care homes,[34] clients with lower Global Assessment Scale (GAS) scores received higher amounts of practical support from residence operators and had lower congruence with housemates than higher-functioning clients. In another study,[35] the most powerful client-level variable predicting residential integration was the individual's level of functioning; here, those with better psychosocial functioning were more involved in facility activities than those with poorer functioning. A study of deaf clients with mental illness[36] found that level of functioning remained significant in a multivariate model predicting who was able to live in commercial housing. In addition, age has been found to be related to independent living outcomes. Younger clients were less likely to reside in structured, non-"normal" community housing in one study[34] and were more socially involved in residence and community activities than older clients in another.[16]

Two programmatic variables appear to be significant in studies of residential services. First, program models providing ongoing support are most successful, as opposed to transitional, time-limited housing models.[37-39] In one study, former rehabilitation clients were more likely to be living independently if they had maintained contact with their caseworkers.[40] Another service use variable, program tenure, may have an influence on residential outcomes, given that clients seem to benefit most from longer periods of services delivery. For example, clients with longer tenure at one urban psychosocial rehabilitation program were more likely to be living on their own in commercially available housing than those with shorter tenure.[41]

Multivariate Model

Combining findings from research on women with those on residential outcomes in psychiatric rehabilitation, a multivariate model was constructed. In this model, women's societal status, role expectations, illness course, and service use were all hypothesized to influence their residential outcomes. This is an expansion of the notion of "social disablements" first explicated by Wing and Morris.[42] In this conceptualization, persons with mental disorders experience primary disabilities related to the illness along with secondary disabilities or "adverse personal reactions" to their primary symptoms. But in addition, a tertiary set of limitations known as social disablements is faced by persons with long-term mental illness and influence outcomes. These social disablements include such things as poverty and stigma imposed by society in reaction to mental illness.

Bachrach[43] suggests that women with psychiatric disorders experience social disablements related to their gender. She proposes that social disablements related to being female and having long-term mental illness interact to create "serious deficits in the care of these women in today's psychiatric service systems" (p. 4).[43] Carrying this notion one step further, the present model assumes that gender influences in all four domains can have both negative and positive effects on women's ability to establish independent living. Thus, the model includes variables representing social disablements related to gender such as more limited income resources and the extra burdens of child care responsibilities. It also includes "social enablements" or variables that may enhance residential independence for women such as later age at illness onset, greater community participation, and greater likelihood of being in a marital or cohabiting relationship. Moreover, the model includes those variables found to be significant in prior research on residential outcomes such as age, level of functioning, and programmatic variables.

In this theoretical model, it is expected that positive outcomes will be associated with certain social statuses (being female, being younger, having greater and more varied income sources), illness and disability features (being higher functioning, experiencing a later illness onset, having fewer psychiatric hospitalizations), social role responsibilities (being married or cohabiting, having children, engaging in social and leisure pursuits), and service use patterns (participating longer in rehabilitation programming, experiencing service continuity, participating in therapy, using transitional residences). Control variables include preprogram residential status, ethnicity, and education.

METHODOLOGY

Sample

The sample is composed of 650 clients who received psychosocial rehabilitation services at a large, urban psychosocial rehabilitation agency. The present analysis uses data collected from these clients and their case files at the time they entered the program (intake), at the end of their participation in the program (closing), and six months thereafter (follow-up). Follow-up interviews were conducted from January 1986 through June 1992. The follow-up interview response rate during this period was 75 percent, with most nonresponses due to failure to locate the ex-client rather than the subject's refusal to participate.

When asked to name their reasons for coming to the program at intake, over three quarters (82 percent) of all clients reported that they needed assistance in finding a job, over half (55 percent) said they needed help with activities of daily living, and around a third (37 percent) said they needed helping staying out of the hospital. Upon program entry, 15 percent were living independently (defined as residing in commercial housing with no in-home supports), 44 percent were living with relatives, 24 percent were living in a supported setting such as a group home or board and care, and 17 percent were living in institutions. At the time of their closing from the agency, 36 percent were living independently, 36 percent were living with parents or family, 22 percent lived in a supported setting, and 4 percent were residing in institutions. At the six-month follow-up interview, 34 percent of former clientele were living independently, 35 percent lived with parents or family, 23 percent lived in a supported setting, and 8 percent lived in institutions.

Two thirds (65 percent) of the clients in this study are male and one third are female; 73 percent are White and 27 percent are minority (of the 174 minority clients, 127 are African American, 26 are Hispanic/ Latino, 9 are Asian, 3 are Native American, and 9 are mixed ethnicity). The average age of clients when they entered the agency was 27 years old. Almost three quarters (74 percent) had a high school or college degree, and a very low proportion reported being married or cohabiting (3.4 percent). The median number of prior hospitalizations at time of program intake for the sample was 4.7; 90 percent of all clients had been hospitalized for psychiatric reasons at least once before entering the agency, and their average age at first admission was 21 years. Around a third (37 percent) of the clients stayed in the program 1 year or less, another third (28 percent) stayed 1-2 years, and a final third (35 percent) stayed 2-20 years; the median length of stay in the program was 505 days or about 1 year and 5 months. Half of the clients (50 percent) had lived in one or more of the agency's transitional residences during their tenure. At the time they entered the agency, the average functional assessment rating using the GAS[44] for clients was 48.6, indicating a group with serious symptomatology presence and functioning impairment. At the time of their closing from the agency, the mean GAS score for the sample was 48.7, indicating that the average functioning level for this clientele remained relatively unchanged during their tenure at the agency. Upon closing, around a fifth (22 percent) went on to agency-affiliated programs while the remainder terminated services completely. During the six-month follow-up period, a quarter (27 percent) were rehospitalized; by the time of the follow-up interview, respondents averaged a lifetime of 5.9 admissions. The majority (61 percent) reported that they were seeing a therapist and their mean age at interview was 27 years, ranging from 16 to 60. Only a tenth (13 percent) reported that they were parents. Regarding income sources, 43 percent reported money from Supplemental Security Income (SSI), 45 percent from Social Security Disability Insurance (SSDI), 32 percent from employment, 29 percent from family, 18 percent from public assistance (PA), 6 percent from savings, 3 percent from the Veterans Administration (VA), and 1 percent from unemployment compensation.

Setting of the Research

The setting of the research was an urban psychosocial rehabilitation agency exclusively serving persons with severe and persistent mental illness. The model used at the agency included psychiatric medication management services, vocational training and job placement, general equivalency diploma (GED) and basic education classes, social skills training and recreational activities, and medical services. Residential rehabilitation services included independent living skills training, assistance with budgeting and money management, classes on cooking and nutrition, assistance with obtaining home furnishings, and help with apartment hunting and dealing with landlords. Transitional residences were available for clients desiring time-limited housing.

Categorical Measures

Among the dichotomous variables, gender was coded as "1" for females and "2" for males. Marital status was coded as "1" for those married or cohabiting and "0" otherwise. Minority status was coded as "0" for White and "1" for all others. Parental status was coded as "1" if respondents reported one or more children and "0" if they were child-less. The housing program use variable was coded as "1" if respondents had lived in one or more agency-owned residences during their tenure in the program and "0" otherwise. Ongoing support was coded as "1" if respondents were supported continuously, through alternative pro-grams affiliated with the agency, even after they completed rehabilita-tion, and "0" otherwise. At follow-up, respondents who reported hav-ing a therapist were coded as "1" on the variable therapy and "0" otherwise. Also at follow-up, the series of eight income sources was coded as "1" if reported by respondents and "0" if not; these included PA, SSI, SSDI, VA, unemployment compensation, savings, money from relatives, and income from employment.

Interval-Level Measures

Age at first hospitalization, age at follow-up, and education level were all measured in years. At time of program exit, tenure at the agency was measured in days. Also at closing, respondents' levels of function-ing were measured using the GAS, a single-item measure ranging from 1 to 100 and completed by respondents' caseworkers. Hospitalization was operationalized as the number of psychiatric hospital admissions since leaving the program. Age at first hospitalization used clients' ac-tual ages, substituting age at program entry for clients who had never been hospitalized. Finally, participation in social and leisure time activi-ties was measured by scores on a slightly adapted version of the Katz and Lyerly Social and Leisure Time Activities Scale (KAS-4)[45] ranging from 0 to 60 with a mean of 35 and standard deviation of 5.5. Cronbach's alpha for this scale was .74, indicating adequate internal validity for this measure of community participation.

Dependent Variable

The outcome measure for this study was whether or not the client was living in commercial or privately owned housing without family members or other in-home supports (except spouses or cohabitants). This is the operationalization of consumers' preferred housing arrange-ments in multiple survey research studies. For example, a review of 26 consumer housing preference studies[46] found that the most preferred arrangement was independent living in a house or apartment. In 20 of the studies reviewed, 70 percent or more of the mental health consumers surveyed expressed this preference. This outcome was assessed as a dichotomous variable coded as 1 if the individual was living in such a situation at follow-up and as 0 otherwise.

Statistical Analysis

Frequency distributions and cross-tabulations were computed to examine variables at the univariate level. T tests were used to assess gender differences in residential outcome followed by multivariate analysis (ordinary least squares [OLS] regression analysis and logistic regression analysis [probit]) to test the proposed model. Since less than 10 percent of data were missing for any given variable, mean substitution was used in the multivariate analyses.

RESULTS

Gender Differences in Independent Living

Given the literature on women and residential rehabilitation, we turn first to the question of gender divergence in rehabilitation outcome. Table 6.1 presents the proportions of males and females living independently at three points in time: intake, closing, and follow-up. There was no significant difference in proportions of males and females living in commercial housing at time of program entry. Thirteen percent of all entering males and 18 percent of all females were living on their own at intake. By the time of program closing, however, a significantly higher proportion of women (43 percent) were living independently than men (31 percent). This significant difference between the genders persisted six months later, with 39 percent of all females living independently and 30 percent of all males doing so at follow-up.

To explore this relationship at the multivariate level, OLS regression analysis and logistic regression analysis (probit) were performed. Table 6.2 presents the zero-order correlations for these analyses. Because the dependent variable is dichotomous, its aggregate interpretation is the

TABLE 6.1 Proportions of Males and Females Living Independently at Three
Time Points

Time Point	% Males Independent	% Females Independent	Chi-Square and Significance
At program entry	13	18	2.7 ns
At program closing	31	43	10.04**
At six-month follow-up	30	39	4.68*

NOTE: ns = nonsignificant.
*p < .05. **p < .001.

probability that an individual was living independently at follow-up.
While OLS and logistic regression provide similar results when the
mean of a dependent variable ranges from 25 to 75 percent,[47] outside
this range the effects of continuous variables are over- or underestimated relative to effects of dichotomous variables.[48] At the time of
follow-up, 33.6 percent of the sample were living in commercial housing
on their own or with a roommate; thus, application of OLS techniques
is not likely to distort the findings regarding continuous variables.
Nevertheless, in the following section, we report and compare the results of the OLS and logistic regression.

Multivariate Prediction of Independent
Living: OLS and Logistic Regression

In these analyses, independent living status was regressed on the
22-variable model described above. Table 6.3 presents OLS b-values and
LOGIT coefficients for the hypothesized model controlling for all nonsignificant coefficients. T values from both methods are presented in
parentheses under each set of coefficients.

Turning first to the results of the OLS regression, we can see that
gender itself is not a major differentiator once other variables in the
model are controlled. Gender, therefore, acts indirectly, and its influence
on the probability of living in "normal" (i.e., commercial) housing is
related to a series of other factors. The model's standardized regression
coefficients (β) indicate each variable's relative contribution to the equation. The greatest effects are due to clients' global level of functioning

TABLE 6.2 Univariate Statistics and Correlations for Variables in the Analysis

Variable	1	2	3	4	5	6	7	8	9	10	11	12	13	14	15	16	17	18	19	20	21	22	23
1. Independent living	1.00																						
2. Sex	.08a	1.00																					
3. Minority	-.06	.02	1.00																				
4. Education	.12b	.01	-.18d	1.00																			
5. Parent	.17d	.28d	.07a	-.04	1.00																		
6. Age at first hospitalization	.16d	.07	-.05	.33d	.16d	1.00																	
7. Tenure	.24d	.06	-.06	.13c	-.05	.09b	1.00																
8. Service continuity	-.03	.04	-.00	.12b	-.02	.13c	.23d	1.00															
9. Global Assessment Scale (GAS) at closing	.38d	.04	-.04	.28d	.09a	.25d	.37d	.14d	1.00														
10. Agency residence	.02	.00	-.09b	-.07a	-.17d	-.19d	.17d	.05	.09b	1.00													
11. Age at follow-up	.16d	.12b	-.06	.35d	.32d	.57d	-.01	.19d	.22d	-.26d	1.00												
12. Therapy at follow-up	.08a	.11b	-.06	.18d	-.00	.03	.08a	.05	.04	-.08a	.16d	1.00											
13. Community participation	.13c	.14d	.01	.05	-.01	.01	.04	.05	.16d	.03	-.02	.04	1.00										
14. Marital status	.14d	.13c	.04	.09b	.31d	.06	-.02	-.03	.06	-.12b	.24d	.07	.03	1.00									
15. Number of hospitalizations at follow-up	-.08a	.11b	-.00	-.04	.02	-.09a	-.08a	-.05	-.27d	.04	-.03	.03	-.11b	-.03	1.00								
16. Income—family	-.13c	-.10b	-.13c	.02	-.13c	-.16d	-.10b	-.05	-.16d	.01	-.19d	-.02	-.00	-.04	-.01	1.00							
17. Income—public assistance (PA)	-.11b	.00	-.01	-.14d	.02	-.15d	-.05	.02	-.12c	.01	-.06	.00	-.06	-.06	.14d	-.01	1.00						

18. Income—Supplemental Security Income (SSI)	-.15d	.02	.09a	-.23d	-.05	-.14d	-.06	.02	-.25d	.00	-.15d	-.03	.03	-.10b	.12c	-.12b	.27d	1.00
19. Income—Social Security Disability Insurance (SSDI)	-.01	.04	-.12c	.14d	.06	.17d	-.11b	.03	-.04	.28d	.06	-.02	.04	.08a	-.07a	.00	-.09b	1.00
20. Income—unemployment	.08a	-.00	.05	.03	.11b	.04	-.02	-.06	.05	.01	.04	-.04	.04	-.02	.04	-.02	-.07a	-.05	1.00
21. Income—savings	.02	-.02	-.07	-.01	.00	-.06	.15d	.05	.01	.10b	-.14d	.00	.06	-.01	-.01	.11b	-.02	-.05	-.14d	.07a	1.00
22. Income—Veterans Administration (VA)	.02	-.12c	.05	-.03	.05	-.01	-.02	.00	.02	-.06	.10b	.01	.00	.01	.04	-.03	-.02	-.09b	-.03	.11b	.01	1.00
23. Income—work	.16d	-.04	-.02	.11b	-.08a	.06	.19d	.18d	.34d	.09b	-.01	-.03	.05	-.02	-.21d	-.02	-.17d	-.16d	-.23d	-.08a	.07a	-.09b	1.00
Mean	.34	1.35	.27	12.5	.13	21.5	714.4	.22	48.1	.50	27.8	.61	35	.48	.30	.18	.44	.46	.01	.07	.04	.32
SD	.47	.48	.44	2.21	.34	6.32715	.41	16.6	.50	7.9	.48	5.2	.18	1.0	.45	.38	.49	.49	.12	.25	.18	.47

n = 650

a. p < .05.
b. p < .01.
c. p < .001.
d. p < .0001.

TABLE 6.3 Multivariate Analyses (OLS and PROBIT)[a] of Model Predicting Independent Living at Follow-Up

Variable	Beta[b]	Logit Coefficient[b]
Global level of functioning at closing	.27****	.02****
	(5.99)	(5.59)
Program tenure (no. of days)	.16****	.00****
	(3.87)	(3.44)
Continuous support received	−.12***	−.38***
	(−3.17)	(−3.01)
Parental status	.11**	.39**
	(2.71)	(2.51)
Community participation	.08*	.02*
	(2.12)	(1.96)
Married or cohabiting	.07†	.46*
	(1.77)	(1.66)
Minority status	−.06†	−.21*
	(−1.74)	(−1.80)
Financial support from family	−.06†	−.20*
	(−1.63)	(−1.71)
Receiving unemployment benefits	.06†	.60†
	(1.62)	(1.48)
In therapy	.06 ns	.17*
	(1.54)	(1.68)
Constant	(−2.34)**	(5.14)**
R^2	.23	

$n = 650$

NOTE: ns = nonsignificant.
a. For both methods, t values are given in parentheses under each coefficient.
b. Controlling for gender; age at follow-up; number of psychiatric hospitalizations; age at first admission; use of transitional residential services; education; and income from Supplemental Security Income benefits, Social Security Disability Insurance, public assistance, Veterans Administration, savings, and employment.
*$p < .05$. **$p < .01$. ***$p < .001$. ****$p < .0001$. †$p < .10$.

at time of leaving the program; those with better functioning were significantly more likely to be living on their own at follow-up ($\beta = .27$). Second, clients with longer program tenure were more likely to be living in commercial housing at follow-up ($\beta = .16$). Third, clients who did *not* receive ongoing support from the agency were those who were more likely to be living on their own at follow-up ($\beta = −.12$). Fourth, clients with children were more likely to be living independently than those who were not parents ($\beta = .11$). Finally, clients who reported higher levels of social and leisure time activities were more likely to be living independently than those with lower levels of community participation ($\beta = .08$). These five variables, controlling for all other variables in the model, account for 23 percent of the variance in residential outcome; each is a significant addition to the model and the entire model is significant ($p < .0001$). Inclusion of a control variable assessing residential status at intake (not shown) in this model raised the R^2 to .29 and had little effect on the significant variables (with the exception of the beta for leisure participation, which dropped to $p = .06$).

Four additional variables approach significance in the model and bear mentioning as trends. First, being married or cohabiting increased the likelihood of living in commercial housing ($p < .08$). This confirms the findings of prior research that suggest a positive relationship between marriage and independent living. Second, White clients were more likely to be living in normal housing than minorities ($p < .08$). This may reflect the well-documented housing discrimination faced by ethnic minorities in the United States.[49] Third, clients who reported that they were *not* receiving income from parents or family were more likely to be living in commercial housing than those reporting this income source ($p < .10$). It may be that clients are more likely to receive financial assistance from relatives if they live with family or in supported settings. Fourth, receiving unemployment benefits was positively associated with living in commercial housing at follow-up ($p < .10$). In addition to the direct effects of unemployment income, this variable may also be acting as a proxy for prior work status.

Turning next to the logistic regression analysis, we see virtually identical results. Comparison of t values indicates that global level of functioning still contributes most to the model, followed by tenure, continuity of support, parental status, and community participation. In addition, marital status, minority status, receiving income from family, and being in therapy at follow-up also were significant in the logit model. Interestingly, comparison of the t values from both methods indicates that OLS regression tended to order the variables in the same relative importance as the logit analysis, with a few minor exceptions. A separate discriminant function analysis using the 22-variable model (not shown) indicated that it correctly classified cases grouped as "independent" or "nonindependent" 74 percent of the time; moreover, the eta squared indicated that this model explained 24 percent of the variance, a figure highly similar to that of the R^2 of .23 obtained in the OLS regression.

Gender and the Model's Predictor Variables

The decline in the importance of gender once the full model was tested suggests the need to examine zero-order relationships between gender and the model variables. The correlations in Table 6.2 present these results. First, women were older than men at follow-up, although this relationship was a weak one ($r = .16$, $p < .0001$). Not surprisingly, women experienced their first psychiatric hospitalization at significantly older ages than men. Also as expected, women were more likely to have children than men. Interestingly, women experienced significantly more hospitalizations than men during the follow-up period, although this relationship, too, was a weak one. As in prior studies, women were significantly more likely to be married or cohabiting than their male counterparts in the program; they also reported engaging in significantly higher levels of community activities than men. At follow-up, women were more likely to be in therapy than men, again a weak relationship. Finally, women were less likely to report VA funding or financial assistance from their families than men. On the other hand, gender was not related to level of functioning, length of program participation, or to occurrence of ongoing support.

IMPLICATIONS FOR MENTAL HEALTH SERVICES DELIVERY

The results of this study indicate that a significantly higher proportion of women than men are able to achieve residential independence when the outcome assessed is living in normal community housing. While there is not a gender difference at the start of rehabilitation, by the time of program termination a higher percentage of women are living independently, and this difference continues for at least six months after the end of rehabilitation services.

However, gender itself is not a significant predictor of independent living when the effects of functioning level, parental status, program tenure, community participation, and ongoing support are controlled. These model variables override the effects of gender, suggesting that they have a more direct effect on the ability to maintain commercial housing. The question remains, however, as to how women experience these five important features that predict residential independence as well as their implications for services delivery.

The fact that women were more likely to be married or cohabiting suggests that social relationships may support their efforts to live independently. This is echoed by the finding that women were more likely to engage in social and leisure time activities in the community. The trend toward women's greater likelihood of being in therapy also is relevant here. Women's relationships with partners and with therapists, and their greater community participation, may have provided a safety net of supportive relationships that promoted their attempts to live in commercial housing. Service providers may want to use this information in helping clients build networks of interpersonal relationships that can continue to support independent living goals even after clients have exited programs.

Women were more likely to have children, and the status of parenthood directly predicted positive commercial housing outcomes in the model. Instead of lowering women's chances of residential independence, parenthood appears to have enhanced them. This may be because parenthood involves social interaction with potentially supportive others such as one's own parents, welfare workers, the child's pediatrician, or the child's teachers. If so, then the fact that women are more likely to be parents, and parents, in turn, are more likely to be living independently, is one example of gender as a social enablement for women mental health consumers. On the other hand, this finding could also be a by-product of structured housing program policies that typically exclude residents with children, forcing them to live with family or on their own. Further study is needed to address this issue. Until then, administrators should review residential policies that exclude consumers with children and consider creating services responsive to the needs of parents, such as on-site child care or parenting training.

Regardless of a client's gender, the importance of degree of functional impairment to residential independence is evident in the strong effects of global functioning on residential status. Clients with higher-functioning levels at the time they ended rehabilitation services were more likely to be living in normal housing without supervision at follow-up. This confirms previous findings regarding the importance of overall functioning to independent living. Similarly, the counterintuitive finding of a negative relationship between ongoing support and residential independence may indicate a prior selection process. That is, clients who are able to live on their own may be less likely to request and receive ongoing services. These findings suggest that the residential rehabilitation services delivered by this agency may benefit higher-functioning clients more than those with greater impairments. Residential programming specifically geared toward helping lower-functioning clients achieve commercial housing may be needed to fill a gap in programming.

The absence of information about satisfaction with current living situation impedes attempts to integrate a consumer perspective into understanding this outcome. While we know that "successful" respondents achieved the goal of living in commercial housing expressed by the majority of consumers in several studies, we do not know whether respondents themselves endorsed such a goal. This is a weakness of the present study. The possibility that some consumers might prefer to live in structured settings to combat loneliness or receive on-site assistance from professional staff remains to be addressed. Women with child care responsibilities may benefit from these kinds of in-home supports, and this question deserves further exploration both by researchers and by those who design residential programming.

This analysis has tested the effects of gender as both a disablement and an enablement for the residential outcomes of women mental health consumers. It may be that the role responsibilities that accrue to women act to promote independent living rather than inhibit it, so that gender functions as a social enablement rather than a disablement. At the same time, however, women had no advantage over men in other significant areas such as global functioning, length of program participation, or service continuity. This suggests that gender and perhaps client-level variables in general will not suffice in predictive models for residential rehabilitation services, as others have noted previously.[50,51] Similarly, a narrow focus on client features may miss some of the important environmental and contextual features that should be addressed in residential program design.

It may be that women's documented poorer performance in the vocational realm[52-55] is counterbalanced by superior residential outcomes following psychiatric rehabilitation. This may mean that specialized residential programming should be developed for men, particularly those who are lower functioning and are isolated from social supports. It is hoped that future research will further test some of the predictive relationships identified in this study so that service designers can capitalize on these associations, making sure to nurture the natural processes that co-occur with residential independence.

REFERENCES

1. Mowbray CT, Chamberlain P: Sex differences among the long-term mentally disabled. *Psychology of Women Quarterly* 1986; 10:383-392.
2. Angermeyer MC, Kuhn L: Gender differences in age at onset of schizophrenia: An overview. *European Archives of Psychiatry and Neurological Sciences* 1988; 237:351-364.
3. Test MA, Burke SS, Wallisch LS: Gender differences of young adults with schizophrenic disorders in community care. *Schizophrenia Bulletin* 1990; 16(2):331-344.
4. Bennett MB, Handel MH, Pearsall DT: Behavioral differences between female and male hospitalized chronically mentally ill patients. In: Bachrach LL, Nadelson CC (Eds.): *Treating Chronically Mentally Ill Women*. Washington, DC: American Psychiatric Press, 1988.
5. Loranger AW: Sex differences in age at onset of schizophrenia. *Archives of General Psychiatry* 1984; 41:157-161.
6. Mowbray CT, Herman SE, Hazel KL: Gender and serious mental illness. *Psychology of Women Quarterly* 1992; 16:107-126.
7. Salokangas RKR: Prognostic implications of the sex of schizophrenic patients. *British Journal of Psychiatry* 1983; 142:145-151.
8. Test MA, Knoedler WH, Allness DJ, et al.: Characteristics of young adults with schizophrenic disorders treated in the community. *Hospital and Community Psychiatry* 1985; 36:853-858.
9. Test MA, Berlin SB: Issues of special concern to chronically mentally ill women. *Professional Psychology* 1981; 12:136-145.
10. Seeman MV: Schizophrenic men and women require different treatment programs. *Journal of Psychiatric Treatment and Evaluation* 1983; 5:143-148.
11. Angermeyer MC, Kuhn L, Goldstein JM: Gender and the course of schizophrenia: Differences in treated outcomes. *Schizophrenia Bulletin* 1990; 16(2):293-318.
12. Goldstein JM: Gender differences in the course of schizophrenia. *American Journal of Psychiatry* 1988; 145:684-689.
13. Angermeyer MC, Goldstein JM, Kuhn L: Gender differences in schizophrenia: Rehospitalization and community survival. *Psychological Medicine* 1989; 19:365-382.

14. Watt DC, Szulecka TK: The effect of sex, marriage and age at first admission on the hospitalization of schizophrenics during 2 years following discharge. *Psychological Medicine* 1979; 9:529-539.

15. Boyer CA: Obstacles in urban housing policy for the chronically mentally ill. In: Mechanic D (Ed.): *Improving Mental Health Services: What the Social Sciences Tell Us.* (New Directions for Mental Health Services, Vol. 36). San Francisco: Jossey-Bass, 1987.

16. Grusky O, Tierney K, Manderscheid RW, et al.: Social bonding and community adjustment of chronically mentally ill adults. *Journal of Health and Social Behavior* 1985; 26:49-63.

17. Earle J, Roach V, Fraser K: *Female Dropouts: A New Perspective.* Alexandria, VA: National Association of State Boards of Education, 1987.

18. Strasser J: Urban transient women. *American Journal of Nursing* 1978; 45:2078-2079.

19. Bachrach LL: Deinstitutionalization and women: Assessing the consequences of public policy. *American Psychologist* 1984; 39(10):1171-1177.

20. Keskiner A, Zalcman MH, Rupert EH: Advantages of being female in psychiatric rehabilitation. *Archives of General Psychiatry* 1978; 28:689-692.

21. Pickett SA, Cook JA, Solomon ML: Dealing with daughters' difficulties: Caregiving burdens faced by parents of female offspring with severe mental illness. In: Greenley JR (Ed.): *Research in Community Mental Health.* Greenwich, CT: JAI, in press.

22. Pickett SA, Greenley JR, Greenberg JS: Off-timedness as a contributor to subjective burdens for parents of offspring with severe mental illness. *Family Relations,* in press.

23. Haas GL, Glick ID, Clarkin JF, et al.: Gender and schizophrenia outcome: A clinical trial of an inpatient family intervention. *Schizophrenia Bulletin* 1990; 16:277-292.

24. Cook JA, Pickett SA: Feelings of burden and criticalness among parents residing with chronically mentally ill offspring. *Journal of Applied Social Sciences* 1988; 12:79-107.

25. Russo NF: Overview: Forging research priorities for women's mental health. *American Psychologist* 1990; 45:368-373.

26. Kutza EA: Benefits for the disabled: How beneficial for women? *Sociology and Social Welfare* 1981; 8(2):298-319.

27. Thurer SL: Women and rehabilitation. *Rehabilitation Literature* 1982; 43:194-197.

28. Glass R: Meeting the program needs of women: Mainstream child care. *Rehabilitation Literature* 1982; 43:220-221.

29. Stevens BC: Dependence of schizophrenic patients on elderly relatives. *Psychological Medicine* 1972; 2:17-32.

30. Jacobson A, Richardson B: Assault experiences of 100 psychiatric inpatients: Evidence of the need for routine inquiry. *American Journal of Psychiatry* 1987; 144:908-913.

31. Kates B: *The Murder of a Shopping Bag Lady.* San Diego, CA: Harcourt Brace Jovanovich, 1985.

32. Lamb HR, Grant RW: Mentally ill women in a county jail. *Archives of General Psychiatry* 1983; 40:363-368.

33. Drake RE, Wallach MA, Hoffman JS: Housing instability and homelessness among aftercare patients of an urban state hospital. *Hospital and Community Psychiatry* 1989; 40(1):46-51.

34. Davies MA, Bromer EJ, Schulz SC, et al.: Community adjustment of chronic schizophrenic patients in urban and rural settings. *Hospital and Community Psychiatry* 1989; 40:824-830.

35. Kruzich JM, Kruzich SJ: Milieu factors influencing patients' integration into community residential facilities. *Hospital and Community Psychiatry* 1985; 36:378-382.

36. Cook JA, Graham KK, Razzano L: Psychosocial rehabilitation of deaf persons with severe mental illness: A multivariate model of residential outcomes. *Rehabilitation Psychology* 1983; 38:265-278.
37. Blanch AK, Carling PJ, Ridgway P: Normal housing with specialized supports: A psychiatric rehabilitation approach to living in the community. *Rehabilitation Psychology* 1988; 33(1):47-55.
38. Boydell KM, Everett B: What makes a house a home? An evaluation of a supported housing project for individuals with long term psychiatric backgrounds. *Canadian Journal of Community Mental Health* 1992; 11(1):109-123.
39. Nagy M: De-congregating a residential program for people with psychiatric disabilities. *Psychosocial Rehabilitation Journal* 1989; 12(4):70-74.
40. Cook JA, Jusko R, Dincin J: *Predicting Independent Functioning in the Community: Results From a 3-Year Follow-Up of Psychiatric Clientele*. Presented at the American Orthopsychiatric Association annual meetings, Chicago, 1986.
41. Bond GR, Dincin J, Setze P, et al.: The effectiveness of psychiatric rehabilitation: A summary of research at Thresholds. *Psychosocial Rehabilitation Journal* 1984; 7:6-22.
42. Wing JK, Morris B: Clinical basis of rehabilitation. In: Wing JK, Morris B (Eds.): *Handbook of Psychiatric Rehabilitation Practice*. London: Oxford University Press, 1981, pp. 3-16.
43. Bachrach LL: Chronically mentally ill women: An overview of service delivery issues. In: Bachrach LL, Nadelson CC (Eds.): *Treating Chronically Mentally Ill Women*. Washington, DC: American Psychiatric Press, 1988, pp. 1-18.
44. Endicott J, Spitzer RL, Fleiss JL, et al.: The Global Assessment Scale: A procedure for measuring overall severity of psychiatric disturbance. *Archives of General Psychiatry* 1976; 33:766-771.
45. Katz M, Lyerly S: Method of measuring adjustment and social behavior in the community: Rationale, description, discriminative validity and scale development. *Psychological Reports* 1963; 13:503-535.
46. Tanzman B: An overview of surveys of mental health consumers' preferences for housing and support services. *Hospital and Community Psychiatry* 1993; 44:450-455.
47. Goodman L: The relationship between modified and usual multiple-regression approaches to the analysis of dichotomous variables. In: Heise D (Ed.): *Sociological Methodology*. San Francisco: Jossey-Bass, 1976.
48. Vanneman R, Pampel F: The American perception of class and status. *American Sociological Review* 1977; 42:422-437.
49. Van Horne WA, Tonnesen TV (Eds.): *Race: Twentieth-Century Dilemmas, Twenty-First Century Prognoses*. Milwaukee: University of Wisconsin, 1989.
50. Cournos F: The impact of environmental factors on outcome in residential programs. *Hospital and Community Psychiatry* 1987; 38(8):848-852.
51. Hull JT, Thompson JC: Predicting adaptive functioning among mentally ill persons in community settings. *American Journal of Community Psychology* 1981; 9(3):247-268.
52. Cook JA, Jonikas J, Solomon M: Models of vocational rehabilitation for youth and adults with severe mental illness. *American Rehabilitation* 1992; 35:243-265.
53. Cook JA, Roussel A: *Who Works and What Works: Effects of Race, Class, Age and Gender on Employment Among the Psychiatrically Disabled*. Presented at the American Sociological Association annual meetings, Chicago, 1987.
54. Vash CL: Employment issues for women with disabilities. *Rehabilitation Literature* 1982; 43(7-8):198-207.
55. Menz FE, Hansen G, Smith H, et al.: Gender equity in access, services and benefits from vocational rehabilitation. *Journal of Rehabilitation* 1989; 55:31-40.

Part II

Special Issues of Empowerment, Severe Mental Illness and Survivors of Trauma, and At-Risk Populations

Part II of this book examines special issues in women's mental health services: empowerment (Section A), severe mental illness and survivors of trauma (Section B), and at-risk populations (Section C). Empowerment, severe mental disorders, and trauma are issues that affect all people, regardless of gender, race, age, or ethnic origin. Men may also be victims of violence; have serious mental disorders; and face social, financial, and geographic barriers to treatment. Nevertheless, as the chapters in Part I of this book have indicated and the chapters in Part II will illustrate, women, as a heterogeneous population, experience a different set of mental health risks than men, particularly women who bear and raise children, who care for their family, or who have suffered trauma.

In addition, systems serving women in need of mental health and/or substance abuse services (or women with comorbid disorders) have generally been fragmented, poorly organized, or nonexistent. For example, jails and prisons historically have not offered parity in the treatment of mental disorders and substance abuse for women compared with services that exist for men. In addition, nursing homes, with a principal population of women, have been overwhelmed with estimates of unmet need for mental health care, particularly for women with serious mental disorders.

The two chapters in Section A of Part II examine consumer involvement in decision making and self-determination, including building collaborative relationships for making life choices in treatment intervention, policy making, and supportive housing. Kalinowski and Penney (Chapter 7) review the development of the ex-patient social movement and discuss empowerment, choice, healing, and recovery. Through selected case studies, the authors illustrate the power dynamics that exist in mental health services and the resulting outcomes of these practices on women. Kalinowski and Penney also discuss internal and external mandates for achieving personal empowerment in mental health services.

Ridgway and colleagues (Chapter 8) propose a highly individualized and participatory approach to the development of supportive housing programs, based on a recognition of the impact of the environment on mental health. They suggest that people should assist in designing their environments to create areas that reflect and reinforce their personal identities. Literature reviewed by the authors suggests that involving residents in the design of their living situations could improve clinical outcomes as well as residential stability and satisfaction. The authors conclude that current models of residential planning and housing development have neglected selected aspects of housing in favor of concerns about productivity, cost, and conventional standards of safety and decency. They suggest that incorporating women's concerns into mental health policy making may ultimately benefit men as well as women.

Section B of Part II consists of eight chapters (Chapters 9 through 16) on women with severe mental illness, including those who have survived trauma. Mowbray and colleagues (Chapter 9) present an overview of the critical issues and problems in life functioning for women with severe mental illness, many of whom have adjoining substance abuse and victimization. The authors conclude that gender itself is a barrier to effective mental health treatment and that greater attention must be given to improving treatment and rehabilitation services to women with severe mental illness.

Blanch and colleagues (Chapter 10) discuss the results of a statewide task force on women with severe mental illness who have parenting responsibilities. They suggest that existing mental health, rehabilitation, and social services programs have largely ignored parenting as an important and valued role for these individuals. They conclude that there is a critical need for improved coordination, services planning, and management between mental health and social services delivery systems to ensure that the needs of both women with severe mental illness and their children are adequately addressed.

Chapters 11 through 16 discuss the epidemiologic, legal, and service system issues of women with severe mental illness who have experienced trauma. Through empirical and case study methodologies, these chapters explore current services delivery deficiencies and suggest strategies for making mental health delivery systems more responsive to women with serious mental illness who have suffered physical and sexual abuse.

In Chapter 11, Alexander and Muenzenmaier discuss the importance of early and adequate identification of co-occurring mental illness, substance abuse problems, and victimization in treatment programs for women. They cite the need to include assertive outreach programs, comprehensive and flexible services, and a treatment philosophy based on competency building and empowerment, in safe and accessible programs within the community.

Stefan (Chapter 12) examines the impact of law on women who have survived sexual abuse in childhood and who have been diagnosed with borderline personality disorder. Through examples of case law, the author discusses how perceptions of women with mental disorders may affect their legal status. She reviews how a diagnosis of borderline personality disorder affects legal outcomes in five areas: law of evidence, family law, disability benefits law, law related to civil commitment and rights in institutional settings, and antidiscrimination law. Stefan also discusses how clinicians, mental health professionals as witnesses, and administrators/policymakers can better understand, support, and provide safety for women who have suffered from childhood sexual abuse and who continue to struggle with mental illness.

Newmann and colleagues (Chapter 13) examine the impact of failing to assess histories of physical and sexual abuse in women with serious mental illness, or to provide appropriate interventions, on service use and costs of care. Their results revealed that women with abuse histories had significantly higher annual mental health costs compared to women with no abuse histories. In addition, the study revealed that one third of 1,600 clients had unknown physical or sexual abuse histories. The authors suggest that case managers and clinicians receive training in assessment for physical and sexual abuse histories.

Harris (Chapter 14) also critiques the existing mental health service delivery systems for failing to acknowledge and respond to the specific clinical and programmatic needs of women diagnosed with serious mental illness who have survived sexual abuse. She recommends routine assessment of current and childhood sexual abuse, educating clinical staff about working with trauma survivors, avoiding inadvertent retraumatization, and changing the case manager's role to include overall coordination of all aspects of treatment with women diagnosed with severe mental illness who are trauma survivors.

The final two chapters in Section B are case studies of individual experiences within mental health services delivery systems. Jennings (Chapter 15) uses a case study of her daughter to illustrate how the current mental health system may fail to acknowledge or respond to individuals whose problems fall outside the prevailing medical paradigm. This chapter illustrates a pervasive and fundamental flaw in mental health systems: the failure to listen to clients, to accept their experiences as valid, and to modify services accordingly.

Bills and Bloom (Chapter 16) use a personal account of a clinician to examine the successful transformation of a women's inpatient unit in a state hospital setting from chaos and violence to a therapeutic milieu through the use of innovative, community-based approaches in caring for victims of trauma. They conclude that the effectiveness of a trauma-based approach depends on leadership, commitment, and vision on the part of both providers and consumers of care.

Section C (Chapters 17 and 18) of Part II presents the specific needs of women with mental illness who are in selected at-risk populations: women with mental illness who are in jails or prisons and older women with mental illness. Veysey (Chapter 17) discusses the relative lack of somatic, mental health, and substance abuse services for women in correctional facilities compared with services that exist for men. To prevent women from becoming more seriously ill when leaving correctional facilities, and to avoid needless punishment for women who have been identified as having special mental health needs, the author suggests the following mental health services be made available within correctional facilities: screening and evaluation, crisis intervention procedures, peer support and counseling programs, parenting programs, integration of services, training programs for professionals, and outcomes evaluation for treatment interventions.

This section concludes with a chapter by Padgett and colleagues (Chapter 18) reviewing mental health needs and services use in community and institutional settings by older women. While the authors maintain that older women represent a heterogeneous population, they emphasize the importance of focusing efforts on primary care providers in the management and delivery of mental health services for older women.

7

Empowerment and Women's Mental Health Services

Coni Kalinowski, M.D.
Darby Penney, M.S.

Writing about mental health services and the empowerment of women using them presents a considerable challenge. This is an area where basic values, personal experience, and spiritual beliefs play a crucial role, and where careful examination of the underlying issues often leads to conclusions that are in diametric opposition to traditional clinical training and traditional assumptions about people with psychiatric disabilities. Furthermore, the issue of personal empowerment is rarely studied by researchers and rarely addressed in professional journals. Information is more likely to be found in personal testimony, unpublished papers, journal entries, Internet communications, and other media outside the professional literature—media at which clinicians and other professionals may look askance.

This chapter will approach the issue of empowerment and women's mental health through an examination of the values and principles of the ex-mental patients' movement, a feminist-influenced social change movement. Recent recipient-led initiatives designed to move the mental health system away from power and control and toward empowerment and collaboration will be discussed, new approaches to clinical practice will be offered for consideration, and the implications for mental health policymakers will be discussed.

THE EX-PATIENTS' MOVEMENT: A POLITICAL
STRUGGLE FOR EMPOWERMENT

While the ex-patients' movement has roots in 19th-century social reform movements and the work of individual ex-patients struggling for justice in that era, the modern movement began in earnest in the 1970s. What was then often termed the "mental patients' liberation movement" took its inspiration from other contemporary collective struggles of disenfranchised peoples, including African Americans and women. Like these movements, the ex-patients' movement was primarily concerned with human and civil rights, with stigma and discrimination faced by its members, and with developing a future in which the larger society would recognize their full humanity.[1]

The early ex-patients' movement developed an analysis of the mental health services delivery system as a top-down, patriarchal system that isolated diagnosed individuals and deprived them of power. Many of the early theorists, writers, and activists were women, many of them influenced by feminist thinking. This is perhaps not surprising, since women are more likely than men to be psychiatrically diagnosed and treated with psychotropic drugs.[2] However, unlike the civil rights movement or the antiwar movement, women have been not only the workhorses of the ex-patients' movement but prominent leaders as well. This has remained true through the years; as Sally Clay has stated, "We are primarily a movement of middle-aged women."[3]

Pioneering activists recognized that the medical model of mental illness, based on the patriarchal view that professional "experts" should control treatment, was a primary source of disenfranchisement. As Susan Stefan has pointed out, "A disease model for emotional distress may carry hidden problems for women and minorities and others whose distress and discontent may be due to their social circumstances, but which the disease model places squarely on deficits in their biological makeup" (p. 198).[4] In an attempt to come to terms with the effect of the medical model on their lives, ex-patient activists embraced the feminist process of consciousness-raising.[5] Consciousness-raising is a group process in which people with some form of commonality share and explore their experiences to draw connections between the personal and the political. As practiced within the women's movement, consciousness-raising helped women recognize that concerns about relationships, sexuality, and feelings of inadequacy were not so much individual problems as they were manifestations of society's systemic oppression of women.

In a parallel way, the practice of consciousness-raising within the ex-patients' movement helped individuals realize that many of the difficulties they encountered were not related to their diagnoses, but were the result of patterns of discrimination and oppression. Ex-patients came to learn that their feelings of isolation, inadequacy, and powerlessness were the result of real practices within the mental health system and real discrimination in the community, not by-products of their illnesses. They came to see that the public at large held a set of negative assumptions about mental patients: "That they were incompetent, unable to do things for themselves, constantly in need of supervision and assistance, unpredictable, likely to be violent or irrational."[5] Consciousness-raising was also instrumental in helping ex-patients recognize their own internalized stigma, their unconscious agreement with society's negative stereotypes of mental patients, and in developing new, more empowering beliefs about their abilities.

The ex-patients' movement continues to work for social, political, and legal equality with other citizens, for the right to self-definition and self-determination, and for person-centered alternatives to disempowering clinical practices. As Judi Chamberlin[5] recounts, groups are united by certain rules and principles: Mental health terminology is considered suspect; attitudes that limit opportunities for mental patients are to be discouraged and changed; and members' feelings—particularly feelings of anger toward the mental health system—are considered real and legitimate, not "symptoms of illness."[6]

Over the past two decades, the ex-patients' movement has evolved from a generally discounted fringe group to one that is a significant political force for change within the mental health field. The feminist values that influenced the development of the ex-patients' movement provide a philosophical base for reforming the mental health system to promote empowerment and recovery for all service recipients regardless of gender. Among the concepts frequently identified as valuable and desirable in the ex-patient literature are empowerment, choice, healing, and recovery.[5-10] Self-help and mutual support are also seen as key ingredients of a process by which people may promote their own healing.[10,11] Applying a feminist analysis, Susan Stefan[4] contends that the mental health system should replace hierarchy with participation and choice, enforced dependency with enhanced control, isolation with connection, models of pathology with models of recovery and strength, and objectification and a primarily biological model with an understanding of people as humans interacting with each other and operating in a social context that has a vast influence on their behavior and mental health.

BEYOND BIOLOGY: MENTAL HEALTH ISSUES IN A SOCIAL CONTEXT

The medical model's characterization of mental patients as people with biological brain dysfunctions has, in many ways, interfered with a full understanding of the lives and needs of people in mental and emotional distress. This model portrays the problem as illness rooted in the individual, treatable primarily by medication, and "takes little account of relationships or social context."[4]

The ex-patients' movement has long recognized that many of the problems of mental patients are the same problems that other poor and marginalized people face: lack of decent housing, lack of access to jobs, inadequate health care services, and isolation from the mainstream of society. A mental health system based on a commitment to empowerment and recovery would focus its resources on these concrete problems so that service recipients could overcome the social barriers that keep them from rejoining the community.

Reliance on the medical model has also kept the mental health system from addressing the link between violence and mental health problems. Recent studies have begun to reveal the extent and the critical nature of this link: Craine et al.[12] found that 51 percent of women reported histories of childhood sexual abuse, Breyer et al.[13] found that 72 percent of female psychiatric inpatients reported physical or sexual abuse histories, and Beck and van der Kolk[14] reported that 46 percent of women who were long-term psychiatric inpatients had histories of childhood incest.

A reformed mental health system that took seriously the connections between violence and mental health problems would examine and discard many of its current practices, and it would address conditions and practices that disempower patients and promote violence. Such conditions include "the 'culture of violence' on some inpatient wards, where staff often provoke patients to violence and use violence or intimidation to control patients" (p. 8),[15] and restraint and seclusion practices that retraumatize individuals who have been victims of violence.

PARTICIPATION AND CHOICE

Self-determination and choice are primary organizing principles of the ex-patients' movement,[5,7-10,16] seen as basic human rights that all people deserve, and as a prerequisite for recovery: People who are not allowed to exercise these rights can become trapped in learned helplessness and despair. There is widespread commitment to the idea that people have a right to choose the services that best meet their needs and that they can do so only if they have access to complete and accurate information. If these values were operationalized within the mental health system, policy making, services design, and individual relationships between recipients and providers would be transformed. Because people who have experienced the mental health system often have profoundly different views on mental health than do professionals, their meaningful participation in decision making can have a significant impact on the way problems are conceptualized and solutions identified, leading to more recipient-friendly outcomes.[17]

For example, the increased participation of service recipients in decisions that affect their lives would almost certainly serve to move people from enforced dependency on the mental health system toward greater control of their own life choices, and might well lead the mental health system to come to grips with the negative effects of learned helplessness and coercion. As Blanch and Parrish[18] found, "Service recipients report that coercive interventions undermine possibilities for recovery and independence . . . recovery appears to be related to having control over one's life. . . . In contrast, involuntary treatment appears to leave individuals feeling hopeless, helpless and believing they will never recover" (p. 7).

If recipients are to regain control over their own lives, professionals will need to learn new ways of working with individuals who use their services. The medical model, as Holmes and Saleebey[19] point out, "gives the professional considerable social control over the client or patient. This sanctioned control, in turn, creates barriers to the very empowerment professional helpers hope to facilitate." As an empowering alternative, the authors advocate a truly collaborative relationship in which the professional "places him- or herself within the same community of the client, which allows the helper and the client to encounter one another as equals working toward the same desired outcome" (pp. 62-63).[19]

CHANGING CLINICAL PRACTICES TO PROMOTE EMPOWERMENT

It is clear that the empowerment of people using mental health services requires a new paradigm of services delivery based on the values of inclusion, self-determination, and the equality and dignity of all people. Few providers or recipients would disagree, yet the revision of services delivery to adhere to these values remains hotly disputed.

The term "empowerment" has come to connote a jumble of concepts and approaches that incorporate the use of less restrictive treatment settings, cost reduction strategies, recipients' rights issues, and attitudinal change. Attempts to incorporate empowerment into practice have generally focused on the increasing client choice and control over services. Invariably, however, clinicians are confronted with situations in which offering improved choices and relinquishing control has not seemed to assist the recipient to direct her life toward desired goals. Such experiences are often disheartening for providers who are committed to the empowerment of the people they serve and have been used by critics of client-directed services to discount the ability of people having psychiatric disabilities to make their own choices.

An explanation for these apparent treatment failures may lie in the conceptualization of empowerment itself. It is sometimes assumed that empowerment is an innate aspect of human existence and that all individuals are equally capable of making choices and directing their lives. This view presumes that once authority is given to the person by external sources, the person can and will assume control and responsibility for her life. In this view, choices are largely determined by external factors such as resources, legal authority, and finances, determinants that are described in this chapter as the "external mandate" for personal empowerment.

Empowerment can alternatively be characterized as a developmental process having both external and internal determinants. This model presumes that people experience an ongoing process of growth and skill development that improves their abilities and understanding regarding choices and the direction of their lives. This process, which we refer to as the "internal mandate" for empowerment, is accompanied by the development of faith, hope, personal value, and meaning.[20-23] While the external mandate will affect the scope of choices and availability of resources, the internal mandate will determine the person's perspective on decision making and self-determination.

The developmental model of empowerment offers an explanation for the treatment failures described above. The individual's internal mandate, consisting of self-determination skills developed to cope with external barriers to empowerment, may or may not support personal empowerment when these barriers are lowered. While it is imperative for mental health services to address external barriers to empowerment, they must also support the person's internal mandate with feedback, encouragement, and evaluative discussion.

Services designed to focus on personal empowerment must begin with the assumption that people make the most advantageous choices that they can, based on their own evaluation of their resources, skills, and experience. Taken together, these choices propel people toward a way of being in the world that reflects their values, interests, identity, worldview, and goals. However, providers have been taught to make judgments and recommendations based largely on community and professional norms, which often reflect the multitude of power biases in our society, and effectively preclude an empowering stance.

Empowering services do not prescribe intervention, but assist people to evaluate their skills and opportunities, to explore their world and personal vision, and to pursue their own goals. To accomplish this, services must:

1. Support the development of a genuine relationship that promotes power sharing and communicates mutual hope, dignity, and respect;
2. Reflect the goals and values defined by the person receiving services;
3. Support the external mandate for empowerment by providing information, opportunity, representation, and choice; and
4. Support the internal mandate for empowerment through discussion, feedback, and serious consideration of the perspective the person brings to decision making and self-determination.

EMPOWERING RELATIONSHIPS

The service provider who wishes to foster personal empowerment must join the person seeking services in a relationship characterized by the communication of respect, value, dignity, and equality. This seemingly obvious and simple task proves to be one of the most challenging aspects of moving from a directive to an empowering stance.

The pervasive prejudice and stigma associated with having a psychiatric diagnosis, sometimes referred to as mentalism, is painfully evident in all aspects of our society. The power difference that exists between those who are psychiatrically labeled and those who are not is acted out repeatedly in interpersonal interaction, policy, attitudes, language, and architecture in what Pierce, writing about the dynamics of racism, termed *macro-* and *micro-aggressions*.[24] Pierce points out that while the effect of accumulated micro-aggressions may be devastating, these micro-aggressions are largely perpetrated unconsciously by individuals and groups who believe they espouse the value of equality, and therefore fail to recognize the offensiveness and destructiveness of their actions and attitudes. Providers of mental health services are not spared from this power dynamic and—despite their best intentions—are a great source of demeaning messages toward individuals receiving services. In fact, it appears that recipients of services often experience greater discrimination within the mental health system itself than in the community at large.[25]

In addition, fear of labeled people, based on myths and stereotypes, has led mental health practitioners into the realm of social control, where intrusive and coercive interventions are demanded to maintain a particular social milieu. Few providers can truly resist the overwhelming social and legal pressures that are brought to bear to "protect the public from the mentally ill." Those who attempt to do so generally find themselves similarly stigmatized, blamed, and discredited.

The tendency to relate to people from a directive stance is further reinforced by professional training, which discourages power sharing with the client and instead emphasizes prescribing the correct treatment, maintaining interpersonal distance, and assigning accurate diagnostic labels. As a result, the attempt to form an equal partnership requires the unlearning of very deeply ingrained behaviors and attitudes, and providers may find themselves unwittingly operating from a traditional autocratic stance. Indeed, it is questionable whether a truly egalitarian relationship is achievable, or whether the most we can hope to accomplish is to approximate power sharing:

Ms. A is a 54-year-old woman diagnosed with schizophrenia who refused medications on an outpatient basis and was repeatedly admitted to an acute inpatient unit for agitation and disruptive public behavior. She felt medication was poison and that "a man coming through the walls" would kill her if she took it. She insisted on living in the projects with friends, and refused to consider a residential program, though the team felt that her friends could not care for her adequately. The treatment team referred to her as "extremely disabled," "non-compliant," and "oppositional," and attributed her refusal of services to "poor judgment" due to her "deeply entrenched delusional beliefs." They put a plan in place to refer Ms. A to the state hospital for long-term institutionalization. However, Ms. A objected strenuously, and the treatment team, knowing they would lose a guardianship hearing, opted to offer her services from an Assertive Community Treatment (ACT) team that operated from a client-directed perspective. Members of the ACT team discussed the situation with Ms. A, and obtained much the same information as the inpatient team had. Because their focus was on empowerment, however, they questioned whether the inpatient team had pejoratively labeled Ms. A due to her unwillingness to comply, and concluded that the team did not have sufficient knowledge of Ms. A's perspective to understand her decisions.

The ACT team concentrated on spending time with Ms. A and addressing issues of importance to her. Over time, members of the team were able to develop a degree of trust and credibility with Ms. A. Many of her fears of being robbed and attacked by the man in the wall, previously construed as "delusional," became comprehensible within the context of her experiences in the housing projects.

It was learned that Ms. A was very close to the small children in the household where she lived, and despite her disability, Ms. A was an important support to them. Her concerns about their safety in the housing project caused her to want to remain alert and vigilant; the medications made her drowsy. Her frequent hospitalizations were not problematic to her, as they offered an opportunity to recover from the strain of living in fear. She and her friends had resisted all previous inquiry into their home life due to fears of retribution from various social service agencies. The team offered the family assistance to move to a more secure environment. Ms. A experienced a decrease in anxiety and frequency of hospitalization, though she continued to refuse medications and retained her original system of beliefs.[a]

This case study illustrates a number of power dynamics common in mental health care. It is the provider (in this case, the inpatient team), operating from a powerful directive stance, who identifies the problem (schizophrenia, agitation, delusions, frequent hospitalization) and decides on treatment that is appropriate (medications and residential programming) and desired outcomes (compliance, reduced delusions, and fewer hospitalizations). Ms. A's divergent interpretation is discounted and construed as a manifestation of her illness.

Often, disagreement between recipient and provider is not even acknowledged. To do so would imply that the recipient retains an opinion about the situation that merits discussion and exploration. Instead, a refusal to approach the situation from the conceptual framework established by the provider is pathologized and dismissed; perceptions and experiences are recorded as symptoms, and strengths go unrecognized and unacknowledged. The provider's choices are given the label "clinical treatment recommendations" to further signify their import, while the recipient's choices are belittled ("poor judgment"). The recipient is expected to comply with the provider's choices, regardless of their relevance to her worldview and daily experience.

The directive clinical stance, by focusing on deficits, further injures the person at a spiritual level through disregard for the value and meaning of relationships. In this example, Ms. A is viewed by the inpatient team as needy and ill, and her relationships are assumed to provide her with unilateral care and support. The people with whom she lives are assumed by the inpatient team to be her caretakers. The depth of Ms. A's commitment to these relationships is overlooked, as if to imply that

Ms. A's diagnosis renders her incapable of love. Ms. A's contributions of emotional support, homemaking, child care, and disability income are devalued, and the inpatient team recommends that Ms. A be removed to a residential program for additional treatment. Coerced relocations, reproductive losses, and forced separation from important others are common experiences among women psychiatric survivors. Little research is available to document the outcomes of these practices, despite the obvious risks of alienation, disconnection, and depression.

It is important to note that the directive stance also disempowers the inpatient team members, who will remain ineffective in assisting Ms. A as long as they are entrenched in the belief that they are most competent to determine what is in her best interest. Feelings of helplessness and futility generated by failed treatment efforts are powerful contributors to staff burnout and are a commonly cited reason for reluctance to work with people having disabilities.

In contrast to the directive approach, the client-directed provider attempts to minimize the power differential that exists between provider and recipient. In this example, the ACT team members affirm that Ms. A is making meaningful choices about her life and try to discover with her why this particular pattern of life choice constitutes her best option at the present time. In this process, they gradually learn about Ms. A's reasoning regarding her choices and come to understand why Ms. A does not share the goals and values of the inpatient team. When services do not appear to be helpful, it is the shared responsibility of Ms. A and the team to work together to identify new approaches and solutions. The recipient is acknowledged to be the expert on her life, and providers refrain from measuring the reality of the person's experience against their own worldview. Instead, the person's perceptions and experiences are discussed in terms of the impact they have on her personal relationships and life goals.

For example, at one point Ms. A inquired of a staff member whether she believed that the man in the wall was real. The staff member responded that she was not sure and described her dilemma: She believed in Ms. A's integrity and saw her obvious distress, but she had never seen the man herself even when Ms. A pointed him out. This led to a productive discussion about Ms. A's dilemma of feeling discounted and disbelieved and ways that staff might be able to better support her.

Research suggests that the combined influences of misogyny and mentalism may create specific barriers to empowerment for the female psychiatric survivor. Women have, for example, been found to be more likely to be chronically institutionalized, to be told that they must stay on medications for life, and to receive neuroleptics for lengthy periods.[26] These differences are believed to contribute to increased iatrogenic chronicity, reduced goals and expectations, and pessimism for vocational recovery among women who have psychiatric diagnoses.

It remains unclear, however, to what extent these differences represent the specific effects of gender biases as opposed to the more general effects of disenfranchisement, as other groups that experience oppression tend to receive similar treatment within the mental health system. For example, African Americans have been shown to be more likely to be institutionalized than Caucasians and are prescribed higher doses of neuroleptic medications.[27-29]

In either case, the goal of supporting empowerment in women psychiatric survivors requires that both provider and recipient commit to an ongoing examination of power issues in all their manifestations, including gender, psychiatric diagnosis, socioeconomic group, and ethnicity. It is a common misconception that women providers will innately possess a greater understanding of these issues, having been subjected themselves to oppressive experiences attributable to misogyny. In reality, people who have been the objects of oppression are likely to have internalized many stereotypic, negative images and beliefs and remain at risk to be the perpetrators of oppressive acts toward others like themselves. This tendency is amplified by the process of professional acculturation, which demands collusion and identification with existing power structures. Thus, women mental health professionals cannot be assumed to be supportive of women's empowerment in mental health services, and they may at times act in a clearly misogynist manner toward women survivors.

Open confrontation of these issues among providers tends to produce extreme discomfort, anger, and defensiveness, as few people relish a glimpse of themselves in the role of the oppressor and most fear the loss of power. It is therefore of utmost importance that administrators and management of mental health services agencies strive to create a work environment in which it is acceptable and safe to discuss issues of power and discrimination, and in which the examination of these issues is an organizational priority.

DESIGNING SERVICES AROUND
THE RECIPIENT'S GOALS

The most direct way to support the person's external mandate for empowerment in mental health services delivery is to engage the person in defining her own service goals, and then to collaboratively design and implement services that directly reflect these stated goals. This approach to services delivery has been termed "client-directed" to distinguish it from "client-centered" services in which the person is consulted about her preferences, but service decisions are ultimately made by the provider or others in what they feel to be the person's best interest.

Objections raised regarding client-directed services tend to be based on real challenges encountered in clinical practice, but often reflect prejudices and negative stereotypes concerning people who are psychiatrically labeled, compounded by the natural anxiety that accompanies a loss of power. Unfamiliarity with power-sharing experiences produces expectations of insurmountable worst-case scenarios that rarely if ever occur in clinical practice. Some of the more common concerns of providers include the following.

1. *"What if the person asks me to do something illegal or unethical?"* It is important to remember that the goal of client-directed services is power-sharing, not reversal of the oppressive power dynamic. Client-directed providers would be likely to respond to such a request with sincerity regarding their concerns about the possible implications and consequences of such a service plan, and honest feedback about the constraints imposed by ethics or laws.

2. *"What if the person has no service goals?"* This is a common challenge in client-directed services delivery that stems from the fact that setting concrete personal goals and implementation of plans is difficult for everyone. The challenge is increased for the individual who may have

limited her personal aspirations in response to institutional expectations, prejudice, or labeling. In client-directed practice, supporting the person to entertain various personal goals becomes the focus of initial services. The process of goal development can be quite lengthy and can involve considerable exploration of the person's past and present interests, personal visioning, discussion of grief over the loss of past goals, and offering varied opportunities.

3. "*What if the person's goal is unrealistic?*" This concern encompasses instances in which the person is perceived as expressing goals that are excessively ambitious, and those in which the goal reflects a divergent interpretation of reality. In either case, the client-directed service provider would refrain from passing judgment on the value of the person's goal, and would instead facilitate a process in which the individual begins to examine her values and motivation, and to break the goal down into "doable" steps.

This is an area in which stereotypes concerning labeled people become especially apparent, as evidenced by lowered expectations, impulses to protect people from failure, and efforts to redefine people's goals within a more acceptable framework. Because they are based on these prejudices, well-intended attempts on the part of providers to advise people regarding their goals are likely to be received as a put-down and to undermine the quality of the relationship with the person receiving services. Experience in client-oriented programs would suggest that fears regarding "unrealistic goals" are largely unfounded. In one study of client-directed services, a review of over 200 charted client goals revealed only one that reflected a divergent belief system about reality. Virtually all reflected rehabilitation goals that could be fully supported by service providers. The most common goals included having one's own apartment, having paid employment (volunteer work was not a frequent goal), and improving significant relationships.[30]

SUPPORT OF THE EXTERNAL MANDATE

In addition to client-directed services planning, support for the external mandate for empowerment includes expansion of resources, options, legal authority, information, and political influence that will enhance the breadth and weight of the individual's choices.[31] In essence, this calls for providers to focus on the community as a recipient of mental health services, and for communities to be inclusive of citizens of all abilities. It also requires a reexamination of the importance of information to personal empowerment.

Planning

People who are receiving services must be included in a meaningful way in planning and directing the system of services, without resorting to tokenism, in which it assumed that "the consumer viewpoint" can be represented by a single individual. When this occurs, the token individual experiences pressure to operate according to the conceptual framework of the majority and is easily outnumbered and outvoted. Outside the group, the individual runs the risk of being marginalized within her group of origin, and she may be seen as a turncoat or someone who has sold out. To avoid this problem, governing boards, task forces, and administration should be composed of a majority of people receiving services, with ongoing efforts to support gender and cultural diversity. Accommodations and supports, including financial support and transportation, may be needed to assist people with disabilities to fully participate in these roles. Women often need the support of safe child care options.

Community Outreach and Development

Community outreach and development is often overlooked, and even actively avoided. In general, service providers in mental health are reflective and introverted, and they tend to organize services by drawing groups of similarly labeled people to a common site for activities or discussion, segregating themselves and the people they serve from community activities. Rarely are service providers trained in community development or to be aware of the barriers that individuals encounter in daily community life.

Community development efforts should include public education, outreach to local businesses, creating visibility in community projects, and participation in employment and housing development activities.

Women's health and mental health services should be designed to use natural community resources, rather than creating segregated programs for people who are psychiatrically labeled. People who use services and their families are often excellent partners and leaders in these efforts.

Information

Information is essential to personal empowerment: An uninformed choice is not really a choice. In a recent survey of former state hospital residents in Maine, over 95 percent of respondents regarded teaching about medications as important, while only 70 percent stated that they always or sometimes received this service from their providers.[32] Contrary to common stereotypes, providing information about medication side effects does not appear to deter people from participating in treatment, but may increase interest and investment in evaluating and adjusting medication regimens.[30] Information about treatment should be made available in an ongoing fashion and through a variety of approaches, including consultation with professionals, written materials, group discussion, and self-help. Women should be made aware that most of the available information about psychopharmacology is limited to the effects of medications on men and that this gap in medical knowledge may have significant implications for treatment. Individuals should have the opportunity to review their clinical records and to discuss them with their providers.

Information about recipients' rights, effective grievance procedures, and access to advocacy and legal services must be available. In addition, organizations should be aware of the potential for retribution against an individual who uses these services, and should foster an organizational milieu in which conflict and criticism are used constructively.

SUPPORT OF THE INTERNAL MANDATE

The internal mandate for personal empowerment refers to the cognitive, emotional, and spiritual perspective that the person brings to the process of directing the course of her life. As recipient and provider of services work together toward service goals, specific issues regarding empowerment will undoubtedly arise. These issues can be used as opportunities to assist people in examining the complex interaction between their external and internal mandates. By doing so, they may attain a greater understanding of their process of choice and a greater mastery of their self-determination. Choice and empowerment, in this way, are continuously integrated into the ongoing processes of goal development, problem solving, and outcomes evaluation.

Issues pertaining to the development of the internal mandate of empowerment tend to cluster in three general areas that encompass knowledge, skills, and spiritual development.

Choice Identification

This aspect of the internal mandate includes knowledge of choices, the ability to develop options, and awareness of the extent to which one's behavior is or can be chosen. These skills also include the capacity to view one's choices and actions in relation to, but separate from, those of others.

Early in recovery, women usually engage in a process of becoming more aware of the impact of misogyny and mentalism on their lives. Women psychiatric survivors have written extensively about the devastation of internalized stigma and the trauma associated with discrimination and traditional treatments.[33-36] Yet this is an area in which providers of services often fail to support the development of the internal mandate of empowerment. Providers confronted with the traumatizing aspects of treatment commonly react with denial, disbelief, or justification for their actions, which only deepens the injury to the recipient. At times, recipients even describe experiences of retribution, including termination of services, overmedication, and hostile attitudes from staff.

It is important for providers to recognize an individual's identification of and reaction to oppression as an essential part of the person's recovery, and to support the development of the person's internal mandate by facing the anger of the recipient, acknowledging the injurious experience, discussing with the person the provider's role as the offender, and taking action to ameliorate existing power differences. It is also important for these steps to be recognized as a necessary part of the recovery and empowerment of the provider, who must become aware of and assume responsibility for her participation in the power dynamics, and unlearn attitudes and behaviors associated with misogyny and mentalism.

Awareness of choice is vulnerable to compromise in settings that focus exclusively on biological approaches to treatment and regard treatment participation as a compliance issue. The biological model attributes psychiatric disability to a genetically determined neurochemical condition. Taken to the extreme, people may come away with the impression that they cannot influence the course of their recovery because they cannot defeat their biological makeup. They may respond with a sense of futility, helplessness, or despondence. This response may in turn be interpreted by staff as further evidence of the biological illness, leading to a downward cycle of hopelessness. Recipients have also recounted experiences in which this sense of helplessness caused them to relinquish existing efforts to monitor and control their own behavior, as for example, a woman survivor of trauma who had come to regard her outbursts of rage as an intractable symptom of mania and stopped her attempts to master cognitive behavioral techniques for anger management.

This is not to imply that services that support empowerment should necessarily discount biological approaches to treatment. Rather, somatic treatments may be seen as one of many tools that a person may choose to employ toward recovery. It is the shared responsibility of the recipient and provider to explore all available options and to evaluate which tools are most effective. This process ultimately yields a repertoire of skills, approaches, and resources, often including somatic treatments, that enhances the person's capacity to manage distress and furthers health and recovery.

In settings where compliance with treatment is highly valued, an individual may come to regard decisions about services not as a choice but as a negotiation tactic:

A 19-year-old woman trauma survivor was developing a proactive crisis plan with her community support team. She was asked about interventions that she found helpful, but found it difficult to identify past treatment experiences in which she had not felt coerced and retraumatized. She was then asked to imagine the ideal crisis response for her. She outlined a plan of intervention that was somewhat unconventional, but achievable. The service team inquired whether she would like to pursue negotiations with the hospital to arrange this plan. The woman replied, "Sure—and I'll go to dual diagnosis group when I'm there." A team member was confused. "Do you mean you'll go because other people want you to, or is it because you find the group helpful for yourself?" The woman now looked confused. After a pause she responded, "I'll do O.T., too."

In this example, the individual involved appears to use her choice about the group (and about occupational therapy) as a bargaining tool to further her goal of an effective crisis plan, and she seems unaware that she could base her choice on her own assessment of her needs.

In this example, the discussions about choice and self-determination that occur during the development of the crisis plan should be linked (with the person's permission and participation) to her work in psychotherapy (regarding her early trauma and retraumatization experiences). Issues of empowerment are particularly critical in serving survivors of trauma, who have often been dominated in early life by the tyrannical demands and threats of the abuser. The development of personal choice is superseded by the need to placate the abuser in the attempt to avoid violence, violation, and sometimes death. Specific aspects of the abuse experience, for example, being accused by the abuser of causing events clearly beyond one's control or being blamed for the abuse, may further confound the person's ability to choose, identify outcomes of her choices, and attribute responsibility.

Competence to Choose

These skills include the capacity to seek and evaluate information pertaining to choices and to ascertain when one has sufficient information to proceed with choice and action. Competence to make choices also requires adequate self-esteem. Providers may need to support the individual in obtaining and evaluating information. For people who have had lengthy institutionalizations, this may include reviewing basic skills that have atrophied with disuse, such as writing letters or using the telephone directory. It should also include opportunities for people to develop more complex skills, such as organizing an informational interview, using E-mail and the Internet, questioning the recommendations of a physician, or consulting with an attorney.

It is important to consider, in addressing information-gathering skills, that much information is passed formally or informally along gender, cultural, and class lines in ways that communicate values and social roles. This shapes the fund of information available to the person and contributes to her approach to information gathering. Most individuals consciously or unconsciously respond to these complex social messages. Women, in particular, may have been taught messages that they should not actively pursue new information and that they will be told what they need to know, or they have been encouraged to adopt a pattern of reliance on others in evaluating information.

The issue of personal competence is often a particularly thorny one for women, who are socialized to be cooperative and dependent rather than self-reliant. Women are traditionally expected to wield power by indirect means, and some may experience considerable discomfort and uncertainty in situations in which they are called on to take charge of their lives or act in leadership roles. Fearing that they are "overstepping their bounds," they may be hesitant to make significant choices:

Ms. B, a 38-year-old woman, had been in a state of paralysis in her life for several months despite ongoing psychotherapy and treatment with antidepressants. Her husband had left with no explanation; she was unemployed and was gradually depleting her savings. She was well informed about her options, and, with a background in business, was very capable of addressing her financial concerns. Yet she felt unable to move forward with her plans to sell the house, file for divorce, and go back to work.

The therapist explored this dilemma with her to no avail. On one occasion, the clinic receptionist mistakenly put a call through to the therapist during her session with Ms. B. Her mechanic was recommending $1,500 of repairs to her car. She apologized to Ms. B for the interruption, and expressed her own irritation: "I hate this car repair business. What do I know about the distributor? I just have to trust them to do the right thing. It makes me feel stupid and powerless, but I need my car, so what can I do?" They resumed the session.

The following week, Ms. B reported that she had seen an attorney and was filing for divorce. Two weeks later, Ms. B reported she had been offered a job that she was seriously considering. The therapist was surprised at the sudden movement in Ms. B's life and inquired about what had initiated these changes. She answered, "Remember your mechanic?

I always thought that I shouldn't do anything unless I knew how it would come out. I assumed everyone was that way, that they had all the answers before they made their decisions. When I heard about you and your car, I realized that everybody has to wing it sometimes—you can't always know everything."

In this example, Ms. B is well equipped with information and skills, but is prevented from choosing and acting due to her intense self-doubt. Though prepared to choose, she does not feel competent, and therefore cannot act. This interchange subsequently led to meaningful discussions in the therapy about Ms. B's strivings to adhere to her family's largely unspoken, perfectionistic, and rigid expectations of "ladylike" behaviors. Her failures were grossly exaggerated by her parents and were doubly punished—first, for the failure itself, and second, because attracting attention was not lady-like. Ms. B learned to be very cautious and meticulous in her decisions, and she was rewarded in school and employment for her attention to detail and her quiet cooperation with others. However, she could not own or value her successes, leading to feelings of unworthiness, worthlessness, and self-doubt. At her best, she felt inhibited from directing her life; under stress she felt increasingly conspicuous and incompetent, and experienced increasing difficulty with choice and self-determination.

Women psychiatric survivors' lack of confidence in choice may be a direct result of highly structured treatment settings. People in most institutional settings have few opportunities for choice; activities, housing, diet, social contact, sleep schedules, and clothing are monitored and regulated. Attempts to choose are discouraged and sometimes punished, while compliance is highly valued and rewarded. Residents of institutions, particularly women residents, are often told that they are not able (or "not ready") to choose and act on their goals. The significance of failure may be exaggerated, and the person may be shamed rather than encouraged and supported to evaluate what she has learned. Over time, the cumulative effects of this process may become indistinguishable from the manifestations of psychiatric disability, through a process similar to learned helplessness. If this iatrogenic effect of institutionalization goes unrecognized, the person may be mislabeled "dependent" or "passive-aggressive," or her difficulties may be attributed to her diagnosis, reinforcing perceptions of the person as incapable, and further undermining confidence and initiative.

Clinicians need to avoid these damaging effects by providing services that offer choices and communicate respect and hope for recovery, rather than treatments that focus on setting expectations and limits. The key role of the provider has been described as offering a reservoir of faith in the person's innate capacity to successfully struggle and recover, and communicating recognition of the person's worth.[37-44]

The Inevitability of Choice

Life invariably demands that we make choices and deal with their outcomes. Issues related to this concept address the development of personal accountability, attribution of responsibility, and the proactive evaluation of choice based on possible outcomes. However, to begin to develop these skills, the individual must also be aware that a choice is being made.

This dilemma is most dramatically faced by the survivor of trauma who experiences dissociative events. The person is usually unaware of choices and behaviors occurring during the dissociative episode, and she finds herself repeatedly confronting circumstances that are unexpected and chaotic. The person's confusion and helplessness tends to be misinterpreted by providers as "excessive dependency" and an unwillingness to assume responsibility for her behaviors. Attempts to "hold the person accountable" will generally fail, as the person is lacking the referents that would allow her to identify cause and effect; for the individual it is as if things just happen.

Choice is difficult to sort out and understand in the presence of dissociation. More recent intervention techniques for complex post-traumatic stress disorders have focused on assisting people to identify their triggers and to learn skills to mitigate their distress and decrease the likelihood of dissociation. Issues of personal responsibility also play out in less dramatic circumstances:

A 50-year-old woman with a diagnosis of schizophrenia and a long history of institutionalization was abruptly evicted from her boarding house after repeatedly threatening to "punch out" her landlord for telling her to turn down her radio. She appeared to be doing well from a psychiatric standpoint, and reported that she had no intention of acting on her threats or harming the landlord or others. She requested assistance from her community support worker in order to move her belongings. Upon getting into the car, the woman announced, "I guess it's back to the hospital." The worker asked why she felt she needed the hospital. "Until you find me a place to live," she responded. The worker explained that the hospital would not admit people to intervene in housing issues, and asked the woman how she would like to proceed in finding herself a new place to live. The woman was surprised, and asked the worker to "get her a hotel." The worker suggested that it seemed to her that the woman was capable of playing an active part in finding her new housing, and offered to help her to check out her options and make arrangements on her own. The woman decided to use the program phone to call several hotels; staff checked in with her frequently. She asked for and received assistance to negotiate the room rate.

In this example, the person expects that the mental health worker will step in to assume responsibility. Instead, the worker expresses her confidence in the recipient's ability to address the issue at hand and offers to be available if needed. While it is tempting to pejoratively label this woman due to her expectation that others will care for her, many people receiving services have come to expect custodial care. Often mental health workers will prearrange housing and services simply because it is more expedient, and institutional settings usually "manage" behavior rather than fostering personal accountability.

This example highlights the differences between traditional treatment and recovery-oriented services. People need to know at the outset that services are intended to reflect their stated goals and that it is the role of staff to facilitate their efforts to achieve those goals for themselves. Individuals should be asked about their prior experiences in treatment and about their current expectations. It should be openly stated that this approach attempts to support and engage people in doing things for themselves and that the provider will actively avoid doing things for the person unless she needs assistance. It also needs to be made clear that this does not mean that the worker will be uninvolved or inaccessible. The key difference between this approach and directive treatment is not in the availability of services, but in the effort to reduce the power difference between provider and recipient.

It is also important to distinguish this intervention from abandonment, which occurs when a provider withdraws support and assistance, in the belief that the person will learn from the experience of facing consequences alone. This is rarely helpful, as it is usually experienced by the person as a hostile rejection, and it fails to engage the person in evaluating her choices. Rather, the person should be involved collaboratively in a discussion of the connections between the person's choices, behaviors, and outcomes should involve the person as a true collaborator in the evaluation process. A genuine, egalitarian relationship between the person receiving services and the person providing them works to permit discussion of difficult issues in a manner that communicates respect and value, as well as mutual personal accountability.

IMPLICATIONS FOR MENTAL HEALTH SERVICES DELIVERY

Services that address empowerment demand a careful examination of the power differences that exist between the person receiving services and others, including providers and the community. Many of these power differences represent pervasive societal influences. For women psychiatric survivors, misogyny and mentalism appear to combine to limit opportunity and promote chronicity. However, little is known about the complex interaction of oppression that is perpetrated based on gender, diagnosis, race and ethnicity, socioeconomic class, age, sexual orientation, or spiritual belief. Marked individual differences in the experience of discrimination further complicate efforts to draw general conclusions. Sincere efforts between those receiving and those providing mental health services to address the issue of power, in a respectful and caring manner, will create the affirming and genuine relationship that is essential to stimulate healing, empowerment, and recovery.

To be effective in supporting empowerment, services must be designed around the goals of the recipient; must support the development of a respectful, egalitarian relationship between the people receiving and providing services; and must support both external and internal determinants that influence the person's ability to direct the course of her life. Such services will be mutually empowering for the provider, recipient, and community; however, they will often call into question traditional therapeutic concepts or approaches. Much work remains to be done in defining and implementing services that promote empowerment. Organizations and practitioners who wish to move in this direction can begin to change the focus of interventions and communications. Some questions that may assist an evaluation of the capacity of services to support empowerment follow:

1. Do services reflect the person's stated goals?
2. Is the person actively guiding all aspects of her services development, implementation, and evaluation?
3. How do services support the person's developmental issues with respect to empowerment (the internal mandate)?
4. How do services address power differences and discrimination faced by the person?
5. Does the person feel that services fit with her self-concept and values?
6. Does the person feel that services build on her strengths and interests?
7. Does the person feel she has access to the information she needs about the program approach, her rights, and her services?
8. Does the person feel that services are flexible enough to accommodate change and struggle?
9. Do recipients feel that they participate meaningfully in the leadership and operations of the service organization?
10. Do recipients feel that the grievance procedure is effective and safe to use?
11. Do community members feel that the boards and other governing bodies associated with the agency reflect the diversity of the community with respect to gender, ethnicity, and other cultural and socioeconomic concerns?
12. Do services use natural networks of support?
13. Do staff feel they are supported in their growth and development with respect to personal and professional empowerment?
14. Does the organization engage in community development efforts?
15. Does the organization actively confront and discourage stigma and discrimination, internally and in the community?
16. Do interpersonal interactions and the physical environment in the organization communicate respect to recipients, staff, and others?
17. Do recipients and staff feel that the program cultivates opportunity?
18. Do services address the spiritual issues that pertain to empowerment?
19. Are resources available to provide effective accommodations for consumers, staff, family members, and community members to participate fully in directing the organization?

ENDNOTE

a. This case study and others in this chapter are from the authors' clinical experiences. Some details have been changed to preserve anonymity.

REFERENCES

1. Blanch A, Penney D, Knight E: "Identity politics" close to home. *American Psychologist* 1995; 50:49-50.
2. Eichler A, Parron D (Eds.): *Women's Mental Health: Agenda for Research.* Rockville, MD: National Institute of Mental Health, 1987.
3. Clay S: Personal communication, 1992.
4. Stefan S: Reforming provisions in mental health treatment. In: Moss K (Ed.): *Manmade Medicine: Women's Health, Public Policy and Reform.* Durham, NC: Duke University Press, 1996, pp. 195-218.
5. Chamberlin J: The ex-patients' movement: Where we've been and where we're going. *Journal of Mind and Behavior* 1990; 11(3-4):323-336.
6. Chamberlin J: *The Right to Be Wrong.* Paper presented at the Choice and Responsibility Conference, Albany, NY, June 21-22, 1994.
7. Zinman S, Harp H, Budd S (Eds.): *Reaching Across: Mental Health Clients Helping Each Other.* Sacramento: California Network of Mental Health Clients, 1987.
8. Campbell J: *In Pursuit of Wellness: The Well-Being Project.* Sacramento: California Network of Mental Health Clients, 1989.
9. Knight E: Self-directed rehabilitation. *Empowerment: News From the Recipient Empowerment Project* 1991; 2(7):1-4.
10. Fisher D: A new vision of healing as constructed by people with psychiatric disabilities working as mental health providers. *Psychosocial Rehabilitation Journal* 1994; 19(3):67-81.
11. Chamberlin J: Speaking for ourselves: An overview of the ex-psychiatric inmates' movement. *Psychosocial Rehabilitation Journal* 1984; 8(2):56-64.
12. Craine LS, Henson CE, Colliver JA, et al.: Prevalence of a history of sexual abuse among female psychiatric patients in a state hospital. *Hospital and Community Psychiatry* 1988; 39(3):300-304.
13. Breyer JB, Nelson BA, Miller JB et al.: Childhood sexual and physical abuse as factors in adult psychiatric illness. *American Journal of Psychiatry* 1987; 144:1426-1430.
14. Beck JC, van der Kolk B: Reports of childhood incest and current behavior of chronically hospitalized psychotic women. *American Journal of Psychiatry* 1987; 144:1474-1480.
15. *Report of the Task Force on Restraint and Seclusion.* Albany: New York State Office of Mental Health, 1993.
16. Penney DJ: Essential elements of case management in managed care settings: A service recipient perspective. In: Giesler LJ (Ed.): *Case Management for Behavioral Managed Care.* Cincinnati, OH: National Association of Case Management, 1995, pp. 97-113.

17. Fisher W, Penney D, Earle K: Mental health services recipients: Their role in shaping organizational policy. *Administration and Policy in Mental Health* 1996; 23(6):547-553.
18. Blanch A, Parrish J: *Alternatives to Involuntary Treatment: Results of Three Roundtable Discussions*. Bethesda, MD: Community Support Program, Center for Mental Health Services, 1993.
19. Holmes G, Saleebey D: Empowerment, the medical model, and the politics of client-hood. *Journal of Progressive Human Services* 1993; 4(1):61-78.
20. Deegan PE: Recovering our sense of value after being labeled. *Journal of Psychosocial Nursing* 1993; 31(4):7-11.
21. Deegan PE: Recovery: The lived experience of rehabilitation. *Psychosocial Rehabilitation Journal* 1988; 11(4):11-19.
22. Clay S: *The Wounded Prophet*. Unpublished, 1994.
23. Clay S: *Empowerment and Recovery*. Unpublished, 1994.
24. Pierce C: Offensive mechanisms. In: Barbour F (Ed.): *The Black Seventies*. Boston: Porter-Sargent, 1970, pp. 265-282.
25. Reidy DE: *"Stigma Is Social Death": Mental Health Consumers/Survivors Talk About Stigma in Their Lives*. Unpublished, 1993.
26. Geller JL, Munetz MR: The iatrogenic creation of psychiatric chronicity in women. In: Bachrach LL, Nadelson CC (Eds.): *Treating Chronically Mentally Ill Women*. Washington, DC: American Psychiatric Press, 1988, pp. 143-177.
27. Lewis DO, Shanok SS, Cohen RJ, et al.: Race bias in the diagnosis and disposition of violent adolescents. *American Journal of Psychiatry* 1980; 137(10):1211-1216.
28. Lloyd K, Moodley P: Psychotropic medication and ethnicity: An inpatient survey. *Social Psychiatry and Psychiatric Epidemiology* 1992; 27:95-101.
29. Adebimpe VR: Overview: White norms and psychiatric diagnosis of Black patients. *American Journal of Psychiatry* 1981; 138(3):279-285.
30. Kalinowski C: *Services on the Client's Terms: Experiences at Stanislaus Integrated Services Agency*. Paper presented at the University of California, Davis, Annual Midwinter Conference, Incline Village, NV, January 31, 1992.
31. Mahler J, Chamberlin J: *Empowering Users of Mental Health Services*. Unpublished, 1980.
32. Ralph RO, Lambert D: *Needs Assessment Survey of AMHI Consent Decree Class Members Interim Report*. Augusta: Maine Department of Mental Health, Mental Retardation, and Substance Abuse Services, April 16, 1996.
33. Morganti BJ: Love is . . . *Journal of the California Alliance for the Mentally Ill* 1992; 3(2):15-16.
34. Deegan PE: Spirit breaking: When the helping professions hurt. *The Humanistic Psychologist* 1990; 18(3):301-313.
35. Blaska B: First person account: What it is like to be treated like a CMI. *Schizophrenia Bulletin* 1991; 17(1):173-176.
36. Collier TJ: The stigma of mental illness. *Newsweek* 1993; 121(17):16.
37. Fisher DB: How community psychiatrists and consumer/survivors can promote mutual empowerment. *Community Psychiatrist* 1994; 8(2):5.
38. Fisher DB: *Towards a Positive Culture of Healing*. Unpublished, 1994.
39. Hogan MF: *Recovery: The New Force in Mental Health*. Unpublished, October 1994.
40. Fisher DB: Hope, humanity and voice in recovery from psychiatric disability. *Journal of the California Alliance for the Mentally Ill* 1994; 5:13-15.
41. Blanch A, Fisher DB, Tucker W, et al.: Consumer-practitioners and psychiatrists share insights about recovery and coping. *Disability Studies Quarterly* 1993; 13(2):17-20.

42. Lovejoy M: Expectations and the recovery process. *Schizophrenia Bulletin* 1982; 8(4):605-609.
43. Deegan PE: *Recovery, Rehabilitation and the Conspiracy of Hope: A Keynote Address.* Paper presented at the Western Regional Conference on Housing and Supports, Portland, OR, June 1, 1992.
44. Deegan PE: *Recovery as a Journey of the Heart.* Paper presented at the Conference for Recovery from Psychiatric Disability, Boston, May 10, 1995.

8

Home Making and Community Building

Notes on Empowerment and Place

Priscilla Ridgway, M.S.W.
Alexa Simpson, M.P.H., M.F.A.
Friedner D. Wittman, Ph.D., M.Arch.
Gary Wheeler, M.A.

THE CHALLENGE TO HOUSE AND SUPPORT HOMELESS AMERICANS

Mental health authorities, blindsided by mass homelessness among persons with psychiatric disabilities in the 1970s and early 1980s, found traditional settings and services inadequate to meet emergent needs. Any solution to homelessness had to provide access to affordable housing. The poorest of the poor, including those with prolonged psychiatric disabilities, had to rely on the public sector to address low-income housing needs the free market would not fill. Housing alone was not enough; many homeless people needed treatment, support services, and rehabilitation. Innovative program models that linked services to housing arose to fill this gap.[1,2] In the past several years, planning, program development, and housing production flourished, and supportive housing initiatives have taken shape in many states.[3-5]

"Supported" or "supportive" housing are generic terms used to label diverse approaches. In some programs, recipients access scattered-

NOTE: This chapter appeared as an article in the *Journal of Mental Health Administration*, 1994, Vol. 21, No. 4, pp. 407-418.

site mainstream housing linked to an individualized, flexible set of services and supports. In other cases, the housing is clustered and includes
apartment houses and single-room occupancy (SRO) hotels, with on-
site or off-site social services, a specialized program of services, or case
management linked to the setting. Some programs house only those
with prolonged psychiatric disabilities or dual diagnoses, others have
nondisabled tenants as well.

In this chapter, we explore decision-making processes driving supportive housing development, and some of the environmental problems that result when the voice of the consumer is not heard. We offer
a series of examples and ideas concerning co-design of personal environments and describe positive outcomes that such processes would
achieve. We then turn to the need for consumer involvement in the creation of social settings and self-help communities, and we describe the
role that the physical environment can play in engendering prosocial
behavior. The chapter concludes with implications for services delivery
and the need for leaders to assume a collaborative stance to create truly
empowering supportive housing programs.

THE POLITICS OF PLACE: PLANNING AND
DEVELOPING SUPPORTIVE HOUSING

Studies have found that homeless people must be engaged and
served on their own terms.[6,7] Homeless mental health consumers often
have little interest in traditional mental health services; they want housing, jobs, and help getting on with their lives.[8] Consumer housing preference needs assessments, first designed and tested in the mid-1980s,[9,10]
are now an accepted tool in planning supportive housing. A recent
meta-analysis of more than 40 studies found the vast majority of consumers would prefer to live in permanent, independent, normative settings with flexible supports; few wish to live with other consumers in
congregate and/or staffed sites,[11] although some variation in preferences occurs based on life experience and differences in local housing
markets.[12,13] Planners now believe they know what consumers want,
based on such sample survey data. Unfortunately, the field continues
to ignore the desires and needs of individuals and denies the opportu-

nity for empowerment that accrues when a person makes choices directly relevant to his or her life.

In fact, decisions about supportive housing are generally not made by consumers but by mental health administrators and specialized staff; public and private developers; local, county, and state officials; and sometimes, one or two consumers representing all consumers. These players put together a real estate deal, and the project sponsor becomes the client of design-build experts—architects, engineers, interior designers, and contractors to renovate or construct residential space. Once design-build professions are involved, their design conventions and hard-line blueprints often leave little leeway for the imprint of potential tenants on the "product." In the open housing market, monied consumers can shop among several options or even help design their own housing; new middle-income housing is designed based on market surveys. In supportive housing, typical market forces do not apply. Potential tenants lack purchasing power, and supportive housing developers commonly stand in as surrogate decision makers, designing housing and support services based on what they believe consumers need, want, or deserve.

These decision makers can lose sight of the human dimension in the complex housing development process. The pressure to get people off the street, external contingencies, and cost concerns have led the field to define "success" in terms of the number of housing units that come online. These units may meet local codes and conventional standards of decency, but many are characterized by a utilitarian industrial-strength drabness and some have the distinct flavor of the institutional settings they were intended to replace. The housing is bland and furnished like the lowest-cost dorm room, with uniform, pre-chosen furniture, wall color, and window treatments. The result is often anonymous and dehumanizing cookie-cutter units.

Mental health systems are developing supportive housing at the rate of hundreds and even thousands of units, but the field often does not recognize the difference between developing a unit of housing and creating a *home*. Housing can be produced in multiples of units, but a home is made one at a time. A home is personal space; to create a home, the voice of the individual tenant must be heard. If development staff fail to listen, supportive housing may simply provide more quasi-institutional space.

Issues of power and control in mental health settings often go unexplored. Until recently, mental health systems have generally expected patients or clients to be passive, while staff create therapeutic milieus in their best interests. Decision making has traditionally been hierarchical and centralized, vested in administrative or clinical authority. Threats of involuntary confinement or expulsion from programs have routinely been used to enforce compliance with program rules and treatment regimes. The mental health field has recently come to recognize the need to empower consumers to promote rehabilitation and recovery. Supportive housing can be an important resource in empowering consumers, if decision makers can quash the tendency to create settings that reinforce dependency and social segregation. The primary goal of supportive housing should not be the development of units of housing or the delivery of units of services. The primary goal should be to empower each individual to develop a home and a sense of belonging in his or her community.

If we want to avoid re-creating quasi-institutional settings, we must remember what we already know. We know behavior is a function of the transaction between the person and his or her environment. We know better than to house people in environments they neither help to create nor control.[14,15] We have a body of knowledge in environmental and social psychology on locus of control and learned helplessness that describes the devastating effects of controlling milieus, including weakening of identity, loss of motivation and competence, passivity, a sense of powerlessness, stress, and psychological and physical symptoms.[16-19] We know that shelter, personal space, and "mastery over the environment" are critical for healthy human life.[20] Yet, when persons labeled mentally ill suffer the effects of controlling environments, these reactions are viewed as "negative symptoms" of mental illness rather than as predictable person/environment interactions.

Our existing knowledge allows us to predict potential outcomes for staff-controlled supportive housing. In the best-case scenario, people will, with very limited resources, personalize their space and make it their own, because it is human nature to create a personal niche. Many tenants will remain passive, or show a slow, general deterioration in their emotional and physical health. Neglect of the environment will also likely occur. We will see continued dissatisfaction and lack of goodness of fit between people and their environment; some people will leave. In the worst-case scenario, we will see active destruction of the newly rehabilitated units, as the authors have witnessed in some California supportive housing SROs.

THE SOLUTION: CO-CREATING
THE LIVING ENVIRONMENT

Instead of imposing a completely preconfigured environment on an individual, planning and development must proceed from the individual outward. "Home making" must not be viewed as some passé "women's work," but as an opportunity to promote empowerment, diversity, and choice. We must involve people as co-creators of their own home and community. Strong consumer involvement in planning, design, and development of settings will ensure "good design"—that is, programs and living situations that consumers want and need.

Planning should start with consumer housing preference studies on a local level. Individual needs can be clustered, and a local plan can be composed of many individual supportive housing plans, in a bottom-up approach. Planners must stop creating settings and programs for an anonymous, generic target population (e.g., "the chronically mentally ill") or subpopulations (e.g., "the dually diagnosed") and acknowledge not just the heterogeneity of the population but also the individuality and humanity of each person. People with psychiatric disabilities have individual values, they come from diverse cultural backgrounds, they may face physical challenges and specific developmental tasks, and they choose different lifestyles, including having intimate relationships and parenting. No one housing type or household configuration will meet these needs. Only once the personal needs and preferences of local consumers have been identified should housing development begin.

Consumers (future tenants) should participate in the actual planning and design of particular projects. Wittman[21] describes a participatory approach to architectural planning that could be used. This approach begins with a *problem definition phase*. Before any firm decisions about facilities are made, project planners ask potential occupants about their wants and needs in the environment and its surrounding area. A conceptual model is built based on presenting needs and concerns.

Issues are clarified by one or more focus groups of 8-12 future tenants who act as ongoing advisers to the process. Any other important constituency groups (such as on-site service providers) are also involved. In the *solution-seeking and generation of design concepts phase*, focus group(s) refine their ideas, preferences, and needs for the setting, which are translated into physical design concepts by the design professional(s). Design proposals are reviewed by the focus group(s). In the *design development and implementation phase*, design professionals and builders follow through on the focus groups' concerns. The groups provide input as detailed design issues surface, as well as whenever changes are contemplated during construction or renovation. Future occupants make more individualized choices concerning interior design, and they are involved in the move-in. A commitment is also made to alter the environment if occupants are found to have important unmet needs.

A similar process was used by Patricia Harrison, a university professor and architect, the Sacramento Housing and Redevelopment Agency, and Loaves and Fishes, a homeless services organization.[22] In a series of workshops, street and shelter homeless people voiced their strong preference for personal living situations. Small (400-square-foot) manufactured units were designed that include distinct living, dining, cooking, and sleeping areas. Linked together, several units form what looks like a cluster of California ranch-style homes. Future tenants wanted to have privacy and a sense of community, so units include front porches that open onto shared green space, and the site plan includes a community laundromat, coffee shop, and other small shops. The potential tenants want to provide their own security and to keep the 60-unit, three-acre project "clean and sober." This design is part of ongoing dialogues and a "1,000 Cottages Concept" to end homelessness in the state's capital.

Can such approaches work with those who are psychiatrically disabled? Imbimbo and Pfeffer[23] conducted a series of workshops with homeless women, most of whom had psychiatric disabilities. One workshop involved brainstorming the meaning of "home" and identifying the kinds of settings, interior design, amenities, activities, feelings, and relationships that the term *home* evokes. A second workshop explored the women's residential histories, and whether they considered their former living situations "home." In the third workshop, each woman designed and modeled her "ideal home" using materials such as construction paper, markers, glue, scissors, and tiny replica trees. The women created imaginative personalized spaces furnished with such things as a sofabed, wall units, knick-knacks, shutters, curtains, big pillows, and a brightly patterned rug.

An architectural planning group, Gran-Sultan Associates, conducted a post-occupancy survey of residents of two newly renovated New York City SROs to help ensure future projects are sensitive to the needs of similar residents.[24] Such surveys could be used proactively before housing is completed. The interviewees all had histories of psychiatric disability; ranged in age from 19 to 64; and had entered the SROs from shelters, the street, or psychiatric hospitals. The survey elicited general reactions to the facility; asked what made (or would make) it feel like a home; critiqued individual and community spaces; and assessed environmental or other supports needed for security, ease of activity (e.g., chores, visiting, program activities), and special needs during periods of emotional distress.

Most of those surveyed liked having individual "apartments," control over their living situation (e.g., "you can decorate, change things," "residents are involved in decisions," "you pay your own rent, buy your own food"), and other features. In-depth questioning revealed that the units were almost universally disliked because they were too small (e.g., most were 90-100 square feet). The units made some respondents feel claustrophobic or like they were in jail. It was very difficult for residents to have visitors; the units had no seating and only enough space for cooking and sleeping. Residents strongly preferred individual baths and kitchens but wanted standard-size refrigerators and stoves, storage, and counter space to stock up on foodstuffs and prepare food easily. Residents also desired increased secure storage, shelving, task lighting, improved sound insulation, personal control over heating and cooling, and more public telephones or individual phone service. Respondents also wanted their units to be more personalized and homelike with softer lighting; nicer decor; and personally chosen wall color, curtains, and linens.

Interior designers who have had training in psychology have developed participatory approaches to the design process that could be adapted for use in supportive housing programs. Torrice[25] works with young people, some of whom have special needs, to create highly personalized environments. He begins by asking the person to envision "a perfect personal space." A process of mapping choices within the available space creates a rough floor plan. Subjective color preferences are determined, and a personal notebook is jointly developed that includes pictures, floor plans, paint chips, carpet samples, and other materials. Through continued dialogue, a plan for the space is refined.

Second author Simpson designs *with* rather than *for* her interior design clients, using an interactive process. The client begins defining needs and preferences by looking at a list of evocative words and a set of "idea books" created from magazine clippings. The client flags any image or word that evokes a strong positive or negative feeling and briefly notates his or her reaction. The client and designer go over the list of words and idea books together. The designer then translates and integrates the "raw data" of preferences into an initial approach to the space plan and makes suggestions concerning style, color, and materials. The media used invite the client to participate in, play with, and change the design as it evolves. For example, proposed floor plans are presented as "user-friendly," colorful, cartoonlike sketches that lend an illusion of three-dimensionality. Hard-line drawings are prepared only as construction documents, after all client-centered decisions have been made. Such involvement in interior design is not intended to help people develop "style" or "good taste," nor would most laypeople be expected to know the technical vocabulary of design.[21] Rather, these interactive processes allow the designer to learn what is meaningful for each client, what he or she believes makes for a good environment, and what the personal meaning of "home" is for that individual.

Some supportive housing developers are apparently attempting to keep costs as low as possible by offering the fewest possible amenities; the smallest square footage allowable; and sparsely furnished, uniform accommodations. Even very small living spaces can be personalized for a few hundred dollars using modular units built of inexpensive materials. A person can select and help assemble or build modular units to meet his or her personal needs for storage, shelving, sleeping, seating, and so on. Modular furniture creates fluid rather than static environments, and it allows a person to reconfigure a setting as his or her needs and interests change, or simply as a function of self-expression and exploration. For small outlays, tenants can personalize aspects of their home such as wall color, floor tiles, carpeting or throw rugs, bed and window coverings, posters, and so on. Even when no budget exists to create personalized environments, options and choices can still be found. Quality donations of new and used furniture and other household goods can be solicited, as Furnish A Future, Inc., has done in New York City, where homeless individuals and families "shop" a huge warehouse full of goods for their new homes.[26] Alternatively, churches, civic groups, clubs, or individuals could be asked to donate a specific amount for a formerly homeless individual to set up a home. This fund would allow an individual to plan, budget, and shop for personal items.

What Outcomes Will Co-Creation Facilitate?

What will happen if the field shifts its focus from the development of units to the co-creation of individual homes? We envision several outcomes: the recovery of a sense of self-identity and self-esteem, the recovery of a sense of security and privacy, improved social status and a sense of having a stakehold in the community, recovered personal efficacy and competence, and increased residential stability resulting from improved person-environment fit. If these outcomes are facilitated, empowerment naturally occurs.

Recovery of Self-Identity and Self-Esteem

Many people who have experienced prolonged mental disorders and homelessness have lost a sense of themselves by being treated as faceless cases or as part of an anonymous mass of those held in mental institutions, jails, or shelters. Stripped of personal possessions and history, they have often been reduced to a survival mode. Yet, even in the state of homelessness, people construct makeshift habitats or "survival niches" as a form of street-architecture.[27]

The creation of personal space is a statement that "I exist." When a person makes choices and creates a self-expressive environment, he or she says, "This is how I want to live, this is who I am in this place, at this time." The living situation can become an outer expression of a recovered sense of personal identity, a mirror to the self. Consumer involvement in co-creation of the setting demonstrates the staffs' respect, in effect saying, "You are valued, you are a unique person whose ideas and needs we hold in esteem. What you think, feel, and desire, matter." The personalized environment can reflect a reclamation of identity that may include family; ethnic, racial, or cultural heritage; important early life experiences; or other sources of pride. It may also provide space for involvement in new interests, activities, and hobbies. Having an environment that allows one to explore and develop more fully into oneself may form the basis for more positive functioning in the social world.

Recovery of Security and Privacy

Personal control over the environment allows an individual to feel secure. Why are security and privacy the most important issues for many supportive housing residents?[24,28] The state of homelessness is profoundly insecure, often brutal. To be homeless is to be in constant danger from the elements, the brutalities of human predators, or harassment by police.[29,30] To recover from the trauma of homelessness, a person may need a safe sanctuary in which to rebuild health and peace of mind. The need for security and privacy may spring from even earlier losses and assaults. Evidence indicates that the loss of family structure or early childhood sexual or physical abuse or other early traumas may set the stage for later homelessness.[30-32] Developmental theory holds that the early security of the home and family bonds give a young person the strength to grow and courage to explore the outer world. Perhaps when early stability and safety is violated, a person is more vulnerable to cognitive disorganization, to further victimization, and to problems in achieving a stable inner- and outer-life.

The process of co-creating a home may provide a vehicle for healing such injuries to self. Supportive housing may give a person the chance to have his or her first experience of a safe home. A stable home base may be a prerequisite for taking on challenges and achieving further growth. A "safe house" allows a person to play out inner dramas and undertake self-healing work. Control of the environment may be especially significant for those recovering from early abuse, because it enables a person to create healthy personal and physical boundaries. Likewise, "clean and sober" housing may give those in recovery from substance abuse the physical, psychological, and personal space needed to heal.[33,34]

The desire for a secure home does not only affect former mental patients; the need for "defensible space" is universal.[35,36] Middle- and upper-class individuals "cocoon" to countervail the stressors in their work and community. People in supportive housing face special challenges when they seek security and privacy. They are often expected to live in close proximity to people whom they have not chosen to live with, and to have their personal idiosyncrasies under continual surveillance by staff. If supportive housing is viewed as a person's home and not program space, respect for privacy increases. Ware and her colleagues[28] found when staff of shared living apartments avoided intruding on residents' social space and bedrooms, but residents had access to staff areas, the "politics of space" that characterized life in other mental health settings was inverted. Residents valued their newfound privacy above anything else.

Security may be such a critical issue for some supportive housing residents because they are, in fact, in danger. When a premium is placed on the number of units developed rather than on helping each person achieve a secure home, settings in dangerous, disorganized neighborhoods are often targeted for redevelopment. When supportive housing is concentrated in areas of abandoned properties, drug dealing, prostitution, liquor outlets, and high rates of crime, what are we saying about the people we serve? Is what was called "ghettoization" a few years ago[37,38] now a public good? Because recovery is difficult or impossible in conditions of constant stress and threat, some leaders in the mental health and drug and alcohol field have made a commitment to develop properties only in relatively safe and stable neighborhoods.[33,39,40] If mental health authorities make the decision to develop supportive housing projects in dangerous areas, they should commit resources to community organizing to clean up and rebuild the social fabric of the surrounding neighborhood as well.

Recovering Social Status and a Stakehold in the Community

Mental illness and homelessness confer a terrible stigma on the individual, with toxic social consequences. Homeless people often report feeling either reviled or invisible in the social world. Supportive housing can help repair the social self. Tenancy in a personally valued environment, especially in the mainstream, socially integrated housing that most mental health consumers prefer,[11] conveys the message of positive social standing. Decent housing helps provide a stable social identity. Anecdotal evidence indicates that good-quality supportive housing tends to promote the redevelopment of informal social support networks, including renewed family contact. Perhaps having the physical space for a social life allows the person to regain a bona fide niche in the social world and to interact with more confidence with others.

Involvement in planning, creating, and shaping the environment will go far toward giving an individual a stakehold in the community and a personal sense of ownership of his or her own home. Having a stakehold should increase personal satisfaction, improve the person's subjective quality of life, and improve the care that is taken of the physical environment. People who have no stakehold lack pride of place, while living in a place one calls "home" gives a person a sense of belonging in the broader community. The return from homelessness and achievement of householder status is an important rite of passage that should be celebrated.[41]

Recovering Personal Efficacy and Competence

Shaping the environment, exploring values, and making selections among options builds a sense of personal efficacy and competence. When the environment is as the individual wishes, it provides direct visual feedback that reinforces a sense of personal power and effectiveness. Interactions between consumers and planners, design-build professionals, staff, and shopkeepers allow consumers to come out of themselves and experience successful transactions with others. Relationships built around the co-creation of the physical space may lead to attempts and success at other relationships and decision-making processes.

To a large degree, having and making choices, especially the layering of multiple choices in the process of everyday life, is synonymous with personal power. "Empowerment" is often found in the details of the mundane world. It comes from controlling access to personal space, from being able to alter one's environment and select one's daily routine, and from having personal space that reflects and upholds one's identity and interests. People who have never spent time in institutions or other environments controlled by externally imposed routine, or who have not been without housing, probably cannot truly understand the joy and relief that having personal control of a living situation brings.[42]

Increased Residential Stability Through Improved Person-Environment Fit

Person-environment fit interests those who design residential services. In attempting to match consumers with environments and configure relevant sets of environmental supports, planners often forget just how subjective personal satisfaction is. If people live in environments that do not meet their definition of "home," they will remain unsettled.[43] When a person feels a subjective sense of satisfaction with a setting, he or she is more likely to function better, be healthier, and settle in.[44] While homeless people may accept a reasonable alternative to the streets, they may not view their housing as their home. Long lease-up periods and the sizable proportion of newly-housed tenants who are found to continue to want to move show that some supportive housing programs are not achieving person-environment fit. Co-creation of the individual environment should greatly increase the likelihood that a sense of person-environment fit is achieved.

Community Building and Co-Creation of Group Settings

The co-creation process must sometimes extend beyond the development of a personal home, to the development of "community." Supportive housing sponsors often seek to "create community" by developing multi-unit housing. As we have noted, most consumers would prefer to live in socially integrated settings rather than in housing designated for those with psychiatric disabilities.[11] In spite of these preferences, many sponsors house people based on their psychiatric label, to achieve cost-efficiency or to access certain funding streams. Sponsors also avow tenants' shared history will lead to mutual support. Yet most sponsors pay little attention to how the physical environments they develop may engender or constrain social life. Simply housing people with similar problems in high density will not create a functional mutual support group. This is how tenants of one SRO setting for formerly homeless women with psychiatric disabilities described their living environments *before* efforts to build a positive group process:

It was a madhouse literally. The women were always bickering, arguing, fighting, acting crazy. . . . It was deserted most of the time, we were cast out, isolated. . . . There were thirty-six women and we didn't have much to do with each other. . . . We had no unity.[45]

Physical settings can encourage sociability or may tend to block social life.[21,46,47] "Sociopetal" settings, which create opportunities for social interaction, usually provide an open circulation plan, offer a variety of social spaces, and are lively and inviting. "Sociofugal" spaces encourage separation and isolation.[47] Wittman[48] describes SRO hotels as prime examples of sociofugal space. SROs lack shared social space; their long corridors of blank walls punctuated by anonymous doorways are visually dull and can be depressing, frightening, and even disorienting to anxious people. In fact, such settings were not designed to serve as a complete living environment but rather as sleeping spaces for urban blue-collar workers, who labored among others and spent their free time in the many restaurants, shops, barber shops, and bars that made up busy neighborhoods. To expect such settings, which are often now surrounded by blighted urban areas, to serve as both individual homes and shared social support settings requires design innovation, significant capitol investment to reconfigure the existing physical space, group work within the milieu, and strong neighborhood organizing to reweave the damaged social fabric of the community.

More than two in three of the psychiatrically disabled SRO residents interviewed by Gran-Sultan Associates[24] felt that several functionally distinct social spaces would improve their SRO housing. Their suggestions included a small lounge for television viewing, a separate game and music room, an outdoor patio, small visiting areas, and quiet areas to sit and read or have a small-group meeting. Interviewees wanted these common areas to be well-furnished and colorful and to have living plants. They wanted bookcases and areas to be well-stocked with equipment and materials. Developers can hardly expect people to increase their level of social interaction and form a self-help community until they provide the social spaces, equipment, and supplies that encourage or allow tenants to do so.

Social settings operate on the basis of formal and informal ground rules. Rather than empowering supportive housing tenants to make decisions about life within their housing, sponsors often issue directives and a list of rules for tenants, ignore group process, and then intervene harshly when rules are broken or incidents show the "community" has broken down. There is a vast difference between living in a milieu based on shared values and one dictated by externally imposed rules for conduct. Rather than disempowering people through dictatorial approaches, some sponsors have developed tenant associations and share decision-making authority with residents about program development and issues such as eviction or acceptance of tenants, the hiring and evaluation of staff, and the like.[41,49,50] Others apply traditional group work methods, using desirable social activities such as a supper club to build a positive group process.[51,52] Some supportive housing programs employ consumers or former consumers to act as staff and positive role models for their peers.[53-55]

Even when empowerment is an avowed goal, tenants and staff may have very different ideas about what this means. Ware and her colleagues[28] studied "evolving consumer households" in Boston, which increased tenants' reliance on group-centered decision making while staff assistance slowly withdrew. Staff suggested that housemates communally budget, manage their money, and make purchasing decisions together. The tenants' idea of empowerment was for each person to control personal finances, make almost all purchases individually, and only share resources based on an "economics of reciprocity," helping one another out only when someone temporarily ran short.

A very few supportive housing programs have invested in developing tenant-driven intentional communities.[49,56] One effort in Santa Clara County, California,[49] created neighborhood-based, 60- to 100-person "communities" of ex-patients living in supportive housing settings. Members were encouraged to participate in community activities but they were never coerced. Staff used group work exclusively and trained community members in mediation techniques to resolve their interpersonal problems. Members participated in outreach, intake and orientation of new members, the hiring and training of staff, self-help, advocacy, and program evaluation. Group life emerged from the needs and efforts of group members.

If peer-based communities are to work, they must be empowerment based—that is, people must live in a community of choice rather than in forced groupings, ground rules should emerge from the group process and not be imposed from without, physical spaces must offer ample opportunities for both personal privacy and a variety of social interactions, group process must be nurtured through a variety of activities and forums, and problem-solving and mediation resources must be available to the group.

IMPLICATIONS FOR MENTAL HEALTH SERVICES DELIVERY

Empowerment cannot be an add-on activity in an otherwise traditional mental health system. Empowerment must permeate all activities—and all stages of supportive housing development—from needs assessment and program planning to the design and co-creation of individually adapted and personalized space and, where applicable, to the evolution of group process in a community of choice.

Full involvement of consumers has some costs, in terms of time and in terms of creating more personalized and, therefore, more varied settings. This approach demands that budgets include sufficient resources to personalize environments and to alter them when people move on and new tenants arrive. The proposed benefits, such as self-esteem and personal satisfaction, are "soft" measures; no formal cost-benefit studies exist that test these ideas. Evaluation of the impact of consumer involvement in co-creating their environment must follow. Increased self-determination may in fact reduce the costs associated with disability in the long run. Even without firm cost-benefit data, leaders must begin to undertake such efforts because they want to see stronger, healthier, more active people who have a better quality of life.

Empowerment-oriented practice requires innovative techniques and new staff roles.[41,57] If consumers are to have homes and not just housing, program developers and the design-build experts they employ must serve as facilitators, consultants, and midwives to consumers' dreams. People need support to move from being passive recipients to active decision makers. Creative, structured, and interactive processes, tools, and techniques must be developed or imported and adapted. Real choices and a variety of concrete options must be made available so that decisions are not made on the basis of limited experience.

If developers create housing that has the amenities most people want, project staff will have more time to spend on personalizing desirable settings. Even so, there is no substitute for the empowering process of active choice-making. If we truly want to foster empowerment, we must give up the idea that we can define "home" for another or dictate how others should live. To facilitate empowerment, we must learn new ways to listen to the voice of consumers, and to listen we must become more humble and flexible. It is hoped that such practice will lead to a time when we no longer think of provider "versus" recipient, or the provider "empowering" the consumer, but rather simply act as people sharing ideas, collaborating, and solving problems together. While no mental health system has the resources to fulfill every dream, it is only by attempting to do so that we open ourselves to the infinitesimal calculus of grace that occurs when each person is honored, when people work together, truly hear one another, and act from the heart.

When we wholeheartedly enter into such processes we can let go of the illusion that we must "empower" consumers. No person can empower another human being. We *can* stop creating contexts that impede personal expression. We can provide processes and supports that allow each individual to reawaken and use his or her own vitality, his or her own creative force, the inner generative energy that allows any human being to heal and grow. Working together, supportive housing can provide the context for real recovery—the recovery of personal identity, the recovery of privacy and personal security, the recovery of valued social roles and social status, the recovery of a sense of being at home in a community that has its basis in deep compassion, hopefulness, and mutual respect.

REFERENCES

1. Ridgway P, Zipple AM: The paradigm shift in residential services: From the linear continuum to supported housing approaches. *Psychosocial Rehabilitation Journal* 1990; 13(4):11-32.
2. Blanch AK, Carling PJ, Ridgway P: Normal housing with specialized support: A psychiatric rehabilitation approach to living in the community. *Rehabilitation Psychology* 1988; 432:47:55.
3. Ridgway P: *Meeting the Supported Housing and Residential Service Needs of Americans with Psychiatric Disabilities: A State-by-State Review*. Boston: Boston University, Center for Psychiatric Rehabilitation, 1987.

4. Cohen MD, Somers S: Supported housing: Insights from the Robert Woods Johnson Foundation Program on Chronic Mental Illness. *Psychosocial Rehabilitation Journal* 1990; 13(4):43-50.
5. Livingston J, Gordon L, King D, et al.: *Implementing the Supported Housing Approach: A National Evaluation of NIMH Supported Housing Demonstrations Projects.* Burlington, VT: Center for Community Change Through Housing and Support, 1991.
6. Morrissey JP, Dennis DL: *NIMH-Funded Research Concerning Homeless Mentally Ill Persons: Implications for Policy and Practice.* Rockville, MD: National Institute of Mental Health, 1986.
7. Ridgway P, Spaniol LR, Zipple AM: *Case Management Services for Persons Who Are Homeless and Mentally Ill: Report from an NIMH Work Group.* Boston: Center for Psychiatric Rehabilitation, 1986.
8. Ball FLJ, Havassey BE: A survey of the problems and needs of homeless consumers of mental health services. *Hospital and Community Psychiatry* 1988; 35(9):917-921.
9. Daniels L, Carling PJ: *Community Residential Rehabilitation Services of Psychiatrically Disabled Persons in Kitsap County.* Boston: Boston University Center for Psychiatric Rehabilitation, 1986.
10. Ridgway P, Carling PJ: *A Users Guide to Needs Assessments in Community Residential Rehabilitation.* Boston: Boston University, Center for Psychiatric Rehabilitation, 1988.
11. Tanzman B: An overview of surveys of mental health consumers' preferences for housing and support services. *Hospital and Community Psychiatry* 1993; 44(5):450-455.
12. Schutt RK, Goldfinger SM, Penk WE: The structure and sources of residential preferences among seriously mentally ill homeless adults. *Sociological Practice Review* 1992; 3(3):148-156.
13. Stuening E, Rafferty M: *Housing Preferences of Homeless People.* New York: New York State Psychiatric Institute, 1987.
14. Ellenberger H: Zoological garden and mental hospital. *Canadian Psychiatric Association Journal* 1960; 5:136-147.
15. Cumming J, Cumming E: *Ego and Milieu: Theory and Practice of Environmental Therapy.* New York: Atherton, 1967.
16. Deci RL, Ryan RM: *Intrinsic Motivation and Self-Determination in Human Behavior.* New York: Plenum, 1985.
17. Fisher S: *Stress and the Perception of Control.* Hillsdale, NJ: Lawrence Erlbaum, 1984.
18. Seligman ME: *Helplessness: On Depression, Development and Death.* San Francisco: Freeman, 1975.
19. Garber J, Seligman ME (Eds.): *Human Helplessness: Theory and Application.* New York: Academic Press, 1979.
20. Maslow AM: *Motivation and Personality.* New York: Harper and Brothers, 1954.
21. Wittman FD: *Architectural Planning and Design in Complex Organizations.* Unpublished doctoral dissertation. University of California, Berkeley, School of Architecture, 1983.
22. Delsohn G: Sacramento's homeless thrive in communal settings. *San Francisco Examiner* 1993; September 19:F4.
23. Imbimbo J, Pfeffer R: *The Olivieri Center: A Study of Homeless Women and Their Concept of Home.* New York: City University, 1987.
24. Olson RV: *Design Issues and Recommendations for an SRO: The Residents' Perspectives.* New York: Gran-Sultan Associates, April 1993.
25. Torrice AF, Logrippo R: *In My Room: Designing for and With Children.* New York: Fawcett, 1989.
26. Good works: The comfort of home. *House Beautiful* 1992; 134(10):40,44.

27. Hopper K: Counting the New York homeless. *New England Journal of Public Policy* 1992, Spring/Summer:771-791.
28. Ware NC, Dejarlais RR, AvRuskin TL, et al.: Empowerment and the transition to housing for homeless mentally ill people: An anthropological perspective. *New England Journal of Public Policy* 1992; Spring/Summer:297-314.
29. Fischer PJ: Victimization and homelessness: Cause and effect. *New England Journal of Public Policy* 1992; Spring/Summer:229-246.
30. D'Ercole A, Struening E: Victimization among homeless women: Implications for service delivery. *Journal of Community Psychology* 1990; 18:141-152.
31. Bassuk EL, Rosenberg L: Why does family homelessness occur? A case-control study. *American Journal of Public Health* 1988; 78(7):783-788.
32. Susser ES, Lin SP, Conover SA, et al.: Childhood antecedents of homelessness in psychiatric patients. *American Journal of Psychiatry* 1991; 148(8):1026-1030.
33. Wittman FD (Ed.): *A Guide to Low Income Housing for Homeless People Recovering From Alcohol and Other Drug Problems.* DHHS Pub. No. (ADM) 91-1739. Rockville, MD: National Institute on Alcohol Abuse and Alcoholism, 1991.
34. Shaw S, Borkman T (Eds.): *Social Model Alcohol Recovery.* Burbank, CA: Bridge Focus, 1990.
35. Sommer R: *Personal Space: The Behavioral Basis of Design.* Englewood Cliffs, NJ: Prentice Hall, 1969.
36. Newman O: *Design Guidelines for Creating Defensible Space.* Washington, DC: U.S. Government Printing Office, 1976.
37. Segal SP, Aviram U: *The Mentally Ill in Community-Based Sheltered Care.* New York: John Wiley, 1978.
38. Lamb HR, Goertzel V: Discharged mental patients: Are they really in the community? *Archives of General Psychiatry* 1971; 24(1):29-34.
39. Knisley MB, Fleming M: Implementing supported housing in state and local mental health systems. *Hospital and Community Psychiatry* 1993; 44(5):456-461.
40. Keck J: Responding to consumer housing preferences: The Toledo experience. *Psychosocial Rehabilitation Journal* 1990; 13(4):51-58.
41. Zipple TZ, Holland P: *Residential Rehabilitation: Supporting Staff and Empowering Consumers.* Workshop presented at the 18th annual meeting of the International Association of Psychosocial Rehabilitation, New Orleans, LA, July 26-27, 1993.
42. Ridgway P (Ed.): *Coming Home: Ex-Patients View Housing Options and Needs. Proceedings of a National Consumer Housing Forum.* Burlington, VT: Center for Community Change Through Housing and Support, 1988.
43. Horwitz J, Tognoli S: The role of home in adult development: Women and men living alone describe their residential lives. *Family Relations* 1982; 31:335-341.
44. Barker RG: *Ecological Psychology.* Stanford, CA: Stanford University Press, 1968.
45. Cohen MB: *Interactions and Mutual Influence in a Program for Homeless Mentally Ill Women.* Unpublished doctoral dissertation. Brandeis University, Florence Heller School for Advanced Studies in Social Welfare, 1988.
46. Spivak M: *Archetypal Space.* Boston: Harvard Medical School, Laboratory of Community Psychiatry, 1970.
47. Osmond H: Function as the basis of psychiatric ward design. *Mental Hospitals* 1957; 8(4):23-30.
48. Wittman FD, Biderman F, Hughes L: *Sober Living Guidebook for Alcohol and Drug-Free Housing.* Berkeley: University of California, Institute for the Study of Social Change, 1993.

49. Mandiberg J, Telles L: The Santa Clara County Clustered Apartment Project. *Psychosocial Rehabilitation Journal* 1990; 14(2):22-23.
50. Culhane DP: Ending homelessness among women with severe mental illness: A model program from Philadelphia. *Psychosocial Rehabilitation Journal* 1992; 16:63-76.
51. Berman-Rossi T, Cohen M: Group development and shared decision making working with homeless mentally ill women. *Social Work With Groups* 1989; 11(4):63-78.
52. Martin MA, Nayowith SA: Creating community: Group work to develop social support networks with homeless mentally ill. *Social Work With Groups* 1988; 11(4):79-93.
53. Harp HT: Independent living with support services: The goal and future for mental health consumers. *Psychosocial Rehabilitation Journal* 1990; 13(4):85-89.
54. Brown MA, Wheeler T: Supported housing for the most disabled: Suggestions for providers. *Psychosocial Rehabilitation Journal* 1990; 13(4):59-68.
55. Wilson SF, Mahler J, Tanzman B: *A Technical Assistance Report on Consumer and Ex-patient Roles in Supported Housing Services*. Burlington, VT: Center for Community Change Through Housing and Support, 1990.
56. Long L, Van Tosh L: *Consumer-Run Self-Help Programs Serving Homeless People With a Mental Illness*. Rockville, MD: National Institute of Mental Health, 1988.
57. Freund PD: Professional role(s) in the empowerment process: "Working with" mental health consumers. *Psychosocial Rehabilitation Journal* 1993; 16(3):65-73.

9

Women With Severe Mental Disorders

Issues and Service Needs

Carol T. Mowbray, Ph.D.
Daphna Oyserman, Ph.D.
Daniel Saunders, Ph.D.
Alba Rueda-Riedle, M.A.

The existence of sex bias in mental health treatment is a long-standing and probably still unresolved issue. For example, early research by Broverman et al.[1] identified the negative perceptions of women held by clinicians and the double bind in which women were placed, in that the expected characteristics of a "healthy" adult varied markedly from those for an adult female. Clinical and practice research has found gender biases in diagnosis[2] and in treatment, which serve to demean women (as dependent, passive, seductive, hysterical, etc.), foster traditional and limited sex roles, and respond to women patients as sex objects.[3]

An awareness of how such biases might affect services to women with long-term psychiatric disabilities is of more recent origin. Test and Berlin[4] were apparently the first to point out that in terms of differential service provision, the "chronically mentally ill are regarded as almost genderless" (p. 136). However, their early review was able to identify research establishing numerous significant differences in major domains of life functioning. While several authors have since elaborated on these problems,[5-7] systematic attention to researching gender differences among persons with long-term mental illness is still clearly lacking. A prior review documented failures to specify the gender composition of research samples or to report on gender differences for several major mental health journals.[8]

In this chapter, we review the most recent literature concerning women with long-term, severe mental illness (SMI), using Test and Berlin's[4] topics as an organizing framework. We begin with a summary of gender differences in demographics and clinical characteristics, and then move on to discuss problems in major areas of life functioning: instrumental roles; interpersonal roles, including social, sexual, marital, and family roles; and physical health, including medications. We then review the literature on two major problem areas for women with SMI: substance abuse and victimization. Finally, we end with some implications for mental health administrators and practitioners, framed from a public health perspective.

GENDER DIFFERENCES IN DEMOGRAPHICS AND CLINICAL CHARACTERISTICS

It seems to be common knowledge for most mental health providers that women far outnumber men in diagnoses of major affective disorders, especially depression. The lifetime prevalence for major depressive episodes in women is 1.67 times that of men—affecting a staggering 21.3 percent of the female population.[9] However, women in fact actually outnumber men in all major psychiatric diagnoses from the *Diagnostic and Statistical Manual of Mental Disorders*, third edition (*DSM-III*),[10] except one—antisocial personality disorder, according to two national epidemiological studies.[9,11] These gender differences upset conventional notions that men have higher rates of anxiety disorders and nonaffective psychoses, such as schizophrenia and schizoaffective disorder and that schizophrenia is primarily a disorder of young males. Despite the over-representation of women in most categories of mental illness diagnoses, it is men who are overrepresented in more intensive treatment programs: Women are more likely to receive outpatient treatment[12,13] and men, inpatient care.[3] Programs oriented toward schizophrenia report an overwhelming majority of males attending.[14]

There are also major gender differences in the demographics of persons with SMI. Several research studies have corroborated the fact that women in treatment with a mental illness diagnosis are significantly older than men[15] and also that women have a later age of onset.[16] The latter gender difference may be particularly marked in schizophrenia.[17] That is, the age of onset for schizophrenia is 27 for females versus 21 for males.[18] Similar though less dramatic differences are found for unipolar depression (25 for females vs. 23 for males) and for bipolar disorder (20 for females vs. 18 for males).[19]

Research also consistently indicates gender differentials in marital status among persons with mental illness: National weighted estimates show that while a minority of men with SMI marry (31 percent to 46 percent married), a majority of women do (55 percent to 75 percent married[20]). In fact, in overall population studies, marriage has consistently been interpreted as serving a protective function in men, while in women its function is more questionable. Married men usually have the lowest rates of mental illness, especially depression, while single (never married) women are often *less* depressed than their married counterparts.[3,21]

Differences in the racial composition of male versus female populations diagnosed with mental illness have been explored, but so far no significant differences have been supported. However, epidemiological data from one site of a major national study indicated a four-way interaction of age, ethnicity, sex, and diagnosis, that is, higher prevalence rates for older Mexican American women and younger non-Hispanic women, especially on alcoholism, drug abuse, phobias, and depression.[22] Clearly, the meaning of gender is socially constructed and varies by culture; it is not surprising that these differential constructions would also affect manifestations of mental illness.

Explanations for gender differences in diagnosis have been posited, but none clearly established. They have included differential vulnerability due to socialization and social roles,[3] environmental factors,[17] hormonal differences,[14] and other biological explanations.[16] However, much of this research is flawed, using small samples that may not be representative, questionable measures of premorbid competence, and treatment outcomes that are confounded with gendered role expectations.

Thus, although often ignored in treatment considerations and research, gender appears to play a major role in the etiology and manifestation of mental illness. While more scientifically sound research is needed as to etiology, at this time the evidence does seem consistent enough to mandate attention to gender differences in persons with SMI, and their implications for mental health services. We now turn our attention to reviewing the research findings that are available concerning women's role performance and problems in functioning.

GENDER DIFFERENCES IN INSTRUMENTAL ROLE PERFORMANCE

Test and Berlin's[4] review of special concerns for women with SMI reported that women experienced significant vocational disadvantages. However, in the few subsequent descriptive studies of persons with SMI that investigated education and employment, no significant gender differences have been found.[15,23,24] This might reflect social change; more likely, it reflects methodological problems (e.g., not controlling for women's older ages and thus greater opportunities for vocational experiences). Holstein and Harding[25] suggest there are measurement problems in assessment of work roles, in that multiple roles are often not considered in measures of social functioning. This was a particular problem for women in their sample in that nearly half of the working women, but none of the men, had additional responsibilities caring for others.

While gender differences in work status may be unclear, those involving vocational rehabilitation services provision are not. Across all types of disabilities, women represent less than one third of the caseloads of vocational rehabilitation programs, with reported earnings at closure only 56 percent of those achieved by men.[26] Similarly, in Fairweather Lodge programs (a psychosocial residential and employment program), fewer females than males are being served (37 percent vs. 63 percent).[27] Cook and Roussel[28] found that women in a large, urban psychiatric rehabilitation program were given fewer job placements than men before "graduating" and that they were retained in the agency longer before getting their first paid jobs. Once in these independent job placements, women received significantly lower salaries. The differential treatment and representation of women in vocationally oriented programs may reflect cultural expectations that vocational performance is more important to men, higher staff expectancies for men's vocational activity,[6] or the availability of primarily masculine jobs (e.g., janitorial, construction). Whatever the cause, this limited attention to their vocational needs would certainly appear to disadvantage women with psychiatric disabilities, especially given the traditional disparities between economic levels of women and men in our society.

The instrumental role of living independently has also received some limited study. In several reports, women with psychiatric disabilities were more likely to be in independent, stable housing than in dependent care or temporary housing.[29] In studying the residential status of clients in a large psychiatric rehabilitation center, Cook interpreted gender effects on housing status to be indirect, primarily due to women's better functioning and the fact that they were more likely to have children. While these results may reflect more positive outcomes vis-à-vis chances for more normative community living for women, they could as well reflect staff biases rating women as more functional because of their perceived compliance and greater experience in housekeeping roles, or they could reflect policies of dependent care facilities, which typically exclude residents with children. Thus, the meaning of gender differences in independent living outcomes for women may be unclear (similar to the vocational arena).

However, in terms of services, there are clear gender differences in obtaining adequate housing. For single women, neighborhoods that contain affordable housing are often unsafe and may contribute to high rates of assault.[8] Women with psychiatric disabilities who are mothers also indicate unmet needs in terms of housing available to support them and their children.[30] Overall, it appears that gender differences in instrumental role performance have received insufficient research attention, and the unique needs women have for work and housing have not been considered in service provision.

INTERPERSONAL ROLES

Social and Sexual Roles

There is a relatively large body of literature linking socialization for female gender roles with depression, suggesting that women are socialized to be nurturing of others, supportive of their needs, and attentive to their desires. Unfortunately, this other-directedness can come at the expense of one's own sense of worth and efficacy.[31,32] While social and sexual roles, friendships, and intimate relationships can be central supports, they can also be key stressors for women. However, we know very little about the interpersonal connectedness of women with SMI. What supports do they receive from friends, neighbors, and acquaintances; who can they turn to when they need help?

A recent study by Test, Burke, and Wallisch[33] suggests that the daily life circumstances of men and women with SMI differ in important ways. Women were more likely than men to be hospitalized for nonpsychiatric reasons. Women were also more likely to be married or divorced, involved in heterosexual relationships, parents, and actively involved in parenting when they were. Men were more likely to be jailed and to commit suicide. Males and females did not differ in the number of friends they were in contact with, but females were more likely to report kissing, dating, and sexual activity. From this and other reports, it appears that women with SMI are likely to be sexually active. Thus, Test et al.[33] report that in their sample of young adults, three quarters of women, but only 40 percent of males, were sexually active. Sexual activity has been documented in both hospital and community settings.[29,34] Unfortunately, over time, stable sexual relationships may be replaced with casual sexual encounters.[35] Women with SMI may also be more at risk of experiencing unwanted sexual advances, harassment, and exploitation. Another recent study focusing on the social and sexual roles of women with SMI found that the vast majority of women self-reported a need for help in dealing with difficult relationships—both in getting their emotional needs met and in dealing with emotional and sexual abuse.[36]

Marital and Family Roles

Marital and family roles are major social roles since marriage and parenting are normative signs of adult status and reflect important developmental tasks.[37-40] Women are particularly likely to view social connectedness and relationships with others as important and self-defining.[31,32] With regard to parenting and family roles, women are more likely to value spending time and being involved with children and serving their emotional and physical needs.[41] Given their normative, social, and developmental centrality, marital and family roles are particularly likely to be central to women's sense of who they are and what is possible for them. Success in this domain may therefore provide women more than men with a sense of worth and competence, while setbacks may be particularly stress-inducing and straining, providing the basis for a variety of negative self-images.[42-44] In relationship to mental illness, developing and maintaining a sense of self as active and responsible may be critical to recovery.[45]

Unfortunately, women with a mental illness appear likely to experience a variety of social stressors in their intimate and family relationships. These stresses may increase vulnerability; thus, for example, married women of low socioeconomic status with young children and no paid employment outside the home are at increased risk of developing a psychiatric disorder.[46] Mental illness in turn may increase stress in social relations. A recent review by Downey and Coyne[47] suggests that marital conflict is likely to be high up to four years after a depressive episode and that divorce is common among depressed women. In addition, women with a mental illness are more likely to marry a spouse with a psychiatric disorder—a situation that increases risk of exacerbation of their own symptoms and severity of marital and family disturbance.

As in other domains related to women and mental illness, information is scarce as to the marital and family roles women with a mental illness carry out and the successes and problems they may encounter. There does seem to be agreement that women with SMI have a greater number of children than average and are more often divorced or not married than the norm, thus raising their chances of raising children as single parents.[34] In their review of the literature, Hammen, Burge, and Adrian[48] suggest that adverse socioeconomic circumstances and lack of resources are part of the life circumstances of women with SMI. The stress of parenting under conditions of poverty, social isolation, and marital discord increases risk of childhood disorder.[49] And in fact a large literature exists suggesting that children of women with SMI are at risk for a variety of behavioral and emotional problems.[47,50-62] In addition, these children make up a sizable minority of children removed from

given more prescriptions for psychotropic drugs,[72-75] regardless of diagnosis.[76] Thus, their side effects should be of particular concern with women patients; for example, tardive dyskinesia has been repeatedly documented to be more frequent and more severe in females.[14] Other research has also indicated health problems specific to or more prevalent in women, such as weight gain, amenorrhea, dysmenorrhea,[4,6] skin and hair problems, problems with lactation,[14] and breast cancer[77]—all possibly side effects of long-term psychotropic medications.

Of perhaps even greater concern than these reports from small clinical studies vis-à-vis health problems is consistent documentation that women with SMI have problems accessing appropriate physical health care services. For a variety of reasons, psychiatric patients in general have been reported to often receive incomplete health care.[78] One study found that psychiatrists have difficulties detecting physical illnesses.[70] There are still reports published of undiagnosed medical problems being misdiagnosed as psychiatric.[79] For women, the fear is that because of preexisting beliefs concerning their tendencies toward hypochondria, health problems in women with SMI may be even more often mislabeled as part of a delusional system than they are in men.[80] In fact, Heyding[70] found that psychiatrists are more likely to miss physical illness problems in women.

Furthermore, in numerous areas, research has found that mental health providers give inadequate attention to gender-specific health problems of women, for example, services related to contraception, family planning, and avoiding sexually transmitted diseases;[5,81] services delivered to pregnant mentally ill women;[82,83] and pelvic examinations.[78] Despite the fact that substantial numbers of women are affected (30 percent according to Post[84]), psychiatrists do not ask women with psychiatric disabilities about medication side effects of a sexual nature (e.g., vaginal dryness), while they frequently ask male patients about ejaculation and other sexual performance issues.[85] Women with a long-term mental illness have been found to be as sexually active as males (39 percent in one report from a large agency providing psychosocial rehabilitation services).[86] Among populations with a mental illness diagnosis, knowledge about AIDS appears woefully inadequate.[87] As might be suspected, mental health service providers are also inadequate in providing information about contraception, family planning, and so on. Given the fact that unwanted pregnancies have significantly more impact on women than men, this lack of attention has vastly different gendered implications.

Thus, the overall physical health status of women with SMI definitely indicates the need for service providers to regularly include this topic in service planning for female clients. However, the literature also indicates that health education and health assessment services in mental health programs are not adequate, perhaps even less so for females. Attitudinal problems as well as competency and skills appear to be involved. Attention to the health of women psychiatric patients warrants more attention in service provision. While the literature on this topic has expanded since Test and Berlin's[4] early review, larger-scale research studies providing more comprehensive information on health status and health care access, availability, and acceptability are definitely needed.

SUBSTANCE ABUSE

While several psychiatric diagnoses are more common in women, substance use diagnoses are not. However, while women use less drugs, a secular trend toward higher female drug abuse rates and earlier onset of drug use among women has been documented.[88,89] Furthermore, the comorbidity of mental illness and substance abuse in women is high: At least 30 percent of mentally ill women also have a substance abuse diagnosis.[90] Additionally, women are more likely than men to become alcoholic after or during depression.[91] Women in substance abuse treatment programs have been found to score higher on levels of depression and anxiety as well as on levels of general psychological distress than men.[92,93] Overall, women's mental health problems may be compounded by feelings of guilt, shame, and anxiety about their addictions.[88]

In terms of the type of substance use, women are more likely than men to abuse licit drugs, such as tranquilizers, stimulants, and sedatives.[94] These are often drugs prescribed to them or to other people they know.[88] In addition, women report having a high incidence of marijuana and cocaine use.[95] With regard to addiction type, women report substance abuse addiction more often than men[88,95] and are more likely to describe sudden, intense onset occurring after a major life event such as an accident, disruption of family life, or sudden physical illness.[88,95] There is evidence to suggest that addicted women frequently come from families in which one or more family members are also addicted or in which drugs were used as a primary coping strategy by one or more family members.[88,95] Therefore, family factors such as existence of drug abusers within the family, extent of the social network, and stress emanating from conflicts within the family should be considered in making sense of women's substance abuse.[96]

Research with minority samples has found a number of subgroup differences. Street drugs and alcohol are the drugs most commonly used by low-income minority women, and prescription drugs are usually more prominently used by middle-class minority women.[96] Differences between minority and non-minority women have also been documented: Minority women overall are likely to start heavy drug use at a younger age than nonminority women.[96] Minority women are less likely than nonminority women to use drugs alone, tending to use drugs with groups or in the company of female friends.[97] These women's environmental exposure to drugs is compounded by relationships with drug-abusing partners and their dependence on family members or public assistance for survival.[88,95,98]

The escalation of drug use, especially among women of childbearing age, is clearly a matter of concern.[99] Substance abuse history increases isolation from non-drug-related relationships that are more likely to provide support with parenting and everyday functioning.[100] The social networks of women with substance abuse problems may be where drug use started and/or is encouraged. In fact, research on family processes has documented that family maladaptive interactions are related to behavior problems especially when drug use is concerned.[101]

Women with both mental health and substance abuse problems present characteristics that are very different from men with the same mental health and drug-abusing histories. However, community-based interventions with women with mental illness do not address the unique characteristics and challenges that women must deal with, especially where parenting is concerned.[102] A small survey of community mental health services in the city of Detroit revealed that less than 15 percent offered services to substances-abusing, mentally ill populations, and even these limited services focused on dually diagnosed individuals in general. There are specialized programs aimed at children and young adults with a mental illness diagnosis, but none of them addresses the unique situation of women dually diagnosed.

It is important to develop programs that take into account gender and cultural-relevant characteristics to more completely help women with mental illness and substance abuse problems.[96] A careful consideration of women's multiple roles and social networks is crucial since these are issues likely to jeopardize women's use of prevention and treatment services. In addition, the characteristics of the services provided (e.g., individual vs. group services), the availability of service supports such as child care and transportation, and expectations about services should be taken into account since researchers have found that women are more likely than men to rely on these when deciding on whether to get help or continue service receipt.[91,103] Finally, women who abuse substances are more likely to experience negative psychological consequences of drug use than are men due to less permissive and accepting cultural norms with regard to women's drug use.[91] As a result, women are less likely to admit substance use and to seek out help.[104] Services aimed at reaching these women need to be developed.

SEXUAL AND PHYSICAL VICTIMIZATION

The victimization of women takes many forms, including physical and sexual abuse by strangers, acquaintances, co-workers, lovers, husbands, and ex-partners. General population surveys reveal that about a third of all married women can expect to experience some form of physical abuse during their marriages.[105] Violence in dating and cohabiting relationships may be even higher.[106] Sexual harassment affects a fourth to half of women employees and students.[107] About one fifth of adult women have been raped.[107] Many women also suffer from the effects of abuse experienced in childhood. Child sexual abuse, defined as any sexual contact from fondling to intercourse, affects 20 to 30 percent of all girls.[108] Physical abuse of girls, with injury or injury potential, affects approximately 10 to 20 percent.[108]

Having a severe mental disorder does not provide immunity from abuse. In fact, the opposite seems to be true. Women outpatients and inpatients have higher than normal rates of all forms of victimization. For example, in 11 studies, child sexual abuse histories were reported by 36-70 percent of the women, and averaged about 50 percent.[108-113] The rates of physical assault, usually by an intimate, are also higher in psychiatric populations, averaging 54 percent across four studies.[109,111,112,114] Recently, we have learned of a very insidious form of abuse—the sexual abuse of women by their therapists, which occurs at alarmingly high rates.[115]

Victims differ from nonvictims on the rates and severity of many psychological problems. The core symptoms for most victims are chronic depression, anxiety, and phobias.[107,113,116] The high rates of abuse in marriage may explain why married women are more depressed than single women.[96] However, physical and sexual assault survivors do not seem to have higher than normal rates of schizophrenia.[116,117]

Rates of post-traumatic stress disorder (PTSD) are especially high in victim groups.[117,118] Many victims alternate between "numbing" (dissociative states) and hyperarousal. There is increasing evidence of physiological changes in the brain from traumatic stress.[119] When abuse occurs in a close relationship, a more complex form of PTSD may result, with the additional problems of difficulties with affect regulation, damaged self-image, idealization of the perpetrator, hopelessness, and somatization.[120] Victims usually experience a profound sense of betrayal, and their basic assumptions about living in a safe world may be shattered.[121] Substance abuse is a common way to cope with anxiety, pain, and depression and may help victims achieve dissociative states.[108,122] The effects of child sexual abuse deserve special attention because memories of the abuse may be partially or completely repressed,[123] personality development can be profoundly affected[124] (and include borderline personality traits or multiple personalities), and these survivors probably experience more isolation and shame than other victims.[125]

Despite the association of victimization with certain types of psychological problems, conclusions about causation are difficult to make. Most studies can be easily misinterpreted because they fail to establish if the problems existed before or came after the abuse. One exception is a study showing that battered women differ little from other women prior to being battered.[126] After the abuse, their rates of suicide attempts, substance abuse, psychiatric emergency room visits, and mental hospitalizations rose dramatically. Fifteen percent entered state mental hospitals and 26 percent attempted suicide. In addition to the likelihood that abuse usually precedes and contributes to depression, anxiety, and other problems, alternative scenarios are also possible. There is anecdotal evidence that offenders choose women who seem vulnerable; to create even greater dependence, some men who batter keep medication from their partners. Others may paternalistically use force to get their partners to take medication or to stop abusing drugs.

The association between victimization and severe mental disorders may also be a false one. Trauma symptoms can mimic mental disorders, especially dissociative symptoms and flashbacks. Psychiatric practitioners have a long history of not believing the reports of victims and seeing them as symptoms of "craziness." Caution is needed, for example, because Minnesota Multiphasic Personality Inventory (MMPI) profiles of battered women can be easily misinterpreted to mean that they are schizophrenic, or have paranoid or borderline personalities.[127] Self-labeling may also occur. Many women seek help because their batterers convinced them that they are crazy after years of isolation and degradation.

Despite increased awareness of women's victimization, detection rates by professionals remain quite low in both inpatient and outpatient settings.[111] Even if detected, the life-threatening nature of the abuse is often ignored.[128] A particularly tragic example is described by Ann Jennings,[129] whose daughter's child sexual abuse was not detected despite many years of psychiatric hospitalization. Even when mental health workers were aware of the abuse, they did not help her to heal emotionally and she eventually killed herself.

Abuse goes undetected because practitioners may lack training or confidence in their ability to handle the issues involved.[130] Male practitioners are less likely to detect abuse, to see it as serious, and to take a thorough history.[131,132] Victims may be reluctant to disclose out of shame or fear of retaliation. Most victims say they would tell if they were asked directly.[133] Emergency room workers and family therapists have learned to conduct assessment interviews away from male partners. Detection rates also increase when a large number of behaviorally specific questions are used. To be avoided are terms like "abuse," "rape," and "assault." Instead, asking about specific behaviors like "hit you with an object" or "forced you to do something sexual" will bring better results. Questioning can also be normalized, for example, "We have learned that many coming here are hurt by people they love, so we ask all our clients these questions."

Steps are increasingly being taken to provide more sensitive care and treatment. For example, private living quarters and alternatives to physical restraints may be especially important for sexual abuse survivors.[134,135] Practitioners are increasingly aware that women may be stalked, harassed, and occasionally murdered after leaving an abusive partner.[136] Safety planning must be the first priority. Victim shelters and hot lines can help the victim or the practitioner with safety planning, including individual and legal strategies. Once safe, the woman can be helped with decision making, problem solving, and trauma recovery.[123] Most treatments help victims reframe their negative symptoms as coping behaviors—as their best attempts to respond to terrorizing events that anyone would experience as traumatic. Interventions may also be needed to help increase the support and sensitivity of the victim's significant others.[135] While retelling of the trauma is often essential for trauma recovery, women with SMI may need special support groups and carefully paced trauma work.[137] Psychotropic medication may actually interfere with accessing the emotions that are needed for recovery.[91] Victims with severe mental disorders need special care. However, there is a "silver lining" to these women's bleak stories because in many cases, recovery from the psychic wounds of victimization can also lead to recovery from a mental disorder.

IMPLICATIONS FOR MENTAL HEALTH SERVICES DELIVERY

In a traditional model of mental health service provision, persons with mental illness periodically experience symptoms that, in turn, can produce impaired community functioning and role performance. The role of the mental health practitioner is to treat the symptoms (e.g., through medication or other therapies) or to minimize conditions that contribute to symptoms (such as stress). Client characteristics (such as lack of motivation) or environment (lack of resources) may present barriers to treatment effects. However, in this examination of gender differences in community functioning and in services receipt, we see repeatedly that gender itself is a barrier to effective mental health treatment. In numerous ways, the review identifies biased treatment based on gendered assumptions (e.g., that women have less need of vocational rehabilitation services) or discriminatory treatment (women are more often served in outpatient services; substance abuse treatment services are less accessible and acceptable to women). Furthermore, gender relates to factors that are more likely to keep women away from treatment: higher rates of health problems, medication side effects, parenting responsibilities, domestic violence, and victimization, which render women isolated and powerless. Related to the fact that women are more affected by the preceding factors, they are also likely to demonstrate increased mental and emotional problems. Their prior treatment and life events also put them at greater risk for psychiatric symptoms in adulthood, for example, due to higher rates of childhood sexual abuse, adult victimization, or greater comorbidity of substance abuse and psychiatric disorders.

Yet again and again in sections of this review, we have concluded that there is insufficient attention in treatment and rehabilitation services to women's special needs. Again and again, we have noted that there is insufficient research addressed to specific problems of women with SMI and to factors that increase or decrease the effects of these problems on community functioning, psychiatric status, and role performance. It is overwhelming how a factor like gender that has such extensive and significant effects on individuals' histories, their problems, their use of services, and service effectiveness could be so greatly ignored for so long a period of time. Since the review by Test and Berlin,[4] now more than 15 years old, attention to gender and progress in treatment of women with SMI has been modest, at best.

The implications for mental health practice are far-reaching, yet simple. Gender and all its implications and ramifications have to be considered in every aspect of service to persons with SMI: diagnosis, assessment, planning, delivery of mental health treatment and rehabilitation, and evaluation of outcomes. This means that clinicians and administrators must be thoroughly familiar with, ever vigilant of, and committed to addressing differences associated with female gender. Initial and periodic training may be needed on many gender-related topics. This involves pre-service training from professional practice curriculums and inservice training in agency settings. Knowledgeable supervisors will be particularly important to ensure that gender sensitivity is practiced through services. Administrators need to review procedures concerning referral, screening, and/or entry to programs to ensure that they are based on meeting women's actual needs, rather than gender stereotypes.

Many of the services gaps identified in our review can be filled by appropriate attention to women's issues within existing program structures. That is, women are more likely than men to use community mental health services, but less likely to view them as helpful. In fact, these women are quite likely to rate the services as being of no help at all. Perhaps this is because these services were not designed with the real-life needs and circumstances of women in mind.[36] Some new programs and service components may need to be added to increase access and effectiveness for women, for example, integrated treatment for women with dual diagnosis, group treatment for victims of sexual assault, respite care or baby-sitting access for children of female clients, and transportation to service locations. This is a question of investing now or paying later in terms of increased dysfunction of women as well as their children and/or other family members. Research is also needed on all the above topics. Journal editors should require authors to report on the gender composition of study samples and to routinely test for gender differences. Good research should regularly incorporate variables in study designs to help explain mechanisms through which gender differences occur. To address possible bias, researchers should use larger samples of clients, representative of those using psychiatric rehabilitation and mental health services, including minority populations, lesbians, and all age groups. Finally, the role of sociocultural context in framing the supports and stresses experienced by women with SMI must begin to be explored. For example, it has been argued that African American women are more likely to give and receive help within extended family networks than are Whites.[138] Yet the ability of family networks to provide support to women with a mental illness has not been explored. Similarly, we do not know the extent to which cultural beliefs about the meaning of mental illness or acceptance of formal support systems may change women's perceived supports and stresses, enable or hinder the uses of community mental health or community support services. Thus, many important topics remain unexplored, hindering our ability to provide effective, gender-relevant services.

Individuals with a mental illness have traditionally been understood primarily in terms of the course of their illness. This narrow focus has meant that their goals, motivations, and life tasks will have been seen as subsumed by their mental illness. After a generation of discourse involving the psychosocial rehabilitation and community mental health movements, the restrictiveness of the previous focus is clear. Individuals with a mental illness occupy sociocultural niches that inform the social and subjective nature of their everyday experiences and the nature of their normative goals as well as color the ways in which mental illness is experienced and expressed.[139-141] An awareness of the significance of gendered roles and needs and its interaction with cultural context has been lacking, with consequent effects being particularly deleterious for women. As did Test and Berlin[4] nearly two decades ago, we once again issue a call to correct this situation.

REFERENCES

1. Broverman I, Vogal S, Broverman D, et al.: Sex role stereotypes and clinical judgements of mental health. *Journal of Counseling and Clinical Psychology* 1970; 34:1-7.
2. Loring M, Powell B: Gender, race, and DSM-III: A study of the objectivity of psychiatric diagnostic behavior. *Journal of Health and Social Behavior* 1988; 29:1-22.
3. Hankin J: Gender and mental illness. *Research in Community and Mental Health* 1990; 6:183-201.
4. Test MA, Berlin SB: Issues of special concern to chronically mentally ill women. *Professional Psychology* 1981; 12(1):136-145.
5. Bachrach LL: Deinstitutionalization and women: Assessing the consequences of public policy. *American Psychologist* 1984; 39(10):1171-1177.
6. Bachrach LL: Chronically mentally ill women: Emergence and legitimation of program issues. *Hospital and Community Psychiatry* 1985; 36:1063-1069.
7. Bachrach LL, Nadelson CC (Eds.): *Treating Chronically Mentally Ill Women*. Washington, DC: American Psychiatric Press, 1988.
8. Mowbray CT, Oyserman D, Lutz C, et al.: Women: The ignored majority. In: Spaniol L (Ed.): *Psychological and Social Aspects of Psychiatric Disability*. Boston: Center for Psychiatric Rehabilitation, 1996, pp. 171-194.
9. Kessler RC, McGonagle KA, Zhao S, et al.: Lifetime and 12-month prevalence of DSM-III-R psychiatric disorders in the United States. *Archives of General Psychiatry* 1994; 51:8-19.
10. American Psychiatric Association: *Diagnostic and Statistical Manual of Mental Disorders*. 3rd ed. Washington, DC: American Psychiatric Association, 1980.
11. Robins LN, Locke BZ, Regier DA: An overview of psychiatric disorders in America. In: Robins LN, Regier DA (Eds.): *Psychiatric Disorders in America: The Epidemiological Catchment Area Study*. New York: Free Press, 1991, pp. 328-366.

12. Wilcox JA, Yates WR: Gender and psychiatry comorbidity in substance abusing individuals. *American Journal of Addictions* 1993; 2(3):202-206.

13. Rhodes A, Goering P: Gender differences in the use of outpatient mental health services. *Journal of Mental Health Administration* 1994; 21(4):328-346.

14. Seeman MV: Gender differences in treatment response in schizophrenia. In: Seeman MV (Ed.): *Gender and Psychopathology.* Washington, DC: American Psychiatric Press, 1995, pp. 227-251.

15. Test MA, Knoedler WH, Allness DJ, et al.: Characteristics of young adults with schizophrenic disorders treated in the community. *Hospital and Community Psychiatry* 1985; 36:853-858.

16. Goldstein JM, Tsuang MT, Faraone SV: Gender and schizophrenia: Implications for understanding the heterogeneity of the illness. *Psychiatry Research* 1989; 28:243-253.

17. Greenwald D: Psychotic disorders with emphasis on schizophrenia. In: Brown LS, Ballou M (Eds.): *Personality and Psychopathology: Feminist Reappraisals.* New York: Guilford, 1993, pp. 144-176.

18. Gottesman II: *Schizophrenia Genesis: The Origins of Madness.* New York: Freeman, 1991.

19. Burke KC, Burke JD, Regier DA, et al.: Age of onset of selected mental disorders in five community populations. *Archives of General Psychiatry* 1990; 47:511-518.

20. *Client/Patient Sample Survey of Inpatient, Outpatient, and Partial Care Programs.* Rockville, MD: National Institute of Mental Health, 1986.

21. Gove WR: Sex differences in the epidemiology of mental disorder: Evidence and explanations. In: Gomburg ES, Franks V (Eds.): *Gender and Disordered Behavior.* New York: Brunner/Mazel, 1979.

22. Burman MA, Hough RL, Escobar JI, et al.: Six-month prevalence of specific psychiatric disorders among Mexican-Americans and non-Hispanic Whites in Los Angeles. *Archives of General Psychiatry* 1987; 44:687-694.

23. Herman SE, Amdur R, Hazel K, et al.: *Clients With Serious Mental Illness: Characteristics and Typology.* Lansing: Michigan Department of Mental Health, 1988.

24. Shtasel DL, Gur RE, Gallacher F, et al.: Gender differences in the clinical expression of schizophrenia. *Schizophrenia Review* 1992; 71:225-231.

25. Holstein AR, Harding CM: Omissions in assessment of work roles: Implications for evaluating social functioning and mental illness. *American Journal of Orthopsychiatry* 1992; 62:469-474.

26. Menz FE, Hansen G, Smith H, et al.: Gender equity in access, services and benefits from vocational rehabilitation. *Journal of Rehabilitation* 1989; 55:31-40.

27. Fergus E: *A Profile of Lodge Program Characteristics by Region.* Paper presented at the Ways of Working Conference, East Lansing, MI, March 26-27, 1987.

28. Cook JA, Roussel AE: *Who Works and What Works: Effects of Race, Class, Age and Gender on Employment Among the Psychiatrically Disabled.* Paper presented at the annual meetings of the American Sociological Association, Chicago, 1987.

29. Cook JA: Independent community living among women with severe mental illness: A comparison with outcomes among men. In: Levin BL, Blanch AK, Jennings A (Eds.): *Women's Mental Health Services: A Public Health Perspective.* Thousand Oaks, CA: Sage, 1998, pp. 99-119.

30. Blanch AK, Nicholson J, Purcell J: Parents with severe mental illness and their children: The need for human services integration. In: Levin BL, Blanch AK, Jennings A (Eds.): *Women's Mental Health Services: A Public Health Perspective.* Thousand Oaks, CA: Sage, 1998, pp. 201-214.

31. Oyserman D, Markus HR: Gender and thought: The role of the self-concept. In: Crawford M, Gentry M (Eds.): *Gender and Thought: Psychosocial Perspectives*. New York: Springer-Verlag, 1989, pp. 100-127.

32. Oyserman D, Markus HR: Self as social representation. In: Moscovici S, Flick U (Eds.): *Psychology of the Social*. Berlin: Rowohlt Taschenbuch Verlag GmbH, 1996.

33. Test MA, Burke SS, Wallisch LS: Gender differences of young adults with schizophrenic disorders in community care. *Schizophrenia Bulletin* 1990; 16:331-344.

34. Mowbray CT, Oyserman D, Zemencuk J: Motherhood for women with serious mental illness: Pregnancy, childbirth and the postpartum period. *American Journal of Orthopsychiatry* 1995; 65(1):21-38.

35. Verhulst J, Schneidman B: Schizophrenia and social functioning. *Hospital and Community Psychiatry* 1981; 32(4):259-262.

36. Cogan J: *Assessing the Community Support Services Needs Women With Psychiatric Disabilities May Have Regarding Relationships*. Burlington, VT: Conference for Community Change Through Housing and Support.

37. Carli L, Traficante D: *The Couple and Choice of Parenthood: An Interpretation Based on the Transgenerational Perspective of Attachment Theory*. Paper presented at the International Society for the Study of Social Behavior and Development (ISSBD), Quebec City, Quebec, Canada, August 1996.

38. Luster T, Okagaki L (Eds.): *Parenting: An Ecological Perspective*. Hillsdale, NJ: Lawrence Erlbaum, 1993.

39. Cohler BJ, Musick JS: Psychopathology of parenthood: Implications for mental health of children. *Infant Mental Health Journal* 1983; 4(3):140-163.

40. Gizynski MN: The effects of maternal depression on children. *Clinical Social Work Journal* 1985; 13(2):103-116.

41. Bloom K, Shoenmakers KM, Masataka N, et al.: *Factors That Affect Child Orientation as a Component of Self Concept*. Paper presented at the International Society for the Study of Social Behavior and Development (ISSBD), Quebec City, Quebec, Canada, August 1996.

42. Bloom K, Delmore-Ko P, Masataka N, et al.: *Child Oriented Self-Schema: Social Perceptions and Cross-Cultural Comparisons*. Paper presented at the International Society for the Study of Social Behavior and Development (ISSBD), Quebec City, Quebec, Canada, August 1996.

43. Markus H, Cross M: The willful self. *Personality and Social Psychology Bulletin* (Special Issue: Centennial Celebration of the Principles of Psychology) 1990; 16(4):726-742.

44. Stott FM, Musick JS, Clark R, et al.: Developmental patterns in the infants and young children of mentally ill mothers. *Infant Mental Health Journal* 1983; 4(3):217-234.

45. Davidson L, Strauss JS: Sense of self in recovery from severe mental illness. *British Journal of Medical Psychology* 1992; 65:131-145.

46. Romans-Clarkson SE, Walton VA, Herbison GP, et al.: Motherhood and psychiatric morbidity in New Zealand. *Psychological Medicine* 1988; 8:983-990.

47. Downey G, Coyne JC: Children of depressed parents: An integrative review. *Psychological Bulletin* 1990; 108(1):50-76.

48. Hammen C, Burge D, Adrian C: Timing of mother and child depression in a longitudinal study of children at risk. *Journal of Consulting and Clinical Psychology* 1991; 59:341-345.

49. Hammen CL, Gordon D, Burge D, et al.: Maternal affective disorders, illness and stress: Risks for child psychopathology. *American Journal of Psychiatry* 1987; 144:736-741.

92. Griffin ML, Weiss RD, Mirin SM, et al.: A comparison of male and female cocaine abusers. *Archives of General Psychiatry* 1989; 46:122-126.
93. McGlashan TH, Bardenstein KK: Gender differences in affective, schizoaffective, and schizophrenic disorders. *Schizophrenia Bulletin* 1990; 16(2):319-329.
94. Kail BL: Drugs, gender and ethnicity: Is the older minority women at risk? *Journal of Drug Issues* 1989; 19(2):171-189.
95. Lex BW: Prevention of substance abuse problems in women. In: Watson RR (Ed.): *Drug and Alcohol Abuse Prevention.* Totowa, NJ: Humana, 1990.
96. Comas-Díaz L, Greene B: *Women of Color: Integrating Gender and Ethnic Identities in Psychotherapy.* New York: Guilford, 1994.
97. Lex BW: Review of alcohol problems in ethnic minority groups. *Journal of Consulting and Clinical Psychology* 1987; 55(3):293-300.
98. Reed BG: Drug misuse and dependency in women: The meaning and implications of being considered a special population or minority group. *International Journal of the Addictions* 1985; 20:13-62.
99. Black M, Schuler M, Nair P: Prenatal drug exposure: Neurodevelopmental outcome and parenting environment. *Journal of Pediatric Psychology*1993; 18(5):605-620.
100. Kearney MH, Murphy S, Rosenbaum M: Mothering on crack cocaine: A grounded theory analysis. *Social Science and Medicine* 1994; 38(2):351-361.
101. Szpocznik J, Santisteban D, Rio A, et al.: Family effectiveness training: An intervention to prevent drug abuse and problem behaviors in Hispanic adolescents. *Hispanic Journal of Behavioral Sciences* 1989; 11(1):4-27.
102. Oyserman D, Mowbray CT, Zemencuk JK: Resources and supports for mothers with severe mental illness. *Health and Social Work* 1994; 19(2):132-141.
103. Kingree JB: Understanding gender differences in psychosocial functioning and treatment retention. *American Journal of Drug and Alcohol Abuse* 1995; 21(2):267-281.
104. Lex BW: Alcohol and other psychoactive substance dependence in women and men. In: Seeman MV (Ed.): *Gender and Psychopathology.* Washington, DC: American Psychiatric Press, 1995, pp. 311-358.
105. Straus MA, Gelles RJ: Societal change and change in family violence from 1975 to 1985 as revealed by two national surveys. *Journal of Marriage and the Family* 1986; 45:465-479.
106. Stets J, Straus MA: The marriage license as hitting license: A comparison of assaults in dating, cohabitating, and married couples. *Journal of Family Violence* 1989; 4(2):161-180.
107. Koss MP, Goodman LA, Browne A, et al.: *No Safe Haven: Male Violence Against Women at Home, at Work, and in the Community.* Washington, DC: American Psychological Association, 1994.
108. Briere JN: *Child Abuse Trauma.* Thousand Oaks, CA: Sage, 1992.
109. Carmen E, Rieker PP, Mills T: Victims of violence and psychiatric illness. *American Journal of Psychiatry* 1984; 141:378-383.
110. Jacobson A, Herald C: The relevance of childhood sexual abuse to adult psychiatric inpatient care. *Hospital and Community Psychiatry* 1990; 41:154-158.
111. Jacobson A, Richardson B: Assault experiences of 100 psychiatric inpatients: Evidence of the need for routine inquire. *American Journal of Psychiatry* 1987; 144(11):908-913.
112. Muenzenmaier K, Meyer I, Struening E, et al.: Childhood abuse and neglect among women outpatients with chronic mental illness. *Hospital and Community Psychiatry* 1993; 44:666-670.
113. Rose S: Acknowledging abuse backgrounds of intensive case management clients. *Community Mental Health Journal* 1991; 27:255-263.

114. Post RD, Willett AB, Franks RD, et al.: A preliminary report on the prevalence of domestic violence among psychiatric inpatients. *American Journal of Psychiatry* 1980; 137:974-975.
115. Pope KS, Bouhoutsos JC: *Sexual Intimacy Between Therapists and Patients.* New York: Praeger, 1986.
116. Gleason WJ: Mental disorders in battered women: An empirical study. *Violence and Victims* 1993; 8:53-68.
117. Hanson RK: The psychological impact of sexual abuse on women and children. *Annals of Sex Research* 1990; 3:187-223.
118. Holtzworth-Monroe A, Smutzler N, Sandin B: A brief review of the research on husband violence: The effects of husband violence on battered women and their children. *Aggression and Violent Behavior* 1997; 2:179-213.
119. van der Kolk BA: The body keeps the score: Memory and the evolving psychobiology of posttraumatic stress. *Harvard Review of Psychiatry* 1994; 1:253-265.
120. Herman JL: Complex PTSD: A syndrome in survivors of prolonged and repeated trauma. *Journal of Traumatic Stress* 1992; 5:377-392.
121. Janoff-Bulman R: *Shattered Assumptions: Towards a New Psychology of Trauma.* New York: Free Press, 1992.
122. Dutton MA: *Empowering and Healing the Battered Woman: A Model for Assessment and Intervention.* New York: Springer, 1992.
123. Williams LM: Recall of childhood trauma: A prospective study of women's memories of child sexual abuse. *Journal of Consulting and Clinical Psychology* 1994; 62:1167-1176.
124. Caffaro JV: Identification and trauma: An integrative-developmental approach. *Journal of Family Violence* 1995; 10:23-40.
125. Finkelhor D: Long-term effects of childhood sexual abuse: Some new data. In: Finkelhor D (Ed.): *Child Sexual Abuse: New Theory of Research.* New York: Free Press, 1984.
126. Stark E, Flitcraft A, Frazier W: Medicine and patriarchal violence. *International Journal of Health Services* 1979; 9(3):461-493.
127. Rosewater LB: Battered or schizophrenic? Psychological tests can't tell. In: Yllö K, Bograd M (Eds.): *Feminist Perspectives on Wife Abuse.* Newbury Park, CA: Sage, 1988.
128. Harway M, Hansen M: Therapist perceptions of family violence. In: Hansen M, Harway M (Eds.): *Battering and Family Therapy.* Thousand Oaks, CA: Sage, 1993.
129. Jennings A: On being invisible in the mental health system. In: Levin BL, Blanch AK, Jennings A (Eds.): *Women's Mental Health Services: A Public Health Perspective.* Thousand Oaks, CA: Sage, 1998, pp. 326-347.
130. Keller EL: Invisible victims: Battered women in psychiatric and medical emergency rooms. *Bulletin of the Menninger Clinic* 1996; 60:1-21.
131. Saunders DG, Kindy P: Predictors of physicians' responses to woman abuse: The role of gender, background and brief training. *Journal of General Internal Medicine* 1993; 8:606-609.
132. Snyder JC, Newberger EH: Consensus and differences among hospital professionals in evaluating child maltreatment. *Violence and Victims* 1986; 1(2):125-139.
133. Craine LS, Henson CE, Colliver JA, et al.: Prevalence of a history of sexual abuse among female psychiatric patients in a state mental hospital system. *Hospital and Community Psychiatry* 1988; 39:300-304.
134. Carmen E, Crane W, Dunnicliff M, et al.: *Massachusetts Department of Mental Health Task Force on the Restraint and Seclusion of Persons Who Have Been Physically or Sexually Abused.* Unpublished report, 1996.

135. Harris M: Modifications in services delivery and clinical treatment for women diagnosed with severe mental illness who are also the survivors of sexual abuse trauma. In: Levin BL, Blanch AK, Jennings A (Eds.): *Women's Mental Health Services: A Public Health Perspective*. Thousand Oaks, CA: Sage, 1998, pp. 309-325.

136. Saunders DG: Prediction of wife assault. In: Campbell JC (Ed.): *Assessing Dangerousness: Violence by Sexual Offenders, Batterers, and Child Abusers*. Newbury Park, CA: Sage, 1994.

137. Redner LL, Herder DD: Case management's role in affecting appropriate treatment for persons with histories of childhood sexual trauma. *Psychosocial Rehabilitation Journal* 1992; 15(3):45-47.

138. Hogan DP, Hao L, Parish WL: Race, kin networks, and assistance to mother-headed families. *Social Forces* 1990; 68:797-812.

139. Griffith EEH: African-American perspectives. In: Mezzich JE, Kleinman A, Fabrega H, et al. (Eds.): *Culture and Psychiatric Diagnosis: A DSM-IV Perspective*. Washington, DC: American Psychiatric Press, 1996.

140. Lin KM: Cultural influences on the diagnosis of psychotic and organic disorders. In: Mezzich JE, Kleinman A, Fabrega H, et al. (Eds.): *Culture and Psychiatric Diagnosis: A DSM-IV Perspective*. Washington, DC: American Psychiatric Press, 1996.

141. Rogler LH: Hispanic perspectives. In: Mezzich JE, Kleinman A, Fabrega H, et al. (Eds.): *Culture and Psychiatric Diagnosis: A DSM-IV Perspective*. Washington, DC: American Psychiatric Press, 1996.

10

Parents With Severe Mental Illness and Their Children

The Need for Human Services Integration

Andrea K. Blanch, Ph.D.
Joanne Nicholson, Ph.D.
James Purcell, M.A.

Parents with severe and persistent mental illness have generally been neglected by mental health policymakers and providers. A national survey conducted in 1990 found that fewer than one third of states routinely collected information about the parenting status of women in their care.[1] Existing policies focused primarily on the medical management of pregnancy, abortion, or labor and delivery. No states reported policies providing for visitation between state hospital patients and their children. Similarly, few states reported programs specifically addressing the needs of this population.

The needs of mothers with mental illness were highlighted in 1981 by Test and Berlin. They noted a general lack of attention to gender-related issues, and they recommended a range of services essential to assist mentally ill women who are mothers in managing daily parenting demands and in coping with the stresses of caring for children.[2] This issue was again documented by Bachrach and Nadelson in 1988.[3]

NOTE: This chapter appeared as an article in the *Journal of Mental Health Administration*, 1994, Vol. 21, No. 4, pp. 388-396.

Bachrach and Nadelson pointed to a failure to identify the special service requirements of women with mental illness, an absence of relevant
services research that might inform service planning, and a lag between
research and practice. They cited the situation of a pregnant woman
who was denied access to housing because of her pregnancy as indicative of a general insensitivity on the part of the service system to the
special service needs of women with mental illness (p. 12).[3] Men with
mental illness may also be parents, although most parents with severe
mental illness identified in preliminary analyses of statewide client
tracking data are women.[4]

Several factors appear to impede the development and implementation of services in support of successful parenting by individuals with
mental illness. The first is, quite simply, that mental health service recipients are not being identified as parents. This may be due to ignorance or oversight on the part of mental health professionals, or to
stigma and an unspoken denial of sexual activity and consequent childbearing, as suggested by Apfel and Handel.[5] Knitzer and Yelton refer to
"institutional doubts about the strengths of parents" and suggest that
both mental health and child welfare workers often question parents'
capacity for growth.[6]

A second factor is that parenting is not generally considered a mental
health issue. Children often come to the attention of child protective
services workers, for example, when they require foster care placement
at the time of their mothers' hospitalizations, or if there are suspicions
of child abuse or neglect. Parenting skills are assessed when children
are deemed at risk for out-of-home placement, rather than as part of a
psychosocial rehabilitation planning process for the adult. Parenting
skills are frequently taught in programs funded through social services,
but rarely in mental health programs. This speaks, perhaps, to a lack of
focus on the life goals of the adult client, a pitfall in mental health planning identified by Anthony, Cohen, and Farkas.[7]

Services for parents with mental illness and their children are also
extremely fragmented. Services are found in different locations, accessed through different mechanisms and funded by different agencies;
programmatic approaches are rarely combined in comprehensive or
flexible ways. The lack of coordination between child welfare and mental health workers reflects the "cross-cultural" barrier to collaboration
suggested by Knitzer and Yelton,[6] who note that there is often substan-

tial skepticism about the capabilities of workers from "other" agencies. Moreover, confusion may be created by the diffusion of role boundaries and struggles for authority over case planning.[8]

The goal of this chapter is to bring public sector and academic attention to the needs and issues facing parents diagnosed with serious mental illness by describing the results of the New York State Task Force on Mentally Ill Parents with Young Children. This task force used consumers as well as mental health and social service professionals to identify the needs of parents with mental illness raising young children, to recommend ways of addressing their needs, and to anticipate and overcome impediments to the implementation of suggested solutions.

The New York State project represents a substantial statewide effort to identify and intervene with a population and set of problems that span organizational boundaries. Many of the issues and strategies identified are consistent with previous analyses of general problems in services integration[9] and in managing programs that involve multiple levels of government.[10] A second goal of this chapter is therefore to describe an initial effort to respond to the needs of parents with mental illness and their children through an intergovernmental, services integration strategy.

THE NEW YORK STATE TASK FORCE

In New York State, persistent efforts by a coalition of mental health advocacy groups eventually succeeded in bringing the issue of parents with serious mental illness to the attention of policymakers at the Office of Mental Health (OMH) and Department of Social Service (DSS). In response, a joint task force was created in June 1992 composed of consumers, researchers, advocates, and professionals from both systems. The task force was charged with the responsibility of studying the prevalence of parenthood among persons diagnosed with serious mental illness, identifying barriers to success, and making recommendations. In particular, the task force was asked to focus on:

1. Reducing family disruption and foster care placements due to parental mental illness;

2. Enhancing the ability of the child welfare system to work effectively with parents diagnosed with serious mental illness and with their children;
3. Developing widespread understanding within mental health programs that patients may also be parents and that this calls for special forms of intervention both for the parents and for their children; and
4. Expanding the capacity of the mental health system, especially psychiatric rehabilitation programs, to support parents diagnosed with serious mental illness.

Task force membership was heavily weighted toward consumer, local government, and provider participation. This composition was important in allowing state-level policymakers to understand and include in their deliberations the complexities of services coordination at the local level.

As a preliminary step, task force staff attempted to gather information about the percentage of persons diagnosed with serious mental illness who have children, and about their current whereabouts. Although no national statistics could be located, relevant data were available from DSS and from OMH evaluations of statewide mental health intensive case management (ICM) and supported housing programs.

New York State DSS data give an indication of the overall scope of this issue. At the current time, there are a total of 63,000 children in foster care in New York State, and another 41,000 children receive mandated preventive services (outpatient services designed to prevent unnecessary out-of-home placements). Data collected in 1991 show that approximately 16 percent of children in foster care (over 10,000 children) and 21 percent of children receiving preventive services (8,600 additional children) have at least one parent with a diagnosed serious mental illness.

Both of the OMH programs serve only persons who have been identified as having a serious and persistent mental illness. Data from these programs suggest that parenting is an important issue among this population. Twenty-two percent of all ICM clients and 25 percent of all supported housing clients have children; of female ICM clients under the age of 35, 45 percent are mothers. While many of these children are ultimately placed in foster care, in many other cases parents retain custody. Twenty percent of ICM and 40 percent of supported housing clients with children currently have custody of one or more minor children.

Data do not currently exist on the cost to the public system of foster care placements due to parental mental illness that could have been prevented, or on the costs of litigation (including court costs, lawyers fees, and multiple evaluations) that are incurred when the state acts to remove children from their parents' care or to terminate parental rights. Anecdotal evidence suggests that both human and financial costs are very high.

The Public Hearing Process

The task force began by holding public hearings to hear firsthand from persons with mental illnesses who were rearing families, from individuals who were reared by a parent with mental illness, and from individuals directly involved in delivering services to them. Almost 100 individuals testified at three sites across the state, including 46 providers, 23 consumer-family members, 6 representatives from local mental health departments, 5 representatives from local social services departments, and 5 others.

Issues generated at the public hearings clustered into three main areas: Services, policies and procedures, and coordination among systems.

Services

Many participants testified about their inability to access needed services due to long waiting lists or a simple lack of services. Needs included housing coupled with family services or supports, day care and early education, specialized clinical services, long-term support services, and respite care for both parents and children. Particular emphasis was given to the need for informal peer support groups for parents with a mental illness, for their children, and for other family members, such as siblings and grandparents.

Many problems were cited concerning the organization and structure of existing services, including the lack of evening and weekend services, the inability to mobilize resources quickly (except for the purpose of investigation), the lack of in-home services, the lack of transportation to services (outside of cities), and the inability of program staff to respond to diversity (including cultural diversity, poverty, limited ability to speak English, etc.). In addition, it was noted that there is often inadequate outreach and/or information about available services.

Policies and Procedures

Testimony suggested that mental health providers generally view people as patients rather than as family members or parents. Intake assessment protocols for adults (in both inpatient and ambulatory care) rarely include questions about parental status or child care responsibilities, nor do providers see it as their responsibility to assist the family with problems caused by the mental health admission (e.g., to arrange needed child care during an inpatient stay), or to communicate with family members (especially children) about a parent's mental illness. Discharge plans do not routinely attend to needed parental supports, nor do mental health providers reach out to DSS at the point of discharge. Few, if any, hospitals make special arrangements to accommodate visitation between parent and child during a parent's inpatient stay.

Testimony also suggested that OMH and DSS policies and procedures reflect inaccurate stereotypes about mental illness. Both systems appear to be uncomfortable with clients' abilities to recognize and define their own needs. This is a difficult issue since workers, especially child protective services workers, may be held accountable by law, the media, and the general public for any incidents that occur after a disposition is made. Strategies need to be developed to support workers who make "risky decisions," and to oppose inaccurate or misleading presentations in the media.

A related issue was that clients are suspicious of services, and they often fear that they will unfairly lose their children. Examples were given of decisions that appeared to the presenters as at best arbitrary regarding custody, visitation, and other parental rights. The family court system was cited as dismissing cases out of hand, setting unrealistic expectations, and not making important distinctions between individual cases.

As a result of real and perceived bias, needed services may not be accessed. To avoid this problem, policies and procedures should be examined to ensure that child placement decisions are made on the basis of criteria that are clearly understood by clients and providers. Staff should be knowledgeable about a range of possible options (including flexible arrangements such as open adoption) and should be trained to assess the potential impact of various options on children.

Confidentiality issues, including providers' perceptions of statutory or other policy restrictions, may also create or exacerbate problems. More attention could be paid to sharing critical information without violating the patient's right to confidentiality. Finally, the need for an ongoing analysis of the impact of social policy on the family unit was cited. Numerous examples were given of how funding and services focus on individuals, rather than on families, and inadvertently drive families apart.

Coordination

Testimony clearly indicated that the OMH adult service system and the DSS child welfare system have limited knowledge about each other and currently lack either motivation or incentives to gain that knowledge. Most adult mental health providers do not understand child protective services law or permanency planning issues, while most DSS workers are not familiar with family systems theory, the impact of mental illness on family interactions, or the differentially disabling nature of different mental illnesses. Moreover, the two systems define and prioritize problems differently, which both impedes communication and encourages a division of responsibility (i.e., "these are *our* kids; these are *your* kids") rather than a sharing of responsibility.

The DSS and OMH adult mental health systems do not routinely engage in joint planning at the systems-, program-, or client-levels. As a result, clients may be deluged with an array of apparently disconnected and uncoordinated services. For example, a mother who testified at the New York City hearing was brought to the hearing by her child's mental health intensive case manager. She told the task force that she was also a client in a DSS preventive services program, where she received parent training and individual counseling. The program had become concerned about her mental status and referred her to a psychiatrist at a mental health clinic. The psychiatrist put her on medication, and also recommended that she be in individual psychotherapy, which she received at the clinic.

Clearly, there is substantial duplication of services in the experience reported by this woman. The child's mental health intensive case manager in reality is the intensive case manager for the entire family, playing a major role in helping to organize the family's life. The preventive services program has a case management function, and the parent training program presumably also has a role in helping the woman to organize the activities of the family. In addition, she is receiving medication from a psychiatrist and individual counseling from both the preventive service program and the mental health clinic.

The task force noted that hundreds of situations of this kind exist and that the provision of duplicative services by multiple systems is counterproductive for clients and unnecessarily costly for the public. The need for better coordination with other human services systems was also cited, particularly the health care and education systems.

Task Force Recommendations and the New York State OMH-DSS Response

A complete listing of recommendations is presented in Table 10.1. Overall, the task force expressed commitment to the premise that although some marginal resources might be needed to implement proposed changes, substantial improvements could be made in the existing service systems without major new program development.

The task force report was well received by OMH and DSS. Both agencies reconfirmed their executive-level commitment to services integration and interorganizational reform by committing staff and resources to move the project into an implementation phase.

The task force identified three overall priority areas for action. The following section summarizes progress to date.

Priority 1: Link mental health and child welfare preventive services for mentally ill parents. OMH and DSS are currently developing a strategy for coordinated financing of "partnerships" between a social services district's preventive services agency and its county-run or contracted mental health outpatient agencies. Specific mental health outpatient programs will be linked with specific preventive service programs, becoming "satellites" of each other. Any services offered by either program can then be offered at either site, allowing clients to choose at which site to be served. Thus, a client reluctant to go to a mental health clinic could receive psychiatric services at the local preventive service program, while a client who prefers to attend a local mental health clinic

TABLE 10.1 Recommendations Offered by Task Force Members

Services
   Increase capacity for in-home services.
   Develop "family services" that do not divide adults from children.
   Increase capacity for off-hour services (not just crisis).
   Provide flexible respite services.
   Develop self-help and support groups.
   Increase supported housing for families.
   Educate parents and children regarding mental illness.
   Provide parental role models and companions.

Policies and procedures
   Revise all regulations, policies, and procedures to incorporate family concerns.
   Increase staff competencies for both DSS and OMH staff.
   Explore ways to share information while respecting client confidentiality.
   Target public day care slots for children of mentally ill parents.
   Explore statutory change regarding termination of parental rights.
   Replicate exemplary practices across the state.
   Require education for children of hospitalized adults.
   Educate providers and courts regarding open adoption.

Coordination
   Merge multiple funding streams, attaching money to families.
   Jointly fund housing and support programs.
   Develop a master strategy for "culture change."
   Co-locate DSS, OMH, and other relevant services.
   Facilitate "co-training" for administrative staff.
   Develop a joint mission statement that focuses on the strengths of parents.
   Improve information sharing at the client level.
   Prioritize DSS-OMH and OMH-DSS referrals.
   Develop financial incentives for completed referrals.
   Provide training for family courts.

NOTE: DSS = Department of Social Service; OMH = Office of Mental Health.

or rehabilitation program could have access to parent training or other child welfare preventive services at that site.

Formal linkages will encourage the delivery of necessary and appropriate services. For example, mental health clients often need access to nonmedical, nonreimbursable services (e.g., transportation, day care), which are readily available through preventive service programs. Similarly, protective services clients may need medication or specialized rehabilitation services best accessed through mental health programs. In addition, services that cannot currently be reimbursed, for example, a mental health clinician testifying in family court, could be reimbursed with preventive services funding. Clients served by both mental health and preventive services programs will receive a single case manager, determined according to the individual's primary problem and/or goals.

Services provided at any of the linked programs will be billed to either the mental health system or the preventive services system, depending on the eligibility of the client and the reimbursability of the services. Software packages to sort eligibility and determine maximal billing practices will be adapted for use in interagency program sites. Linking an open-ended, mandated funding stream (preventive services) to mental health services has the potential to expand access to mental health services at no cost to the counties, or to save counties money without a reduction in services. It is expected, at minimum, to reduce or eliminate duplicate case management and counseling efforts and costs. Moreover, improved support services are expected to lead to fewer foster care placements and fewer mental health emergency room visits.

Short-term, 24-hour respite care for children who are at risk of foster care placement due to family dysfunction or, in this case, due to parental hospitalization, is currently reimbursable on a per diem basis with preventive services funding. OMH is exploring the possibility of adding respite care to the list of allowable services in mental health outpatient programs, which would allow counties to bill Medicaid for this service (saving money for the state through increased federal participation, at no additional cost to the county). Respite care would be tied directly to a parental mental health crisis and to imminent risk of foster care placement for the child and would be limited in duration. Record keeping requirements, forms, and case management standards and planning will be examined and altered to facilitate coordination and eliminate duplication.

Priority 2: Develop a statewide information dissemination and peer support strategy. OMH and DSS have launched a major effort to raise awareness about the needs of mentally ill parents and their children among mental health and social service providers and the general public. To this end, the task force report has been widely distributed, articles have been written for several state and national publications, the issue has been placed on the agenda of several statewide and national conferences, and a focus on parents with mental illness has been added to a number of OMH and DSS planning documents.

OMH and DSS are also funding and jointly overseeing a statewide support program for parents with mental illness through the Mental Health Association in New York State. The Parents With Psychiatric Disabilities Support Project will stimulate the development of self-help and mutual support groups for parents with mental illness (and other family members), provide training for mental health and social services professionals, and provide ongoing information and referral.

Priority 3: Revise regulations, policies, and procedures to reflect greater sensitivity to the needs of parents with mental illness raising children. Both agencies have begun an ongoing process of re-examining regulations, policies and procedures, and training programs to ensure that the issues of parents with mental illness are addressed. Specific actions to be taken by OMH will include revising outpatient regulations to include parenting programs and day care in the sections on continuity of care, thus encouraging mental health adult outpatient providers to develop linkages with family support services. Parental status and related needs will be added to OMH's uniform inpatient and outpatient case records, to prompt clinicians to explore these issues. In addition, OMH is exploring the feasibility of expanding available day care options, establishing separate visitation rooms for parents receiving inpatient care at state facilities, and assessing the responsiveness of inpatient units in general hospitals to the needs of parents. To date, three psychiatric centers have created visiting rooms for children to visit their hospitalized parents.

OMH has also issued a policy to encourage the development of supported housing programs that will provide access to persons with mental illness and their minor children. Program designs must demonstrate the availability of necessary services for family members (especially children) through other funding sources. Several new housing projects following these guidelines have already been developed.

DSS has also started to review policies for intake, case eligibility for preventive services and foster care, case assessment, and planning to ensure sensitivity to the needs and capacities of parents with mental illness. Parent-child visitation and discharge planning practices, including family court practices, are being reviewed, as are criteria for visitation and for reuniting children with their afflicted parent. DSS also plans to issue a policy clarification on confidentiality requirements for child protective, preventive, and foster care cases.

IMPLICATIONS FOR MENTAL
HEALTH SERVICES DELIVERY

Parents diagnosed with serious mental illness pose a classic interorganizational challenge to mental health and social service administrators. Because the issue has largely been invisible to both systems, it is difficult to convince policymakers of its importance. In New York, neither OMH nor DSS would have chosen to make this a priority without strong and persistent advocacy efforts. Administrators and service providers who are interested in this issue should be prepared to encounter widespread indifference to their concerns.

Administrators and service providers should also be prepared to encounter discriminatory attitudes, particularly from the press, but also from some providers. At times during the task force process, it was implied or even stated that people diagnosed with severe mental illness should not marry or have children, because they are too fragile psychologically, carry a genetic predisposition toward mental illness, or are incapable of providing a stable family environment. Similarly, many people with psychiatric diagnoses were reluctant to publicly acknowledge their histories for fear that either they or their children would experience discrimination. Local self-help programs and providers who have gained the trust of their clients are key to organizing effective advocacy efforts.

Ongoing dialogue between all levels of the mental health and social services systems will be necessary to get a balanced view of the issues and for joint efforts to succeed. Facilitating such a dialogue is a challenge. Most of the providers who testified at the public hearings were children's mental health providers. Few child protective services workers and few adult mental health providers chose to testify, despite efforts to encourage their participation. Discussion revealed that while children's providers almost inevitably have contact with the child's parents, the reverse is seldom true. Moreover, child protective services workers often feel that they are seen as unnecessarily cautious and heavy-handed in child protective actions. Building trust and communication between the two systems will therefore be critical for any service provider or administrator interested in developing a more effective interagency response to this set of issues.

The statewide task force process in New York State was instrumental in identifying needed changes in policy, financing, and organizational structures. The issues raised were consistent with previously identified barriers to shifting children's mental health services to a family-centered system of care, including a focus on the individual as the unit of service; a focus on only a portion of the range of necessary services; a lack of attention to informal support networks; and the neglect of resources and expertise of family members.[11]

Addressing these issues will involve county government, agency heads, clinicians, clients, and advocates. In New York State, working groups are being convened to develop and implement needed changes at the program- and client-levels. This process will undoubtedly be difficult, particularly in areas where existing services are scarce or where relationships between local mental health and social services agencies are already strained. Simultaneously, state-level program managers are addressing finance, policy, and regulatory issues. It is hoped this multi-level process will forge a stronger link between structural changes and changes in services delivery than have often occurred in past services integration efforts.[12]

Two major administrative issues remain to be addressed. First is the need to develop a new form of "transorganizational management," which emphasizes the development and operation of interdependent systems and operates through joint decision making, goal-directed planning, and the mutual action of disparate parties.[12] Few mental health or social services administrators are trained in this kind of management, nor do incentives generally exist to encourage cooperative planning and management.

A second need is to develop a rigorous evaluation of services integration efforts. Past recommendations by services researchers have included the creation of new approaches to assess the effectiveness of comprehensive sets of services, approaches which bring attention to complex program processes and components, and link program and family characteristics with outcomes.[11] The success of a services integration approach to this set of problems will ultimately depend on the capacity to demonstrate improved outcomes for parents diagnosed with severe mental illness and their children, including reduced number and

length of out-of-home placements, reduced need for mental health interventions for the children involved, improved parenting skills, and
increased satisfaction on the part of both parents and children. It will
also be necessary to carefully evaluate the cost-effectiveness of an integrated approach to services delivery. Although the New York State task
force was successful in identifying impediments to effective services
delivery for this population, fiscal and management concerns will finally determine the implementation of new services delivery strategies.

REFERENCES

1. Nicholson J, Geller JL, Fisher WH, et al.: State policies and programs that address the needs of mentally ill mothers in the public sector. *Hospital and Community Psychiatry* 1993; 44:484-489.

2. Test MA, Berlin SB: Issues of special concern to chronically mentally ill women. *Professional Psychology* 1981; 12:136-145.

3. Bachrach LL, Nadelson CC (Eds.): *Treating Chronically Mentally Ill Women*. Washington, DC: American Psychiatric Press, 1988.

4. White C, Nicholson J, Fisher WH, et al.: *Describing Chronically Mentally Ill Mothers: A Comparison of Demographic, Clinical Characteristics and Service Use Patterns of DMH Case Managed Women With and Without Dependent Children*. Paper presented at the annual meeting of the American Public Health Association, Washington, DC, November 1992.

5. Apfel RJ, Handel MH: *Madness and Loss of Motherhood: Sexuality, Reproduction, and Long-Term Mental Illness*. Washington, DC: American Psychiatric Press, 1993.

6. Knitzer J, Yelton S: Collaborations between child welfare and mental health. *Public Welfare* 1990; 48:24-33.

7. Anthony WA, Cohen M, Farkas MD: *Psychiatric Rehabilitation*. Boston: Center for Psychiatric Rehabilitation, 1990.

8. Grunbaum L, Gammeltoft M: Young children of schizophrenic mothers: Difficulties of intervention. *American Journal of Orthopsychiatry* 1993; 63:16-27.

9. Woy RJ, Dellario DJ: Issues in the linkage and integration of treatment and rehabilitation services for chronically mentally ill persons. *Administration in Mental Health* 1985; 3:155-165.

10. Agranoff R, Lindsay VA: Intergovernmental management: Perspectives from human services problem solving at the local level. *Public Administration Review* 1983; 43:227-237.

11. Friesen BJ, Koroloff NM: Family-centered services: Implications for mental health administration and research. *Journal of Mental Health Administration* 1990;17:13-25.

12. Agranoff R: Human services integration: Past and present challenges in public administration. *Public Administration Review* 1991; 6:533-542.

11

Trauma, Addiction, and Recovery

Addressing Public Health
Epidemics Among Women
With Severe Mental Illness

Mary Jane Alexander, Ph.D.
Kristina Muenzenmaier, M.D.

The conceptual models we use to organize experience and action powerfully affect assessment, treatment, and hope for individuals who use public mental health services. This chapter is focused on how those who work in and use public mental health systems can affect the epidemics of violence against women and children and the trauma-related addiction that frequently results. These closely related problems, addiction and childhood sexual abuse, seriously complicate how effectively women and those who treat them can access and use clinical and community supports. It is imperative that public mental health systems recognize the effects of childhood trauma and develop systemic and clinical responses that address the day-to-day risks faced by many women with severe mental illness.

NOTE: This work was supported (in part) by the Center for the Study of Issues in Public Mental Health, NIMH grant P50MH51359. The opinions expressed in this chapter are those of the authors and do not necessarily reflect the views of the Center.

215

First and foremost, professionals must bring their awareness of victimization and substance use into the public mental health system by making a consistent effort to identify and acknowledge these experiences that daily affect women's mental health. Next, there are treatment approaches for the long-term effects of victimization that have begun to meet with success, but these have typically excluded women with severe psychiatric disabilities. Successful approaches must be adapted for women with severe mental illness, and they must be made available in a context of advocacy and empowerment for the individuals who need these services. Safe housing and access to job opportunities are important components of the support needed by women with severe psychiatric disabilities as they recover from addiction and heal from their experiences of trauma and abuse. Prevention models must be incorporated into psychiatric treatment services to address health risks such as exposure to HIV infection that are elevated among women with severe mental illness and addiction. Finally, but not least important, serious attention must be given, within the context of public mental health services, to creating constructive solutions for ending the violence against women and children.

RISKS TO WOMEN IN A COMMUNITY-BASED SYSTEM OF CARE

There is a growing awareness of the impact on women and children of the public health epidemics of addiction and violence. Women are twice as likely as men to contract AIDS through drug-related behavior: Two thirds of HIV+ women inject drugs themselves or have a sex partner who does.[1] Twelve million American women now alive will be abused in their lifetimes;[2] between 14 and 25 percent of American women have been, by stringent, legal definition, raped;[3] and in community-based samples, from 20 to 30 percent of American women report that they were sexually victimized as children.[4] The ways that victimization has been ascertained, the stigma attached to it, and the difficulty of legally establishing rape make it likely that these figures underestimate violence, rape, and childhood abuse.

Although the United States has moved since the early 1970s toward a community-based system of psychiatric services, there is little empirical data about the daily stresses and risks faced by women with severe mental illness in their communities. Chances are high that they live in poor neighborhoods, participate in alcohol or drug subcultures, are socially isolated and lonely, and have poor judgment skills that place them in and make them more vulnerable to the consequences of dangerous, compromising, or exploitative situations.[5,6] They are surely affected by the public health epidemics of our times.

ABUSE AMONG WOMEN WITH SEVERE MENTAL ILLNESS: PREVALENCE AND EFFECTS

On the basis of direct interviews about their experiences of abuse, women in psychiatric settings are at even higher risk for childhood physical and sexual abuse than women in community samples. Studies in which participants are directly asked about physical and sexual abuse experiences yield rates of sexual abuse ranging from 20 to 54 percent among mentally ill women in inpatient psychiatric settings,[7-13] and from 22 to 50 percent in outpatient psychiatric settings.[14-18] As many as 81 percent of psychiatric inpatients[12] and 68 percent of psychiatric outpatients[16] report having experienced *either* physical or sexual abuse at some time during their lives.

Trauma history among women with severe mental illness is associated with higher rates of psychiatric symptomatology, including depressive, and psychotic or seemingly psychotic symptoms,[10,17,19,20] suicidal symptoms and repeated attempts at suicide,[10,21] severe and persistent psychotic disorders,[9] borderline personality disorders,[10,22] and panic disorder.[23] Women who have severe mental illness who are homeless and with histories of abuse report higher levels of depressive and psychotic symptoms than their counterparts without histories of abuse.[24] Higher rates of substance abuse are found among women with trauma histories than among those without, in psychiatric emergency rooms,[20] acute psychiatric admission units,[19] and admission units in state psychiatric hospitals that serve patients with more refractory psychiatric problems.[13,25] Women with trauma histories also have higher rates of medical problems than women without, especially dysuria, vaginal discharge, chronic abdominal pain, gastrointestinal distress, and recurrent headaches.[26]

Alcohol and drug problems that co-occur with severe mental illness are associated with high rates of rehospitalization;[27,28] residential instability and homelessness;[29,30] exposure prior to age 17 to sexual abuse and familial violence, including physical abuse;[31] and repeated adult victimization.[32] Comparable rates of co-occurring alcohol or drug problems and severe mental illness have been found among men and women,[33-35] and in some studies, rates of drug abuse or dependence as high as 75 percent have been found among women with severe mental illness.[36,37]

Many of the symptoms and behaviors associated with childhood abuse, such as suicidality, lack of impulse control, and substance use, place women at further risk for physical and sexual exploitation and violence as adults. Among both patient and community samples, women with sexual abuse histories are more likely than those without to be victimized as adults.[32,38] If they use drugs, they may be engaging in "survival sex," in which a woman barters sex for necessities such as a place to stay or food, frequently with a man she knows but who is not her partner. Women engaging in survival sex often get high to have sex or have sex to get high, and they are frequently victims of assault.[39,40] Women who engage in this type of sexual activity also have frequent unprotected sex with multiple partners; are more likely to have had recent and unprotected sex with a man who is HIV+, who injects drugs, or who also has male sex partners; and are more likely to have had forced sex with a partner.[40] Although people with severe psychiatric disabilities are generally less sexually active than the general population, studies of men and women with severe mental illness in a variety of treatment settings show that about half were sexually active in the prior six months; about half of those who were sexually active engaged in sex with multiple partners during that time, and up to a quarter of those who were sexually active traded sex for money or goods.[41-43]

Increasingly, the model of post-traumatic stress disorder (PTSD) has been applied to link the experience of "extraordinary events" that involve "actual or threatened serious injury or death, or a threat to the physical integrity of the self or others, and are experienced with fear, helplessness or horror" to a cluster of symptoms of present distress. PTSD symptoms include intrusion (the person reexperiences the event through intrusive thoughts, flashbacks, nightmares, and physiological reactivity to reminders), hyperarousal (hypervigilance, exaggerated startle response, irritability, difficulty in concentrating or sleeping), and constriction (emotional numbing—inability to feel close to others, to experience positive emotions, or to enjoy pleasurable activities). Symptoms must be present for a month or more and cause significant distress or impairment for PTSD to be diagnosed.[44] Typically, combat, accidents or natural disasters, and rape have been considered the etiologic traumas for PTSD.

A further development of the trauma model, the concept of complex PTSD allows a client and clinician to "connect the dots" between long-term exposure to trauma, such as childhood physical or sexual abuse or neglect, and present dissociative or psychotic symptoms, suicidality, self-mutilation, substance use, or other maladaptive behaviors to form a coherent picture of the severe impact of long-term abuse on personality and identity. Herman proposes that these long-term effects include problems in regulating emotion, and changes in consciousness, self-perception, interpersonal relationships, perceptions of the perpetrator, and finally, in systems of meaning.[45] Equally important, the trauma model recognizes that the client's recovery of autonomy, safety, and self-determination are essential to healing.

Women are more vulnerable to PTSD, particularly to PTSD of long duration, than men. Among a random sample of young enrollees in an urban health maintenance organization (HMO), women, although they were less likely to have been exposed to traumatic events than men, were more likely to develop a PTSD diagnosis following exposure.[46] Furthermore, women were more than four times as likely as men to develop PTSD symptoms that lasted for more than one year.[47]

Substance use, which occurs frequently among both men and women with PTSD,[15,45,48] may serve as a way to cope with the anxiety and depression of PTSD. The heightened risk of victimization among women using alcohol and drugs suggests that something akin to a treacherous positive feedback loop operates between addiction and PTSD. Women who experience the stress of psychotic symptoms, alcohol or drug problems, or tenuous housing can experience prolonged flash-backs that can be mistaken for hallucinations, and their crises may be labeled as psychotic episodes. Similarly, dissociation may be easily misidentified as psychosis. Individuals with trauma histories and psychotic diagnoses might have complex PTSD. Alternatively, a dissociative disorder might co-occur with complex PTSD. Treatment mistakes can follow from a failure to take into account the constellation of problems experienced by women seeking psychiatric services. These include inappropriate prescription of antipsychotic medications, which may compound the problems of dissociation, and treatment being ineffective because it is not focused on the trauma to the woman remaining caught in the intrusion, constriction, and hypervigilance of complex PTSD. As treatments are developed further for people with severe mental illness and trauma histories, researchers will need to explore why these relationships exist and to distinguish among these aspects of complex PTSD.[49] Even at this early point in the development of treatments, failure to ask about trauma or to incorporate into assessment and treatment the trauma model that facilitates effective organization of symptoms and problems is a major barrier to some women's hope for recovery.

Typically, however, neither trauma nor alcohol and drug problems, key risk factors that complicate psychiatric disability and recovery, are identified and addressed in treatment in the mental health sector.[17,50] Clinicians are rarely trained in how and when to ask about sexual abuse and substance use, particularly among women, nor are they trained in how to listen to the answers, and frequently they are lacking in methods of incorporating this information into effective treatment. Therefore, sexual abuse and substance use are still rarely assessed routinely at admission, despite their high rates of occurrence and co-occurrence, and the serious complications they add to severe mental illness especially when not identified.

This is beginning to change. Several states require that questions about physical and sexual abuse histories be asked at intake; the Veterans Administration is beginning an initiative to improve the identification of PTSD and trauma history among its primary care physicians. We would hope that as providers become more aware of the prevalence and consequences of early and recurring trauma, they will ask these questions, and listen to the answers, with more frequency and care.

ASSESSMENT OF SEXUAL ABUSE

The most basic aspect of assessing trauma or addiction involves asking clear, detailed questions about childhood and adult experiences that have not been asked in the past, identifying symptoms that might be related to trauma, and connecting them to the trauma. However, neither researchers nor clinicians should expect a person to label herself as "a substance abuser" or "an alcoholic," or her experiences as "abusive." Acknowledging these problems and experiences is painful, and may be taboo in some cultures. Therefore, the interview should not begin with a question that is phrased in general terms such as: "Were you ever sexually abused?" This type of question requires the respondent to quickly review her memories and decide whether to label herself as a victim of sexual abuse, and it places a significant burden on both her memory and decision processes. Meyer, Muenzenmaier, Cancienne, et al.[51] have developed and psychometrically validated an instrument to assess trauma history for individuals with severe mental illness in an outpatient setting.

All of these questions should be asked with the clear message and understanding that the client may choose not to answer them. Interviewers should be sensitive not only to the client's answers, but to her discomfort, reluctance, or clear refusal to answer. The interviewer should communicate that this issue can be addressed at another time. The very fact that the questions have been asked indicates an openness to discuss the client's experiences of abuse or trauma.

Because trauma survivors frequently experience their contacts with psychiatric services as revictimizing, there has been some movement toward changing policies with respect to restraint and seclusion when a person becomes agitated or out of control. It is important to establish with the patient the conditions that give her some control over these procedures so she can provide for her own safety during this encounter with the mental health system. These include questions like: "When you are agitated, what helps calm you down?" "Do you want a female rather than a male attendant with you?" "Is a quiet room helpful?" "What ways of being given medication are OK?" "If you need to be restrained, is it OK to be face down or face up?"[52]

The timing of specific questions about abuse depends on the interviewer's judgment and the client's readiness to respond. When a client is self-mutilating, is acutely suicidal, or is decompensating, due to flashbacks or a dissociative experience, questions about experiences of abuse might be useful in helping her to connect the symptoms to circumstances. This might be particularly useful to a person who is already participating in a treatment program where she is doing trauma work. If the interviewer thinks a person is too fragile at admission, or the client herself considers the questions too intrusive, questions about abuse should be asked at another time. Here it is important to give control over her experiences, both past and present, back to the client. Timing requires even more judgment in an inpatient setting, but the questions should be asked once the patient is stabilized, and this opportunity should be used to engage women who might not otherwise use mental health services and to prepare them for the discussions that will take place in a psychoeducational group.

The critical point about assessment is that clinicians be trained about the role of trauma in the lives of women with severe mental illness. They need to become comfortable in asking about trauma, and, as important, in listening to the answers empathically. Failure to do so may compound the impact of the disbelief and devaluation that frequently surround early attempts to tell someone about the abuse.

IDENTIFYING ALCOHOL AND SUBSTANCE USE PROBLEMS

Alcohol and drug problems are also not generally well identified in mental health agencies, since providers tend to identify and treat the conditions within their specialty areas.[53] In a study of an admission cohort in a state psychiatric facility, none of the women with current or past alcohol or drug problems had received treatment for them, compared with 77 percent of the men.[31] It is crucial, then, that providers come to know about the serious effects of substance use and violence toward women with severe and persistent mental illness, and develop and disseminate adequate treatment approaches that address them. Until they do, women will continue to depend on high-intensity/high-cost services like long-term and acute inpatient services and emergency rooms to temporarily resolve continuing crises of depression, suicidality, addiction, revictimization, and personality disorders that co-occur with trauma histories.[52]

Women's need for alcohol or drug treatment is frequently extreme before it is recognized. Because providers tend to treat what they know, women who seek services in mental health and general health settings are likely to receive services for mental health problems or physical complaints, and they are generally not asked about alcohol or drug use.[53] In fact, women receiving treatment in mental health clinics and emergency rooms have more severe symptoms due to drinking than men in those settings.[54]

As with questions about trauma, identity-based questions about alcoholism are not very useful. Asked, "Are you an alcoholic?" a woman is likely to say no. Questions should also be relevant for a person who is disabled by a severe psychiatric illness, for instance, "Do you often wake up with such a hangover that you can't get to your job training program?" "Do you sometimes forget or skip taking your medication because you were drinking?" rather than questions about drinking while driving.[55,56] In the same vein, researchers should work with women with severe mental illness and the clinicians who treat them to discover gender-specific indicators of alcohol or drug problems. This would broaden the basis for identification and highlight those indicators in wide use that presently fail to identify women who have a drinking or drug problem.

It is not necessary to establish a *Diagnostic and Statistical Manual of Mental Disorders*—fourth edition (*DSM-IV*) substance-related disorder diagnosis to determine whether a person with severe mental illness has alcohol or drug use problems that should be treated. Brief and direct questions about recent, regular use of alcohol or substances have been found to be as useful as a structured diagnostic interview in targeting substance use problems among individuals using state psychiatric hospitals.[57] Despite their shortcomings in under-identifying women's drug and alcohol problems, use of readily available screens such as the DAST, CAGE, and MAST[55] can help to establish that alcohol or drug use may be relevant in addressing a woman's problems and that the clinician is open to further discussion of these issues as a relationship of trust is established.

TREATMENT APPROACHES FOR
TRAUMA SURVIVORS WITH SEVERE
MENTAL ILLNESS: GENERAL GUIDELINES

Despite the growing awareness of the high rates of early sexual trauma for women with severe mental illness, these findings are not well integrated into their clinical assessments, and services that address their trauma are not yet well developed or readily available. Only 10 to 20 percent of severely mentally ill women whose abuse histories were identified in inpatient or outpatient psychiatric settings reported that these traumas were adequately addressed in treatment[13,17] even when trauma assessment was clinically mandated.[58] In fact, gender-specific treatment for individuals with severe mental illness is just beginning to emerge as providers try to meet the complex service needs of women with severe mental illness who are also homeless and have trauma histories.[2,50,59] Gender-specific services, and a feminist orientation to treatment, have evolved over the past decade in agencies that treat addiction,[60-63] but these initiatives do not address the specific clinical issues that must be incorporated into services for people with severe psychiatric disabilities.

While individual psychotherapy provides the basis for trauma work, the shared experience of a group allows participants to overcome the isolation, shame, guilt, secrecy, and stigma of childhood sexual abuse.[64-68] A range of time-limited groups addressing victimization and abuse experiences has been shown to be effective in alleviating trauma-related distress among women who are not severely mentally ill.

Stress inoculation, assertiveness training, or supportive psychotherapy, combined with information groups, improved self-concept and diminished fear, anxiety, and symptom scores on the SCL-90 of participating adult rape survivors, compared with those on a waiting list.[69] Delayed treatment for rape trauma has been found to be as effective as immediate treatment.[70] Among women with early trauma histories who participated in a randomized trial of a cognitive behavioral skills training group, parasuicidal behavior and anger decreased, and self-rated adjustment improved after six months compared with a standard treatment control group. After one year of treatment, interviewer-rated adjustment also improved and use of inpatient days decreased for the skills training group.[71]

However, because of their fragility and cognitive limitations, women who have histories of psychosis, who are acutely suicidal, who currently use substances, or who have been diagnosed as having borderline personality disorder are generally excluded from trauma groups.[72] Research also suggests that women with complex sequelae to early sexual abuse may not benefit from traditional group work.

In a study of an interpersonal group intervention for trauma survivors without severe mental illness, high dissociation and high emotional lability were associated with nonresolution of PTSD symptoms. Furthermore, overall group outcomes were poorer where a group member had these characteristics and a diagnosis of borderline personality disorder.[73] In process groups of both high and low intensity for fairly high functioning survivors of father incest, women with initially higher levels of distress and depression and less education had poorer outcomes.[74] In a one-year, closed-membership process-oriented group for trauma survivors, women with prior psychiatric hospitalization were more likely to drop out of the group and were less likely to experience improvement in their psychiatric symptoms, trauma-related symptoms, self-esteem, sexual problems, or locus of control than those who had never been hospitalized.[75]

The high rates of trauma histories among women with psychiatric, addiction, and social problems make it imperative that we adapt group models for trauma that work for women with complex and severe psychiatric disabilities. Groups can be made more accessible and safe for women who are severely dysfunctional by altering the cognitive level of the content, the intensity of the approaches, and the structure of the group.[72] For instance, a woman's need to leave or to skip a session(s) because she feels overwhelmed or flooded by the group experience can be reframed as a choice. This legitimizes her need, makes the group more available to women who are easily overwhelmed, and fosters the woman's autonomy and control of the treatment process.

THE PSYCHOEDUCATIONAL GROUP MODEL FOR ABUSE SURVIVORS

There are few well-specified protocols, and virtually no outcomes data, available to help clinicians incorporate individuals with major psychiatric disability due to psychotic disorders like schizophrenia, rapidly cycling bipolar disorder, co-occurring substance abuse, severe borderline personality disorder, or suicidal symptoms into a trauma group. Some approaches for these underserved populations are being developed.[59,76] The psychoeducational group model for abuse survivors, which we describe in the next section, is an adaptation of workshop models for family education,[77] a fairly complicated model that was developed for relatively high-functioning patients. The psychoeducational group model has been in practice in an outpatient state psychiatric facility in cycles of 12 one-hour sessions.

In general, this model adapts the key principles of trauma recovery, empowerment, and reconnection with others[45] to people with co-occurring trauma histories and severe psychiatric disabilities. Having been victimized and isolated, a survivor must regain power over her own life and body, and she must reestablish viable connections with others. In the psychoeducational treatment model, the focus is on resilience and her ability to survive, rather than on her deficiencies. Knowledge and skills provide the means to develop independence. Other survivors and group leaders are partners in this work, so each group member experiences some relief to see that she is not alone. Because the group provides participants with opportunities to break down the isolating barrier of shame and to rebuild social trust, it is a powerful tool for each participant to reestablish autonomy and control over her own life.

Stage-oriented treatment—where the treatment focus matches the client's readiness—is central to doing group work with women whose psychiatric disabilities are complicated by addiction problems and/or trauma histories. In this psychoeducational model, the group facilitators act as allies in establishing safety and empowering each participant to establish her locus of control within herself. Generally, groups should be highly structured and limited to a short cycle (about 10 to 12 sessions), with participants free to repeat the cycle as often as they choose. Like current approaches to addiction treatment that build in the expectation of relapse and address relapse prevention as part of treatment, this model incorporates the understanding that recovery from trauma is a nonlinear process that requires a consistent focus on personal and environmental safety. As with addiction recovery, this process has a long timeframe, and there should be an understanding that clients will return to past coping strategies like self-harm, addiction, rage outbursts, depression, and dangerous behavior that exposes them to revictimization.

Staff and survivors who facilitate groups for trauma survivors should have a personal style and theoretical orientation that allow them to interact empathically and in partnership with clients. Prescriptive approaches that target problems or pathology for treatment tend to be too narrow and nonempowering for trauma survivors. Staff should be comfortable in sharing knowledge with group participants and in teaching them skills that foster their independence. In terms of a knowledge base and experience, staff who facilitate these groups should understand PTSD and the ways in which trauma complicates treatment for women who have severe psychiatric disabilities. They need to be able to deal with psychotic symptoms that may be triggered in the group.

A public health perspective can help staff to effectively recognize and address the wide range of contextual factors that trauma survivors bring to a clinical setting: How can a woman commit to consistent participation in a trauma group if she is actively abusing alcohol or drugs? Does a woman have physical symptoms that affect her ability to participate in a group or to incorporate new coping skills into her life? Does she have access to a physician? Is she homeless? Does she participate in survival sex to obtain shelter? Does she live in an unsafe shelter situation? To what extent do the norms of her culture stigmatize or rationalize her abuse experiences? Does her social network or culture support the assertiveness and independence that this treatment framework develops?

Just as trauma survivors should not work in isolation, neither should staff who work with them. It is key that the group have two facilitators, one of whom can (and probably should) be an abuse survivor. The co-leaders should receive support from each other as they monitor their own and group members' actions and reactions. While it is preferable to have same-gender leaders for a group, we have found that an empathic and nonhierarchical personal style is more important, especially in public mental health agencies where staff resources may be scarce. Equally important to the group's ability to establish a sense of safety and trust are the co-leaders' reliability and commitment to the group in terms of their own timeliness and attendance. Staff also need support in supervision to deal with countertransference, especially boundary issues. Each group facilitator must feel safe and must handle her or his own rescue fantasies, issues of control, or feelings of being overwhelmed by the trauma or participation in revictimizing the client by minimizing the trauma or by blaming her.

Group participants must also be in regularly scheduled individual therapy sessions so they can receive support as they process some of the issues that arise in the group. Co-leadership of the trauma group allows closer monitoring of participants' reactions to content material. Co-leaders can increase the sense of support by reinforcing participants' increased understanding, reframing, or coping. Leaders also provide a source of feedback for one another and support during and across sessions.[78]

For each individual, the goals of this educational approach are to establish some awareness and control over symptoms and experience, and to understand the connection between the trauma and the flash-backs she experiences in the present. This occurs as the woman becomes aware of her symptoms and the objects, events, and experiences that trigger them. She learns that some of her symptoms were coping strategies that permitted her to survive her traumatic experience. Concretely, group members are encouraged and helped to develop and learn to use their own resource lists of people on whom they can rely. In these ways, participants focus on developing cognitive skills for safety and coping, rather than on processing their individual abuse experiences.

In fact, members are discouraged from disclosing the details of their abuse experiences at this stage, since disclosure could trigger flash-backs, or dissociative reactions among the group. Sometimes participants' or group leaders' current needs may move the group into a supportive psychotherapy mode, perhaps by bringing in process issues related to the prior week. It is important to monitor the group process and ensure that a psychoeducational model is maintained. Disclosure about issues related to the trauma is acceptable, such as processes related to disclosure to family members, or circumstances, stimuli, and reactions around the event. Work directly related to the trauma event(s) generally occurs in parallel individual therapy, or frequently, much later on. Safety remains basic in these first groups for women with severe mental illness, and this may well be a stage they return to frequently. Group members learn from each other—those who are coping well at one point may later need the support of other women as they find their needs for safety growing again.

As women participate in this basic psychoeducational group, they may participate in other groups that offer training in skills like relaxation and assertiveness. Groups using nonverbal modalities such as visual art and body movement, which allow participants to experience their bodies, may can be offered and repeated, depending on the participants' preferences and readiness. Each skill that a woman gains to help her eventually deal with the trauma also increases her ability to participate in the more structured initial pychoeducational process. For instance, the ability to stay grounded also enhances her control over her memory and dissociation. However, it is essential that a woman have the coping skills necessary to ensure her safety before she begins to work through the dissociated trauma and to acknowledge her memories. Some women with severe mental illness may not be able to establish enough safety skills to be able to work on processing their memories of their trauma experiences. Still others will revisit the very early stages of recovery from trauma and will need to rely on other women in these groups to help them reestablish safety.

Table 11.1 outlines the curriculum for each session of the psychoeducational group model for abuse survivors. Safety is the main focus of the 12-week group and is incorporated into all of its aspects. At the first meeting, basic information about the group and ground rules for the group are discussed. Ground rules are important to establishing safety, and they are repeated in every session. They include confidentiality regarding what goes on within the group, the right of any participant not to talk, and each participant's responsibility for letting the group leaders know if she becomes upset. After ground rules are reviewed, each session includes a "check-in" about participants' reactions to the last session, and their safety since then. Each session also ends with a check-in about this session.

After the first check-in, there is a short presentation of educational material, followed by a discussion that includes the content itself as well as symptoms or triggers that surfaced. Material is presented in a way that clarifies the concepts and promotes discussion. Group members build a sense of mutual concern and support as they share their thoughts and experiences of the material. Over the 12-week curriculum,

TABLE 11.1 Content of Curriculum

Session 1	Basic information about the group
Session 2	Staying safe in group
Session 3	Staying safe in other environments
Session 4	What are abuse and neglect?
Session 5	Disclosure
Session 6	Reactions of society to disclosure
Session 7	Reactions of family to disclosure
Session 8	Physical and emotional effects of abuse
Session 9	Coping as a child and as an adult
Session 10	New coping skills
Session 11	Avoiding revictimization
Session 12	Wrap up and debriefing

common myths about the rare occurrence of abuse and the culpability of survivors in being abused are debunked. The group hears about and discusses family and cultural values that support the secrecy of abuse; the effects of secrecy and disclosure on the survivor and her family; the physical scars, shame, and guilt that accompany abuse and secrecy; coping skills that no longer work and those that never worked; new coping skills that will help participants to control the content and rate of their remembering, such as identifying cues that trigger memories, relaxation techniques, and use of anti-anxiety medications; and avoiding revictimization by developing and learning to use support and resource lists of helpful and nonhelpful individuals. In the wrap-up session, participants discuss their experience of the group and its utility, and any feelings or reactions that might not have been adequately addressed during the prior 11 weeks.

After the material is presented and discussed, there is a safety check where the group leaders restate rules about safety and make sure everyone can handle the content and discussion of the session. Each session has its own wrap-up where cards containing a statement about the focus of the session are handed out and read out loud. Statements could be: "You deserve to feel and be safe" or "It's OK to say NO" or "Sexual abuse is common." The group consistently provides an emphasis on strengths and on participants' ability to survive their traumas.

The time required to cover a topic may vary depending on the composition of the group, the functional level, and reactions of the group members. So while group sessions should be highly structured, they must also be flexible. For instance, sessions might be of shorter duration to allow for shorter concentration and ability to sit in the session; some participants might be allowed to arrive late, or leave and return later as their reaction to the material warrants. These accommodations support the woman to stay in the group and reinforce her growing sense of autonomy and safety by asking her to take some control over the process and her experience.

Women who had been diagnosed as having schizophrenia, major affective disorder, PTSD, or borderline personality disorder have participated in a group that was conducted along these lines. Independent of diagnosis, they reported that they appreciated the support offered by the group, found it helpful, and appreciated the opportunity to be with other women who had experienced abuse. All wanted to continue. Some stressed that they had not been asked about abuse histories before and that the group enabled them to connect their different experiences of symptoms to the abuse. One woman with a serious alcohol problem felt that no one, including herself, had understood her alcohol use before.

IMPLICATIONS FOR MENTAL HEALTH SERVICES DELIVERY

Integrated, comprehensive approaches have evolved over the past decade in the mental health sector to provide support and treatment for co-occurring mental illness and alcohol or drug use problems. These incorporate assertive outreach, comprehensive services, flexibility, case management, and stagewise treatment that accounts for client motivation to participate in abstinence-oriented interventions and group substance abuse interventions, especially for clients lacking in motivation.[79,80] As these innovative models are disseminated into the treatment culture, gender-specific findings about sexuality, relationship, victimization, depression and empowerment, and assessment of co-occurring problems will be necessary if services are to effectively address gender-specific treatment needs.

Program components cited as important for women in the addiction, psychiatric, and trauma literature include adequate and early identification of associated problems and a treatment philosophy based on competency building and empowerment in safe, accessible, community-based treatment.[2,59-63,79-83] For women with these three tightly interconnected problems, services should be multidisciplinary, comprehensive, and coordinated to address the broad range of their needs as they progress toward and remain in recovery.

Women and those who provide treatment must recognize that recovery is a lifelong and nonlinear process. Trauma survivors are at high risk to engage in unsafe behavior, such as substance abuse, risky sex, and self-harm. In particular, trauma survivors need to understand what abuse is in their adult lives, and how it affects their psychiatric symptoms, their addictive behavior, and their living circumstances. Placed in a trauma context, their substance use can be framed as a way of self-soothing that has become self-harmful. They are likely to be revictimized because of the risks they take while high or to get high, and because the addiction subculture is dangerous and exploitative. Personal elements of relapse prevention that are important for women with substance use problems and victimization histories include learning to identify and develop resources to deal with stress, learning to structure leisure time to maintain abstinence, and using individual and group work to address issues of destructive relationships that compromise recovery. Systemically, they must have access to safe and supportive residential space.[59] They must be encouraged to develop strategies that use available resources like restraining orders and hot lines[60] to diminish or resolve their risk for violence from a partner.

The psychoeducational model for abuse survivors outlined in this chapter, and other programs described in this volume,[59,76] begin to demonstrate how the knowledge base regarding recovery from trauma can be adapted so women with severe psychiatric disabilities may gain skills that allow them to establish control over their memories and trauma-related symptoms. Essential to each of these programs is a long-term commitment to support and empower abuse survivors in their individual recoveries and in their roles as advocates for effective services.

The denial that surrounds abuse, the lack of control that accompanies addiction, and the stigma and disability associated with severe mental illness foster among survivors an extraordinary sense of unreality, powerlessness, and isolation. Their needs for validation, autonomy, and connection are as extraordinary. The psychoeducational approach to treatment described in this chapter aims to empower individuals in their own recoveries: Women actively control their own treatment; the reality of abuse experiences is acknowledged; symptoms are framed and explained as coping strategies for survival in extraordinary circumstances. Survivors report that this type of empowerment to actively participate in their own recovery is vital.[84]

Self-help models based on shared decision making and peer support extend the concept of recovery beyond addiction problems to psychiatric diagnoses. Some rely totally on indigenous leadership. Others incorporate the presence of a professional, or rely intermittently on professional leadership because the acuity of participants' mental health problems in some inpatient settings affects the stability of indigenous leadership.[85] These groups, such as Double Trouble, supported by the Mental Health Empowerment Project, provide participants with strong common bonds and have led to positive outcomes.[86]

Services operated by consumer-survivors also play a major role in the larger process of social change. The self-confidence of group leaders increases, and these empowered individuals then serve as role models for group participants with similar disabilities. Consumer-survivors who are employed in paraprofessional and professional capacities in mental health agencies also serve as role models and diminish stigma by their presence in the workplace. The active and significant presence of consumer-survivors in policy-making groups is necessary to ensure that the consumer-survivor perspective is incorporated in the service system. In New York State, the Mental Health Empowerment Project has established that advocacy is part of the recovery process in mental health consumer self-help movement. In Maine, significant grassroots efforts have been made to incorporate and include the consumer-survivor voice in the development of that state's trauma services.

An exclusive focus on limited outpatient visits to accomplish poorly conceived short-term goals is likely in the long run to increase the dependence of these women on intensive inpatient and crisis services and to impair their ability to function in their daily lives. As states restructure public systems of care, demonstrated effectiveness and efficiency of trauma-focused interventions will be critical for their continued development and support.

Women with severe mental illness, substance use, and victimization histories need physical health care, a recognition of their adult sexuality, preventive education regarding pregnancy and sexually transmitted diseases, and help in dealing with role loss, including their roles as parents. In New York State in 1991, 16 percent of children in foster care (or more than 10,000 children) and 21 percent of children receiving preventive services (another 8,600 children) had at least one parent with severe mental illness.[87] Women with custody of their children need special supports to prevent intergenerational victimization, or extreme overprotectiveness because of the parent's magnified concerns about safety. Noncustodial parents also need skills to cope adequately with the complexities of their relationships with their children and with their children's caretakers in and outside of the foster care system.

Health or mental health agencies participate in revictimizing abuse survivors when they fail to recognize that survivors' symptoms may be related to prior victimization and fail to provide treatment options for them. Standard routines ostensibly designed for safety can also retraumatize abuse survivors. Inpatient settings need to consider alternatives to locked wards, four-point restraints that place a person in a spread-eagle position, restraint and/or being stripped by male attendants, reflexive use of medications in response to what might be flashbacks, and a general lack of physical safety. Psychiatric emergency services should also incorporate sensitive procedures regarding use of restraints, removal of clothing, and isolation that rape crisis programs in medical emergency rooms have had in place for several decades.[7]

As public and private insurers continue to pay close attention to efficacy of treatment—that is, both cost and benefit—clinicians and researchers must pay closer attention to what does and does not work, for whom, and why, particularly among individuals whose psychiatric disabilities are severe. The public mental health systems that primarily serve this group must continue to accommodate both biological and environmental models of psychiatric disability. As survivors' confidence in recovery grows, clinicians and researchers must also take seriously the task of untying the knot of severe psychiatric disability and addiction. We can begin if we acknowledge and address the experiences of trauma survivors.

REFERENCES

1. Rouse BA (Ed.): *Substance Abuse and Mental Health Statistics Sourcebook*. DHHS Pub. No. (SMA) 95-3064. Washington, DC: Superintendent of Documents, U.S. Government Printing Office, 1995.

2. American College of Obstetricians and Gynecologists: *Domestic Violence*. Technical Bulletin 209. Washington, DC: American College of Obstetricians and Gynecologists, 1995.

3. Koss MP: Rape: Scope, impact, interventions and public policy responses. *American Psychologist* 1993; 48:1062-1069.

4. Finkelhor D, Hotaling GT, Lewis IA, et al.: Sexual abuse in a national survey of adult men and women: Prevalence characteristics and risk factors. *Child Abuse & Neglect* 1990; 14:19-20.

5. Test MA, Berlin SB: Issues of special concern to chronically mentally ill women. *Professional Psychology* 1981; 12:136-145.

6. Harris M: Treating sexual-abuse trauma with dually diagnosed women. *Community Mental Health Journal* 1996; 32:371-385.

7. Carmen E, Reiker P, Mills T: Victims of violence and psychiatric illness. *American Journal of Psychiatry* 1984; 141:378-383.

8. Cole C: Routine comprehensive inquiry for abuse: A justifiable clinical assessment procedure. *Clinical Social Work Journal* 1988; 16:33-42.

9. Beck JC, van der Kolk BA: Reports of childhood incest and current behavior of chronically hospitalized psychotic women. *American Journal of Psychiatry* 1987; 144:1474-1476.

10. Bryer JB, Nelson BA, Miller JB, et al.: Childhood sexual and physical abuse as factors in adult psychiatric illness. *American Journal of Psychiatry* 1987; 144:1426-1430.

11. Jacobson A, Herald C: The relevance of childhood sexual abuse to adult psychiatric inpatient care. *Hospital and Community Psychiatry* 1990; 41:154-158.

12. Jacobson A, Richardson B: Assault experiences of 100 psychiatric inpatients: Evidence of the need for routine inquiry. *American Journal of Psychiatry* 1987; 144:908-913.

13. Craine LS, Henson CE, Colliver JA, et al.: Prevalence of a history of sexual abuse among female psychiatric patients in a state hospital system. *Hospital and Community Psychiatry* 1988; 39:300-304.

14. Rosenfeld A: Incidence of a history of incest among 18 female psychiatric patients. *American Journal of Psychiatry* 1979; 136:791-795.

15. Herman JL: Histories of violence in an outpatient population. *American Journal of Orthopsychiatry* 1986; 65:137-141.

16. Jacobson A: Physical and sexual assault histories among psychiatric outpatients. *American Journal of Psychiatry* 1989; 146:755-758.

17. Muenzenmaier K, Meyer I, Struening E, et al.: Childhood abuse and neglect among women outpatients with chronic mental illness. *Hospital and Community Psychiatry* 1993; 44:666-670.

18. Rose SM, Peabody CG, Stratigeas B: Undetected abuse among intensive case management clients. *Hospital and Community Psychiatry* 1991; 42:499-503.

19. Brown GR, Anderson B: Psychiatric comorbidity in adult inpatients with childhood histories of childhood sexual abuse. *American Journal of Psychiatry* 1991; 148:55-61.

20. Briere J, Zaidi LY: Sexual abuse histories and sequelae in female psychiatric emergency room patients. *American Journal of Psychiatry* 1989; 146:490-495.
21. Linehan MM, Armstrong HE, Suarez A, et al.: Cognitive-behavioral treatment of chronically parasuicidal borderline patients. *Archives of General Psychiatry* 1991; 48:1060-1064.
22. Wagner AW, Linehan MM: Relationship between childhood sexual abuse and topography of parasuicide among women with borderline personality disorder. *Journal of Personality Disorders* 1994; 8:1-9.
23. Stein MB, Walker JR, Anderson G, et al.: Childhood physical and sexual abuse in patients with anxiety disorders and in a community sample. *American Journal of Psychiatry* 1996; 153:275-277.
24. D'Ercole A, Struening E: Victimization among homeless women: Implications for service delivery. *Journal of Community Psychology* 1990; 18:141-152.
25. Alexander MJ, Craig TJ, MacDonald J, et al.: Dual diagnosis in a state psychiatric facility: Risk factors, correlates and phenomenology of use. *American Journal on Addictions* 1994; 3:314-324.
26. Friedman MJ, Schnurr PP: The relationship between trauma, post-traumatic stress disorder, and physical health. In: Friedman MJ, Charney DS, Deutch AY (Eds.): *Neurobiological and Clinical Consequences of Stress: From Normal Adaptation to PTSD.* Philadelphia: Lippincott-Raven, 1995, pp. 507-523.
27. Drake RE, Wallach MA: Substance abuse among the chronic mentally ill. *Hospital and Community Psychiatry* 1989; 40:1041-1045.
28. Osher FC, Drake RE, Noordsy DL, et al.: Correlates and outcomes of alcohol use disorder among rural outpatients with schizophrenia. *Journal of Clinical Psychiatry* 1994; 55:109-113.
29. Center for Mental Health Services: *Making a Difference: Interim Status Report of the McKinney Research Demonstration Program for Homeless Mentally Ill Adults.* Rockville, MD: Substance Abuse and Mental Health Services Administration, U.S. Department of Health and Human Services, 1994.
30. Belcher JR: On becoming homeless: A study of chronically mentally ill persons. *Journal of Community Psychology* 1989; 17:173-185.
31. Alexander MJ, Haugland G: *Substance Use and Trauma History in an Inpatient Admission Cohort: The Need for Services.* Poster session presented at the ninth annual NYS Office of Mental Health Research Conference, Albany, NY, December 4, 1996.
32. Russell DEH: *The Secret Trauma: Incest in the Lives of Girls and Women.* New York: Basic Books, 1986.
33. Dixon L, Haas G, Weiden PJ, et al.: Drug abuse in schizophrenic patients: Clinical correlates and reasons for use. *American Journal of Psychiatry* 1991; 148:224-230.
34. Toner BB, Gillies LA, Prendergast P, et al.: Substance use disorders in a sample of Canadian patients with chronic mental illness. *Hospital and Community Psychiatry* 1992; 43:251-254.
35. Pristach C, Smith CM: Medication compliance and substance abuse among schizophrenic patients. *Hospital and Community Psychiatry* 1990; 41:1345-1348.
36. Caton CLM, Gralnick A, Bender S, et al.: Young chronic patients and substance abuse. *Hospital and Community Psychiatry* 1989; 40:1037-1040.
37. Ananth J, Vanderwater S, Kamal M, et al.: Missed diagnosis of substance abuse in psychiatric patients. *Hospital and Community Psychiatry* 1989; 40:297-299.
38. Briere J, Runtz M: Post-sexual abuse trauma. *Journal of Interpersonal Violence* 1988; 2:367-379.

39. Goodman LA, Dutton MA, Harris M: Episodically homeless women with severe mental illness: Prevalence of physical and sexual assault. *American Journal of Orthopsychiatry* 1995; 65:468-478.

40. Simoni JM, El-Bassel N, Schilling RF, et al.: *The Perils of Survival Sex for Women on Methadone.* Paper presented at the Conference on Psychosocial and Behavioral Factors in Women's Health, Washington, DC, September 20, 1996.

41. Cournos F, Empfield M, Horwath E, et al.: HIV seroprevalence among patients admitted to two psychiatric hospitals. *American Journal of Psychiatry* 1991; 148:1225-1230.

42. Cournos F, Guido JR, Coomaraswamy S, et al.: Sexual activity and risk of HIV infection among patients with schizophrenia. *American Journal of Psychiatry* 1994; 151:228-232.

43. Kelly JA, Murphy DA, Bahr R, et al.: AIDS/HIV risk behavior among the chronic mentally ill. *American Journal of Psychiatry* 1992; 149:886-889.

44. American Psychiatric Association: *Diagnostic and Statistical Manual of Mental Disorders* (4th ed.). Washington, DC: American Psychiatric Association, 1994.

45. Herman JL: *Trauma and Recovery: The Aftermath of Violence—From Domestic Abuse to Political Terror.* New York: Basic Books, 1992.

46. Breslau N, Davis GC, Andreski P, et al.: Traumatic events and post-traumatic stress disorder in an urban population of young adults. *Archives of General Psychiatry* 1991; 48:216-222.

47. Breslau N, Davis GC: Post-traumatic stress disorder in an urban population of young adults: Risk factors for chronicity. *American Journal of Psychiatry* 1992; 149:671-675.

48. Helzer JE, Robins LN, McEvoy L: Post-traumatic stress disorder in the general population: Findings of the Epidemiologic Catchment Area Survey. *New England Journal of Medicine* 1987; 317:1630-1634.

49. Rosenberg SD, Drake RE, Mueser K: New directions for treatment research on sequelae of sexual abuse in persons with severe mental illness. *Community Mental Health Journal* 1996; 32:387-400.

50. Alexander MJ: Women with co-occurring addictive and mental disorders: An emerging profile of vulnerability. *American Journal of Orthopsychiatry* 1996; 66:61-70.

51. Meyer IH, Muenzenmaier K, Cancienne J, et al.: Reliability and validity of a measure of sexual and physical abuse histories among women with serious mental illness. *Journal of Child Abuse and Neglect* 1996; 20:213-219.

52. Carmen E, Crane B, Dunnicliff M, et al.: *Report and Recommendations of the Massachusetts Department of Mental Health Task Force on the Restraint and Seclusion of Persons Who Have Been Physically or Sexually Abused.* Massachusetts Department of Mental Health Task Force on the Restraint and Seclusion of Persons Who Have Been Physically or Sexually Abused, January 25, 1996.

53. Wilsnack S, Wilsnack R: Epidemiology of women's drinking. *Journal of Substance Abuse* 1991; 3:133-157.

54. Weisner C, Schmidt L: Gender disparities in treatment for alcohol problems. *Journal of the American Medical Association* 1992; 268:1872-1876.

55. Lehman AF: Heterogeneity of person and place: Assessing co-occurring addictive and mental disorders. *American Journal of Orthopsychiatry* 1996; 66:32-41.

56. Drake RE, Alterman AI, Rosenberg SR: Detection of substance use disorders in severely mentally ill patients. *Community Mental Health Journal* 1993; 29:175-192.

57. Eilenberg J, Fullilove MT, Goldman RG, et al.: Quality and use of trauma histories obtained from psychiatric outpatients through mandated inquiry. *Psychiatric Services* 1996; 47:165-169.

58. Dixon L, Dibietz L, Myers P, et al.: Comparison of DSM-III-R diagnoses and a brief interview for substance use among state hospital patients. *Hospital and Community Psychiatry* 1993; 44:748-752.
59. Harris M: Modifications in services delivery and clinical treatment for women diagnosed with severe mental illness who are also the survivors of sexual abuse trauma. In: Levin BL, Blanch AK, Jennings A (Eds.): *Women's Mental Health Services: A Public Health Perspective.* Newbury Park, CA: Sage, 1998, pp. 309-325..
60. Hagan TA, Finnegan LP, Nelson-Zlupko L: Impediments to comprehensive treatment models for substance dependent women: Treatment and research questions. *Journal of Psychoactive Drugs* 1994; 26:163-171.
61. Wilke D: Women and alcoholism: How male-as-norm bias affects research, assessment and treatment. *Health and Social Work* 1994; 19:29-35.
62. Finkelstein N: Treatment programming for alcohol and drug-dependent pregnant women. *International Journal of the Addictions* 1993; 28:1275-1309.
63. Reed BG: Developing women-sensitive drug dependence treatment services: Why so difficult? *Journal of Psychoactive Drugs* 1987; 19:151-164.
64. Mennen FE, Meadow D: A process to recovery: In support of long-term groups for sexual abuse survivors. *International Journal of Group Psychotherapy* 1992; 42:29-44.
65. Brandt LM: A short-term group therapy model for treatment of adult female survivors of childhood incest. *Group* 1989; 13:74-82.
66. Herman J, Schatzow E: Time-limited group therapy for women with a history of incest. *International Journal of Group Psychotherapy* 1984; 34:605-616.
67. Courtois CA: *Healing the Incest Wound: Adult Survivors in Therapy.* New York: Norton, 1988.
68. van der Kolk B: *Psychological Trauma.* Washington, DC: American Psychiatric Press, 1987.
69. Resick PA, Jordan CG, Girelli SA, et al.: A comparative outcome study of behavioral group therapy for sexual assault victims. *Behavior Therapy* 1988; 19:385-401.
70. Frank E, Anderson B, Stewart BD, et al.: Efficacy of cognitive behavior therapy and systematic desensitization in the treatment of rape trauma. *Behavior Therapy* 1988; 19:403-420.
71. Linehan MM, Heard HL, Armstrong HE: Naturalistic followup of a behavioral treatment for chronically parasuicidal borderline patients. *Archives of General Psychiatry* 1993; 50:971-974.
72. Stone WN: *Group Psychotherapy for People With Chronic Mental Illness.* New York: Guilford, 1996.
73. Cloitre M: *Reduction of Revictimization in Female Child Abuse Survivors—Assessment and Treatment.* Paper presented at the Conference on Psychosocial and Behavioral Factors in Women's Health, Washington, DC, September 20, 1996.
74. Alexander PC, Neimeyer RA, Follette VM, et al.: A comparison of group treatments of women sexually abused as children. *Journal of Consulting and Clinical Psychology* 1989; 57:479-483.
75. Hazzard A, Rogers JH, Angert L: Factors affecting group therapy outcome for adult sexual abuse survivors. *Journal of Group Psychotherapy* 1993; 43(4):453-468.
76. Bills LJ, Bloom SL: From chaos to sanctuary: Trauma-based treatment for women in a state hospital system. In: Levin BL, Blanch AK, Jennings A (Eds.): *Women's Mental Health Services: A Public Health Perspective.* Newbury Park, CA: Sage, 1998, pp. 348-367.

77. Courtois CA: *Workshop Models for Family Life Education: Adult Survivors of Childhood Sexual Abuse.* Milwaukee, WI: Families International, 1993.
78. Sampson DF: Personal communication, June 24, 1996.
79. Osher FC, Drake RE: Reversing a history of unmet needs: Approaches to care for persons with co-occurring addictive and mental disorders. *American Journal of Orthopsychiatry* 1996; 66:4-11.
80. Drake RE, Mueser KT, Clark RE, et al.: The course, treatment, and outcome of substance disorder in persons with severe mental illness. *American Journal of Orthopsychiatry* 1996; 66:42-51.
81. Abbott AA: A feminist approach to substance abuse treatment and service delivery. *Social Work in Health Care* 1994; 19:67-83.
82. Burman S: The disease concept of alcoholism: Its impact on women's treatment. *Journal of Substance Abuse Treatment* 1994; 11:121-126.
83. Center for Substance Abuse Treatment: *Practical Approaches in the Treatment of Women Who Abuse Alcohol and Other Drugs.* Rockville, MD: Substance Abuse and Mental Health Services Administration, 1994.
84. Huckeba H: Testimony. In: J Chassman (Ed.): *Proceedings From a Forum on Individuals Diagnosed With Serious Mental Illness Who Are Sexual Abuse Survivors.* Albany: New York State Office of Mental Health Community Support Programs, June 1995, pp. 12-17.
85. Caldwell S, White KK: Co-creating a self help recovery movement. *Journal of Psychosocial Rehabilitation* 1991; 15:92-95.
86. Markowitz FE, DeMasi ME, Carpinello SE, et al.: *The Role of Self-Help in the Recovery Process.* Paper presented at the sixth annual National Conference on State Mental Health Agency Services Research and Program Evaluation, Arlington, VA, February 1996.
87. Blanch AK, Nicholson J, Purcell J: Patients with severe mental illness and their children: The need for human services integration. In: Levin BL, Blanch AK, Jennings A (Eds.): *Women's Mental Health Services: A Public Health Perspective.* Thousand Oaks, CA: Sage, 1998, pp. 201-214.

12

Impact of the Law on Women With Diagnoses of Borderline Personality Disorder Related to Childhood Sexual Abuse

Susan Stefan, J.D.

This chapter examines the impact of the law on a substantial group of women whose attempts to survive and cope with childhood sexual abuse result in certain behaviors, attitudes, and reactions that are diagnosed as *borderline personality disorder*.[1]

The impact of the law on women diagnosed with borderline personality disorder is pervasive and almost wholly negative. These women are constructed as disabled by the law when it is to their disadvantage to be considered disabled. At the same time, the law erases their disability when it would provide them with some material benefit or protection. This is true across many areas of law, from family law to disability benefits law to mental health law. For these women, the law is itself disabling, a source of disability. It is not, except in rare instances, a source of remedy or empowerment.

NOTE: This chapter is dedicated to Laura Prescott and J. W. for their courage and honesty. I acknowledge the research assistance of Kristina Beard, Beth Wolt, and Adam Stein, and the advice and suggestions of Joel Dvoskin, Laura Ziegler, Laura Prescott, and Professors Mary Coombs, Martha Mahoney, and Wes Daniels.

The diagnosis of borderline personality disorder was first adopted by the American Psychiatric Association in 1980. About 76 percent of people diagnosed with borderline personality disorder are women.[2, a] Considerable research supports the proposition that "sexual abuse is common and etiologically significant in borderline personality disorder."[3-7] This connection has also been noted in case law.[8-10] The diagnosis is especially indicative of early childhood sexual abuse in women who cut themselves, attempt suicide, and/or engage in substance abuse.[3,6,11,12]

Girls who are sexually molested by their relatives often grow up into angry, untrusting women who engage in struggles for power and control over their lives with figures of authority such as doctors, social workers, and case managers.[13] Although these women can also be desperately needy, they receive little sympathy from health care professionals, especially mental health professionals, who characterize them as "enraging,"[14] "mistresses of manipulation,"[15] "hard to manage,"[15,16] and "incit[ing] 'counter-transference,' hatred and rejection."[7] Unlike other diagnoses related to rape or sexual abuse, for example post-traumatic stress disorder (PTSD), the diagnosis of borderline personality disorder carries significant negative connotations and has even been characterized as "an epithet" or "name-calling" by some mental health professionals.[7,17]

The diagnosis describes not only individual behaviors but also interaction between people—the need for reassurance, the struggles for power, the "splitting" or "manipulation" all take place in an interpersonal context. The most negative interactions often occur between the person described as having borderline personality disorder and the people she perceives as having power and control over her. This includes those who called her someone with "borderline personality disorder" in the first place.

In this way, behaviors that reflect women's struggle to reassert their own worth and control over their lives, such as angrily challenging figures of authority, or behaviors that may permit them to survive and overcome tremendous odds, such as cutting themselves,[b] become defined as *dysfunctional*. In fact, the very identity of these behaviors as the struggle of a sexually abused child to redefine her place in the world is transformed into a set of pathological symptoms.

At the same time, many women diagnosed with borderline personality disorder do not conform to professional, legal, and popular images of mental illness. For the most part, they are not psychotic,[7] and they do not hallucinate or have delusions. When in the community, many do exceptionally well in school and in jobs,[18] including owning their own businesses.[19] Yet they are frequently seen at emergency rooms, often institutionalized,[2,20] regularly prescribed antipsychotic drugs, and spend a substantial amount of time in seclusion and restraints.

Being diagnosed with any mental disorder, and with borderline personality disorder in particular, may also lead to legal consequences that operate to rob women who were sexually abused as children of what they most need: their credibility, when they need to speak and be believed; their children, when they need to establish nonabusive connections with the next generation; power over their bodies and lives, when they need to establish autonomy and control; and most of all, the identity of their actions and interactions as part of an ongoing struggle to endure their pain and manage their lives.

Case law shows that women who are diagnosed with borderline personality disorder and/or exhibit patterns of conduct associated with early childhood sexual abuse are likely to be considered mentally disabled and, on the basis of this disability, are subject to (1) involuntary institutionalization; (2) involuntary antipsychotic medication; (3) loss of child custody and termination of parental rights; and (4) being discredited as witnesses in litigation generally, and particularly in litigation charging rape or sexual abuse. This is in substantial contrast to legal treatment of women diagnosed with PTSD, another diagnosis often associated with sexual abuse.

Women with diagnoses of borderline personality disorder are generally not, however, considered sufficiently mentally disabled to (1) receive disability benefits; (2) be qualified for special education benefits; (3) mitigate criminal charges against them; or (4) toll the statute of limitations in civil actions, such as actions to recover damages from their abusers. Ironically, women with diagnoses of borderline personality disorder are also likely to be seen as too disabled to prevail in civil rights litigation charging discrimination on the basis of disability. Again, women with diagnoses of PTSD are more likely to be considered disabled in these circumstances and receive benefits the law grants on the basis of disability.

Therefore, this pattern is not simply about the legal detriment many women suffer when they are known to have a diagnosis of mental illness, nor is it about the social and legal aversion to any woman who behaves aggressively. Rather, it describes a conjunction of the mental health and legal systems in which the aversion to women (especially powerless women) behaving in extreme, angry, and entitled ways is expressed as a pejorative diagnosis. The diagnosis is in turn used by the legal system to support rulings that could not be legally justified absent the aura of expertise and scientific neutrality associated with diagnoses.

For example, a mother's parental rights could not be terminated simply because she was hostile, uncooperative, and acted like a "know-it-all" with social workers.[21] However, many states have laws that permit termination of parental rights because of mental illness, and when hostility, lack of cooperation, and "know-it-all-ness" are cited as symptoms of borderline personality disorder, they can be used to support termination of parental rights.[21]

Judges also reach many of these adverse results simply by applying statutory standards faithfully across different areas of law. Some areas of law, such as family law, apply to all citizens whether they are disabled or not. Other areas of law, such as disability benefits law, by definition apply only to people with disabilities. When women who behave in the ways associated with borderline personality disorder are placed in legal categories populated by people presumed under law to be well and whole, such as "witnesses" or "mothers," they fare poorly because their unstable or "crazy" behavior is highlighted. On the other hand, when they are placed in categories dominated by presumptively mentally ill people, such as people claiming disability benefits on psychiatric grounds, they also fare poorly, because their functional and "normal" behavior is highlighted.

These results reflect the inability of the law to understand and conceptualize the dominant reality of these women's lives: dramatic cycles of accomplishment and agency alternating with vulnerability and crisis. The law assumes that individuals have a stable identity: We are either consistently functional and mentally healthy, or else we are perpetually disabled and dependent.[c] The truth is that most of us fit somewhere along a spectrum between severe mental disability and serene mental health. The range between competence and craziness is particularly exaggerated in the lives of women struggling to overcome the effects of childhood sexual abuse, who skid up and down the spectrum of normality like jazz riffs, graduating with highest honors from college while slashing their arms bloody,[18,22] holding down responsible jobs between suicide attempts and numerous psychiatric hospitalizations.[20,23,24, d]

These women are both oppressed and achieving: victims who refuse to be passive; powerless women who are nevertheless intensely demanding and angry; women whose behavior is extremely disturbing yet who are not psychotic. They fit neither the legal image of mentally ill people nor that of mentally healthy people. They fall into a wide legal abyss between these two categories. Because this is done one case at a time, the overwhelming impact of the law on the lives of thousands of women is lost. This chapter is an attempt to present the picture as a whole and to suggest corrections both specific and systemic.

The next section will summarize the wide range of ways in which perceptions of mental disability may affect a person's legal status and outcomes of litigation. The chapter will then examine in depth how a diagnosis of borderline personality disorder may affect legal outcomes in five areas of law: the law of evidence, family law, disability benefits law, the law relating to civil commitment and rights in institutional settings, and antidiscrimination law.

BACKGROUND: THE LAW AND MENTAL DISABILITY

Benefits Conferred by Law Based on Disability

The law's perspective on mental disability is ambivalent and contradictory. The law provides some benefits on the basis of mental disability. In certain instances, it excuses criminal acts;[25,26] provides special education with individualized plans including therapy and treatment;[27] tolls the statute of limitations to allow legal action to be brought after the statute would have expired;[28-30] provides housing or housing subsidies;[31] provides economic subsidies in the form of disability benefits such as Veteran's benefits, Social Security Disability Insurance (SSDI), and Supplemental Security Income (SSI);[32] provides medical benefits in the form of Medicaid;[33] protects people diagnosed as mentally disabled from abuse;[e] and prohibits discrimination against them.[34-36] The law also provides, in theory, that material a woman divulges to her therapist, or her medical or psychiatric records, will be kept confidential.[37] These benefits, however, do not for the most part inure to women diagnosed with borderline personality disorder, either because the law does not regard them as sufficiently disabled (as in the case of special education, mitigation of criminal charges or sentences, housing subsidies, and disability benefits) or because it regards them as too disabled (as in discrimination law).

Penalties Imposed by Law for Disability

The law is also hostile in many ways to mental disability. Mental disability is, in and of itself, a legally sufficient reason for courts and juries to doubt credibility.[38-41] This can be a crushing blow to the person's autonomy; doubts about credibility often result in family, police, employers, and courts dismissing and disbelieving claims of sexual abuse and harassment. The law has always reflected popular suspicions of fabrication in the area of mental disability,[42] and it is most suspicious of fabrication when the disability is connected to a reported history of sexual abuse.[43]

A diagnosis or history of mental illness is sufficient in some states to remove children from the custody of their mother;[44-50] in other states, while not presumptive, it weighs heavily in judicial considerations of parental competence.[44,51] Persons with diagnoses of mental illness make up the vast majority of people hospitalized against their will;[f] only persons with mental illness can be forced to submit to intrusion on their body in the form of electric shock treatments, psychosurgery, and psychotropic medication. In these legally disadvantageous circumstances, women with diagnoses of borderline personality disorder are commonly considered to be severely mentally disabled. Their diagnosis makes them suspect witnesses and parents, and they are frequently subjected to involuntary institutionalization and medication against their will.

LEGAL TREATMENT OF WOMEN WITH DIAGNOSES OF BORDERLINE PERSONALITY DISORDER

Witnesses and the Issue of Credibility

One of the most painful aspects of childhood sexual abuse is that children are frequently told they will not be believed if they report the abuse, and indeed, they are frequently disbelieved. As adults, women with diagnoses of borderline personality disorder are disbelieved as witnesses in a courtroom because the diagnosis itself is specifically equated with a propensity to lie and distort the truth.

Both federal and state rules of evidence generally permit the introduction of evidence as to a person's "character for truthfulness."[52-55] Expert testimony, including psychiatric expert testimony, is admissible to establish an individual's character for truthfulness.[g] However, experts may not testify as to whether a witness was lying or telling the truth on any particular occasion. As noted above, merely being diagnosed with any mental illness is often sufficient to raise a question about credibility. In addition, some courts have admitted expert testimony that a witness's prior sexual abuse may make her prone to invent or fabricate charges of sexual abuse. In one case, an expert witness testified that "if she had been sexually abused as a child, she might see sexual abuse everywhere."[56]

Courts routinely permit a witness's testimony to be impeached (i.e., attacked) on the basis of a diagnosis of borderline personality disorder. Expert testimony equating a diagnosis of borderline personality disorder with a tendency to lie or distort reality is common in a variety of cases.[56-62]

Many of the cases in which the diagnosis of borderline personality disorder is used to discredit a witness are related to a woman's attempt to seek civil damages for being sexually abused or criminal punishment for the abuser. Defendants charged with rape attempt to discredit the complainant's credibility by claiming that borderline personality disorder causes women to fabricate charges of rape.[58-61]

Although rape defendants also try to discredit the testimony of women with diagnoses of PTSD, there is a crucial distinction between challenges to the testimony of women diagnosed with PTSD and those diagnosed with borderline personality disorder. In the case of women with PTSD, prior sexual abuse is said to trigger false charges of sexual abuse because the victim confuses reality with flashbacks.[63-65] Women with borderline personality disorder are alleged to deliberately make false accusations. Thus, the borderline personality diagnosis becomes a way of introducing testimony that the witness is lying—testimony that would otherwise probably be impermissible.

Similar difficulties arise when women seek justice against abusers in civil court, typically in litigation for damages. When a woman sued her father for abuse that took place in her childhood, the Texas Supreme Court ruled that she had filed too late, unless she could produce independent evidence that the abuse took place. In ruling, the court noted that the plaintiff had been diagnosed with borderline personality disorder and cited the testimony of experts that "people with this disorder are prone to distort the truth."[59]

Another court, holding that the mental health records of a woman who complained to a medical board that her psychiatrist had sex with her must be examined by the court, noted that her diagnosis of borderline personality disorder was "significant to the issue of whether any sexual misconduct occurred. . . . In view of the characteristics of the borderline patient, C.B.'s condition is more than peripherally involved in this case."[60]

In a typical case charging improper sexual relations by a psychiatrist with his patients, the psychiatrist argued that patients who were "borderline personalities" were "unable to distinguish between fact and fantasies."[61] The court did not challenge this characterization; rather, the psychiatrist lost because the court found he "presented little credible evidence that the four complaining witnesses were in fact 'borderline' personalities."[61]

In a case where a nurse sued her neurologist for improper sexual advances and won a substantial verdict, the judge vacated the jury's award of damages. The court found that the evidence against the defendant was "unreliable," in part because the plaintiff "had been suffering from borderline personality disorder for many years which was characterized by periodic hallucinations and delusions, difficulty with male relationships, and 'hate feelings' towards others."[23]

Although mental health professionals often tell pejorative anecdotes about their clients diagnosed with borderline personality disorder, and sometimes these anecdotes even get published,[66] no studies have been done substantiating any relationship between the diagnosis of border-line personality disorder and propensity to tell the truth.[h]

Under the law, courts are not permitted to admit expert testimony for which there is no scientific basis. The Supreme Court recently held that a judge must "ensure that any and all scientific testimony or evidence admitted is not only relevant but reliable."[67] In deciding whether to admit expert testimony, the judge must conclude that the subject of an expert's testimony constitutes "scientific . . . knowledge. The adjective 'scientific' implies a grounding in the methods and procedures of science. Similarly, the word 'knowledge' connotes more than subjective belief or unsupported speculation."[67] Expert testimony that presumes to link borderline personality disorder with a tendency to lie or fabricate evidence should be challenged by the attorneys representing clients with this diagnosis. The attorney must also educate the judge and jury (also through expert testimony) as to the better substantiated aversion of the mental health profession to women with the diagnosis of border-line personality disorder.[2,68,69] For example, in one study, nurses presented with identical fact patterns regarding hypothetical patients responded far more negatively when the patients were identified as being diagnosed with borderline personality disorder than when identical behavior was attributed to patients with schizophrenia.[69]

Expert witnesses are generally not allowed to testify as to whether a specific witness is lying or telling the truth, because this usurps the function of the fact-finder in the case.[70] Yet in many cases involving women with diagnoses of borderline personality disorder, mental health professionals' testimony essentially operates to undermine the credibility of the woman and redefine her reality. This is particularly true in family law cases.

Family Law

To a woman with a history of childhood sexual abuse, family relationships take on an intense importance. For some women, having a child is a way of breaking the cycle of abuse, starting over, and giving a child the love and safety that she never had. Yet the state frequently intervenes in the parental relationships of women with diagnoses of mental disability, especially those who are poor or have been institutionalized. The law permits state agencies to monitor the mother, order her to do a variety of things, and make recommendations to terminate her relationships with her children if she does not comply.

Judges, in their turn, frequently apply the legal standards—parental "unfitness" or the "best interest of the child"—in a way that assumes people with mental illness cannot be fit parents or equates the best interest of the child with not having a parent diagnosed with mental illness. Although any mental illness is suspect, women with borderline personality disorder are particularly vulnerable, because the testimony of treating professionals and caseworkers is often adverse and hostile as a result of mutual antagonism and power struggles. The negative testimony of treating professionals and caseworkers, often seen as neutral experts by the court, is extremely harmful to the mother and is frequently given more weight than her actual behavior toward her children.

Termination of Parental Rights

The Supreme Court has recognized that parents have a constitutional right to associate with and rear their children.[71] Therefore, the state must meet a difficult standard before it may terminate parental rights. The state must show abuse or serious neglect by the parent, and it must usually also show that substantial efforts were made to reunite the parent and child.

Although the statutory standards are supposed to focus solely on whether the parent has abused or neglected the child, many state statutes specifically permit termination of parental rights if the parent is unable to discharge parental responsibility because of mental illness.[48] Occasionally, a woman will argue that borderline personality disorder, or personality disorders in general, are not mental illnesses.[72] These arguments universally fail; as more than one court has noted, "Borderline personality disorder is a form of severe mental illness."[49,50,73] With very few exceptions,[74,75] reported termination cases involving women with diagnoses of borderline personality disorder are decided adversely to the mother.[20,45,48-50,76-84]

In fact, in one case, the mother's positive efforts, compliance with court orders, and determination to retain her parental rights were recharacterized as symptoms of her illness:

During the termination proceedings, Dr. Wunderman opined that the mother was "addicted" to the termination proceeding, and that she had completed the required parenting course, visited her children at the scheduled times, and appeared in court "as a means of escaping a feeling of tremendous emptiness, tremendous loneliness, tremendous nothingness that the borderline personality disorder does feel."[77]

In most cases, borderline personality disorder is not presumed to create such positive behavior. Rather, the cases often involve the presumption that the diagnosis itself is shorthand for unfitness to parent.[81]

In fact, the diagnosis obscures and erases the heroic struggles of women to keep their children against incredible odds. Court decisions recast these efforts as failures without identifying the strength of the woman undertaking them or the harrowing circumstances in which she lives. *In re J.P.*[73] is a classic example of such a case.

In re J.P. involved the children of Velma Hunt, a woman diagnosed with mental retardation and borderline personality disorder. Hunt probably had undiagnosed dissociative identity disorder.[i] She was illiterate and had kidney problems severe enough for her to receive disability benefits. While growing up, she had been physically and sexually abused by members of her family.[j] After she became an adult:

> the father of her son was abusive toward her, throwing her down the stairs when she was pregnant and giving her a black eye. He beat on her because she would not give him her money. Newsome was *also* [sic] abusive and drank alcohol.[73] (emphasis added)

One reason cited by the court for terminating her parental rights was that she had been ordered "not to reside with [the father of her son] because of his physical abuse of her, but she continued to reside with him for some time after the children were removed."[73] The court blames Hunt for this, even though she had in fact separated from Newsome, after which he "broke into respondent's apartment, battered her severely, and caused significant damage to her apartment."[73] After this, the court finds, "Respondent allowed [sic] Newsome to continue to reside with her, which was in violation of the lease. She was evicted soon after."[73] Despite the violent aftermath of her first separation, she separated from Newsome again and went to live with her sister. Her sister's husband subsequently beat her severely enough to "send her to the hospital."[73]

A second reason for terminating Hunt's parental rights was that "she refused to cooperate with Crosspoint,"[73] the community support agency providing her services. Elsewhere in the opinion, however, we find the department's child welfare specialist testifying that "personnel at Crosspoint told her they did not want to work with respondent."[73]

A third reason was that she refused the services of a representative payee for her Social Security disability payments, which the Social Security Administration had never required and which she did not believe that she needed. In addition, it was noted that she had given her children money, which state workers saw as an attempt to bribe them to behave, though Hunt said it was "because she loves them."[k]

Scattered throughout the opinion is the evidence of Hunt's accomplishments. She separated from her abusive boyfriend twice, in spite of his life-threatening violence when she left him. She found housing, began taking literacy classes,[l] missed only one visit with her children, learned how to use the bus, and completed parenting classes.[73] Throughout the entire opinion, there was no suggestion that she had ever been abusive to her children.

Nor was there any suggestion that she had ever been offered any treatment, therapy, or even understanding or sympathy for her history of childhood sexual and physical abuse. One of the state's experts, Dr. Traver, recommended that she be seen by a psychiatrist and receive "counseling for anger control and inappropriate social behavior."[73] She went to the psychiatrist, who testified that she "would not benefit from counseling but recommended a socialization program."[73] This was apparently not provided.

In the end, the court found that Velma Hunt had "made little progress over the approximately 2½ year period between the adjudication and the termination hearing,"[73] and it terminated her parental rights to her children.

Like Velma Hunt, many of the mothers diagnosed with borderline personality disorders are not accused of abusing or neglecting their children. Rather, their rights are terminated because of the diagnosis of borderline personality disorder, which is demonstrated by "symptoms" bearing little relationship to the ability to parent. For example, one court found that "moving residence to residence, job to job, relationship to relationship demonstrates her borderline personality disorder."[72] In that case, the more salient difficulty may have been the mother's "angry outbursts at caseworkers" and what the court characterized as "her projection of blame for her problems onto others."[72]

The mother's anger, which is rarely directed at her children but often at the caseworkers who wield such power over her life, is a recurring theme in these cases.[20,21,72,73,78,80,85,86] In one case, the court found as a fact that the mother had a "moderate to severe borderline personality disorder."[21] The accuracy of the diagnosis was "supported" by the "respondent's hostility, lack of cooperation, 'know-it-all' attitude, and her unwillingness to recognize the needs of her children."[21]

The court found that because of her borderline personality disorder, the mother was:

> not likely to benefit from counseling, is not likely to respond to treatment, be it counseling or psychiatric effort, [and] that such persons [with borderline personality disorder] are resistant to social services and are very unlikely to recognize or deal with their problems, and that the [mother] is in that category.[21]

In *In re J.P.*, Velma Hunt "threatened a representative of the Illinois Department of Child and Family Services with a knife," apparently when the representative arrived to take her children away.[73] This incident was used as an illustration of her "affective instability," which means her moods are not stable and "no one knows how she might react to situations."[73] There is no record that Ms. Hunt was violent or threatened violence against anyone except a man who beat her severely and the caseworker who took her children from her.

In case after case, the mother's conflicts with her social worker emerge as central to the loss of her children.[20,21,73,80] Here, the issues of power and control are particularly salient. Professor Martha Mahoney has suggested that if these women had access to a neutral mechanism to appeal actions and decisions of social workers in these cases, many fewer assaults of social workers might take place.

The negative testimony of experts regarding the diagnosis of borderline personality disorder is also crucial to the termination of parental rights in these decisions. Indeed, in many cases, the majority of the decision is devoted to the testimony about borderline personality disorder.

Only one termination of parental rights[75] case was discovered in the course of this research involving a sympathetic expert witness. Even in this case, the expert testified that the mother did not have a borderline personality disorder, and that if she did, it was not substantial. More important, he also testified that:

> even if appellant were a borderline personality . . . people with such personality traits are not uncommon and frequently are very successful. People in the "caring professions," such as nurses, frequently possess borderline personalities. The key . . . is the person's ability to function.[75]

Too often, however, the mother's ability to function is overshadowed by her diagnosis. For example, the Maine Supreme Court relied on a mother's diagnosis of borderline personality disorder, in conjunction with a single instance of violence directed against her boyfriend in the presence of her children, to affirm termination of parental rights.[78]

In other cases, the mother's ability to function is genuinely affected by the very legal processes associated with separation from her children.[20,87] In one case, the caseworker noted:

> First, it appears that much of the mother's inappropriate and angry outbursts have been due to her being separated from the minor . . . she has never been abusive to the minor . . . the mother copes very poorly under stress, and both the Court process as well as being separated from her child have put her under tremendous pressure and stress, and appear to have escalated her mental health problems.[20]

Because of this, the caseworker, who had previously recommended reunification, recommended that the child not be returned home "until these issues subside."[20] Since "these issues" were the separation from her child and the court proceedings, the social worker effectively created a catch-22, one that is quite common in these cases.

The only appellate case rejecting expert testimony recites circumstances equally applicable to most other cases:

> The trial court's decision to terminate the respondent's parental rights was based largely, if not exclusively, on the testimony of three psycholo-

gists retained by the Department of Social Services. . . . For example, Mr. Pape, after interviewing [the mother] and performing only two psychological tests . . . diagnosed her as having "borderline personality disorder." From such a diagnosis, Mr. Pape concluded "that there's a real possibility of neglect of physical and emotional needs in this case. . . . " The record contains merely the speculative opinions of the psychologists regarding what might happen in the future.[74]

In this case, as in most of the others, there was little evidence of actual neglect or abuse of the child. While the cases abound in generalizations about borderline personality disorders, descriptions of discord between the mother and the social worker, and the mother's failure to accept therapy or admit illness, many lack any detailed, factual examination of the context in which the mother's life takes place and her interactions with her children in that context—in other words, an appreciation of her struggle and the odds she faces, and an assessment of her strengths and her needs as she describes them.

What Martha Mahoney has written of battered women is even more true of women with histories of childhood sexual abuse in family law cases: These women "seldom come to court in ways that show them as one of many like themselves."[88] Thus, "the woman's responses seem unique and problematic because there is no context demonstrating the commonality of their experience."[88]

In the case of women with diagnoses of borderline personality disorder, their voices are not heard at all. Their experiences and stories come to us in the cases mediated through the perspective of the mental health professionals who interpret their behavior. The focus of the mental health professional is on deficits, not strengths, and his or her interpretation of a woman's behavior is located in generalizations about pathology rather than the individual context of her life. For example, one court quoted an expert's testimony that a mother had "moderate to severe borderline personality disorder which interferes with treatment because people similarly afflicted are unwilling to change."[82]

These kinds of generalizations in testimony are subject to the same kinds of legal challenge as expert testimony that people with borderline personality disorder are liars. There is simply no validated scientific research about the parenting ability of women with diagnoses of borderline personality disorder. It should therefore be excluded under the requirements of *Daubert v. Merrell-Dow*.[67]

In addition, prohibiting adverse actions based on unfounded stereotypes about disabilities is explicitly why Congress passed the Americans With Disabilities Act (ADA).[36] Title II of the ADA prohibits a state agency from making decisions on the basis of stereotypes about a disability and prohibits statutory enactments that categorize in discriminatory ways on the basis of disability.[36, m]

Title II of the ADA also requires that parents with disabilities be given an equal opportunity to benefit from any services offered by a state agency, such as reunification services. This obligation includes modifying those services to accommodate a parent's disability.[n] Some states that provide reunification services statutorily permit child welfare agencies to exclude parents with mental disabilities from receiving those services if, because of their mental disabilities, the parents would not benefit from the services.[89] In other states, the agency is excused from its statutory duty of diligent reunification efforts if the reason for termination is the parent's mental disability. These statutes appear to be directly contrary to the ADA's prohibition of discrimination on the basis of disability. Rather than following the mandate that disabilities must be accommodated, these statutes expressly exclude parents with mental disabilities—and only parents with mental disabilities—from reunification services on the basis of their disabilities. These statutes should be challenged under the ADA.

While state courts have generally found that the ADA applies in proceedings to terminate parental rights,[83,90-93] courts also tend to find that the agency has complied with the ADA's requirements after consideration that is cursory at best.[o] At least one court, however, has signaled a willingness to take the requirements of the ADA seriously:

> This statute presents novel and thorny challenges to the Department which hopefully will be seen as a fertile opportunity for new and creative approaches, so that physically and mentally challenged persons may participate and have a chance truly to benefit from state services like parenting assistance. It may well be, as Appellant argues, that the Department must do a great deal more in adjusting its programs to make them meaningfully accessible to the handicapped.[92]

The ADA's requirement of reasonable accommodation means that reunification services must be tailored to the mother's individual requirements rather than using the "boilerplate" reunification plans employed by many agencies. These plans enforce attendance at parenting classes; often require psychological counseling; and are applied to all parents suspected of abusing and/or neglecting their children, regardless of whether the parents have the means or opportunity to attend the classes or will benefit from the kind of counseling provided. Courts rarely inquire as to the appropriateness of the services to the mother's needs, yet failure to meet the requirements often spells death to parental rights.

Reasonable accommodations require looking to what the mother actually needs and tailoring the process of assisting her to her individual situation. Courts have the equitable power to order agencies to provide such specific services. For example, in *Arkansas D.H.S. v. Clark*, the Arkansas Supreme Court upheld a lower court order that the Arkansas Department of Human Services pay for Ms. Clark's Prozac and for bus tokens the family needed to go to counseling the agency ordered.[94]

Most important, however, both child welfare agencies and courts need to recognize that many women who have responded to sexual abuse in childhood with mistrust of authority and anger at coercion will react negatively to the imposition of a variety of demands and services on them, especially when those demands and services are boilerplate and inappropriate to their needs. A sense of the dynamics of many of these situations is conveyed by the court's language in one case:

> The appellant and anyone in her home in a potential parental role were ordered to cooperate 100 percent with the therapeutic services designated by DSS. . . . The appellant and anyone in her home having a potential parental role were ordered to participate 100 percent in a parenting class and cooperate 100 percent in any additional services recommended by DSS.[72]

In case after case, the court focuses primarily on a mother's failure to meet agency-imposed requirements rather than a mother's actual relationship with and behavior toward her children.[20, 73, 74, 84] While this is potentially harmful to all mothers, a mother diagnosed with borderline personality disorder is particularly likely to be hostile and skeptical toward these requirements, especially those that involve explicit or implicit acknowledgment of mental illness. Because the likelihood of resistance is higher, the likelihood of termination based on that resistance—rather than her unfitness as a parent—is correspondingly higher. The cases confirm that this is indeed the outcome in most parental termination proceedings involving mothers diagnosed with borderline personality disorder.

Child Custody

Child custody is different from termination of parental rights in that custody disputes usually take place between parents, or a parent and other relatives, whereas termination of parental rights directly involves the state and usually results in children being placed in the foster care system.

The legal standard used in determining child custody arrangements is "the best interest of the child."[95] This standard is subjective enough to permit judges to make determinations based on value judgments, assumptions, and stereotypes about what constitutes a child's best interest. Judges applying the "best interest" standard have awarded custody of children to fathers who killed their wives.[96] Recently, a Florida court awarded custody to a father who killed his first wife in preference to the child's mother who was a lesbian.[97] In another case, a court denied custody to a father in a wheelchair because he could not show love.[98] Thus, child custody cases provide ample opportunity for the manifestation of biases and stereotypes.

Stereotypes associated with mental illness are so overwhelming that even if there is no adverse evidence about the woman's parenting abilities whatsoever, a diagnosis of mental illness or history of past hospitalization often spells defeat for the mother. Although depression is sufficiently familiar that a woman may escape serious stigma, borderline personality disorder is not. Many court decisions assume that, by itself, such a diagnosis spells intolerable risk:

> In this case, the father's expert witness testified that the mother *had a borderline personality disorder which made her a risk as the custodial parent* and recommended that the father be awarded custody. The court disagreed with this assessment, however, apparently relying on the testimony of the court-appointed expert and the mother's expert, both of whom testified that the mother did not suffer from a borderline personality disorder. . . . In fact, the mother suffered from a single episode of depression, which was treated with medication.[99] (emphasis added)

These cases suggest that it is the diagnosis of mental illness that moves the court to deny custody to mothers, rather than the behavior that resulted in the diagnosis. This is because fathers who engage in more problematic behavior than the mothers, but remain undiagnosed, are often awarded custody. For example, in one case, the court upheld an award of custody to the father, noting, "There was evidence from which the court could have found that Wife had been diagnosed as having major depression and borderline personality disorder."[100] Evidence in the case also showed that the husband was violent toward his wife and was involved in drug dealing, while evidence about his wife was that she stayed in bed late, became easily agitated, and her ability to concentrate and carry on conversations was impaired.[100]

The tendency of mental health professionals to disparage their clients with diagnoses of borderline personality disorder is reflected in the testimony of treating professionals in child custody cases. In one such case, the mother's treating professional testified that she was "extremely manipulative" and "would lie, cheat, and steal."[62]

Changes in child custody are even more difficult to achieve under law, requiring the party seeking to alter the custodial arrangement to prove "a material change in circumstances."[101-103] Yet in several cases, courts changed custody from the mother to the father based in large part on diagnoses or behavior that took place before the original custody decree, and even before the divorce itself. For example, in one case, a court ordered that the parents would alternate custody every six months. This took place for three years, with no complaints about the mother's behavior or parenting abilities. The husband then moved for a modification of the order based on the mother's history of psychiatric hospitalization and "self-mutilating impulses"[101]—a history that predated both the custodial decree and the divorce itself.[101] The court granted the husband's motion for change of custody, because "in her medical records, Stewart was diagnosed as having suicidal tendencies and potential mental disorders.... Exposure to these characteristics can certainly affect a child."[101] There was no evidence offered that Stewart had exhibited any of these behaviors since the divorce, or of any adverse effect on her child. Nevertheless, she lost all contact with her child except a week at Christmas and six weeks over the summer, and she was ordered to pay child support.[101]

In another case, custodial arrangements ordered by the court were altered based in part on the fact that the mother had been diagnosed "as having a borderline personality disorder approximately *seven years before* the final custody hearing, and there was evidence that, prior to the birth of Cameron, Ms. Jones had attempted suicide on three occasions" (emphasis added).[102, p]

The best interest standard also applies to decisions regarding visitation. Courts have power to condition visitation on the mother's entering psychiatric therapy. In one case, subsequently reversed, a court conditioned the mother's visitation with her child on her undertaking therapy, ostensibly for her borderline personality disorder. It was abundantly clear to the appellate court, however, that the lower court was more concerned with the mother being an acknowledged lesbian.[104]

The *Daubert* considerations with regard to expert testimony raised in the previous section are equally valid in the context of child custody litigation. In addition, arguments may be raised regarding the confidentiality of any diagnosis, mental health treatment, or records. These concerns have met with mixed responses from the courts; the best interests of children are generally held to trump parents' rights to confidentiality of their treatment records.

The ADA is, for a variety of reasons, a far less likely vehicle to defeat discrimination in the child custody context than in cases involving termination of parental rights. Although the reunification activities and services of city and state child welfare authorities are clearly subject to the ADA, the decision of a state court judge awarding or modifying child custody between competing parents is probably not, and certainly not in federal court. A doctrine known as the Rooker-Feldman doctrine would prohibit a federal court from altering a child custody determination, even on ADA or other federal grounds.[105] As a practical matter, absent explicit and egregious discrimination,[106] a mother must rely on sympathetic expert testimony to explain to the judge the meaning and context of a diagnosis of borderline personality disorder.

Disability Benefits Law

Veterans' Benefits

Women veterans who are diagnosed with borderline personality disorder are automatically precluded from receiving Veterans' benefits. This is because of a regulation providing that although mental disabilities such as PTSD may be deemed service-connected and thus compensable,[107] personality disorders are conclusively presumed never to be service-connected.[103] Thus, even if a woman in the armed forces was subject to repeated rapes[108] or sexual harassment, if the resulting diagnosis was borderline personality disorder, she could not receive Veterans' benefits. If, instead, the resulting diagnosis was PTSD, the woman would be entitled to disability benefits if the rapes were service-connected.[109,110] Armed service personnel can, however, be discharged from the military because of diagnoses of borderline personality disorder.[108, q]

Social Security Benefits

The standard that must be met to receive disability benefits under either SSI[r] or SSDI[s] is that an individual must:

> have a physical or mental impairment of such severity that [she] is not only unable to do previous work but cannot, considering age, education, and work experience, engage in any other kind of substantial gainful work which exists in the national economy.[111]

The regulations that are used to determine whether a mental disorder is severe enough to be considered a disability contain language that seems to virtually track the diagnosis of borderline personality disorder. The regulations state that the required level of severity for mental disorders is met by:

A. Deeply ingrained, maladaptive patterns of behavior associated with one of the following:

   . . .

   6.   Intense and unstable interpersonal relationships and impulsive and damaging behavior;

   AND

B. Resulting in three of the following:
   1.   Marked restriction of activities in daily living; or
   2.   Marked difficulties in maintaining social functioning; or
   3.   Deficiencies of concentration, persistence or pace resulting in frequent failure to complete tasks in a timely manner (in work settings or elsewhere); or

> 4. Repeated episodes of deterioration or decompensation in work or work-like settings which cause the individual to withdraw from that situation or to experience exacerbation of signs and symptoms (which may include deterioration of adaptive behaviors).[112]

Despite the apparent similarity between behaviors associated with borderline personality disorder and the regulatory requirements for determining eligibility for benefits, women with diagnoses of borderline personality disorder are rarely granted disability benefits.[113]

A variety of reasons explain the failure of women diagnosed with borderline personality disorder to receive benefits on the basis of disability. Women in general appear to have difficulties related to gender in applications for social security benefits. Some studies show that administrative law judges tend to assume more readily that female claimants are "exaggerating their symptoms or turning emotional problems into physical problems."[114]

In addition, there is some evidence judges are reluctant to hear. "In one case, an applicant wanted to share with the judge his traumatic childhood experience of abuse. The judge interrupted the applicant and told him that these incidents were too old to be relevant."[114] When judges do hear the evidence, they may disbelieve it. In one case involving a woman diagnosed with borderline personality disorder, the administrative law judge:

> found that Ellingson schemed for eight years to obtain attention and government support and services. At the heart of the scheme, according to the ALJ, is Ellingson's "story" that she was sexually abused by family members.[115]

To receive benefits, a woman's disability must be continuous for at least 12 consecutive months. The cycling crisis/competence characteristic of many women diagnosed with borderline personality disorder may result in denial of disability benefits (as well as erratic treatment from mental health providers who perceive mental disabilities in more static terms).[116] Women with diagnoses of borderline personality disorder who obtain benefits generally are granted them on the basis of disability relating to either concurrent physical disabilities or substance abuse.[113-118]

Civil Commitment and Rights in Institutional Settings

To legally deprive an individual of her liberty on the basis of mental illness, a court must find that she is both mentally ill and, as a result of that mental illness, dangerous to herself or others.[119,120] Courts uniformly find borderline personality disorder to be a mental illness for the purpose of civil commitment.[121-123, t] Generally, the self-destructive behavior of a woman with a history of sexual abuse is more than sufficient to convince a judge that she is dangerous to herself, and many of these women are involuntarily committed to psychiatric facilities.

Judges rarely consider the impact of the process of commitment itself on these women. These are women who, because of their experiences with abuse by trusted authority figures, have difficulty with authority and with trust, and who react extremely negatively to intrusions on their privacy or attempts to dominate or control them. Yet the process of involuntary commitment often involves strangers showing up at the door unannounced to take an individual away in handcuffs to a mental hospital. The process of involuntary commitment itself may be sufficiently retraumatizing to send a woman over the edge and thus confirm the prediction that she was dangerous, when she was actually only rendered dangerous by the intrusions and interventions of the law. In one case, a woman was dragged naked out of her bathroom and into the street by ambulance personnel, despite testimony of her friend and the police who were on the scene that she had been calm.[124] In another case, a survivor of the Holocaust died of a heart attack after police serving commitment papers broke down her door and dragged her struggling into the street.[125] Even less dramatic detentions by their nature involve invasions of privacy and loss of control in the form of forced psychiatric examinations. Invasion of privacy, loss of control, and removal from familiar and perhaps safe surroundings may cause far more serious emotional problems than those that initially motivated the commitment proceedings.

Some clinicians who specialize in the treatment of borderline personality disorder counsel strongly against the use of coercion, including involuntary commitment, forced medication, and four-point restraints.[7,17] Yet, once committed, many of these women remain hospitalized for weeks, months, even years[123,126]—time that even their treating physicians often admit produces no success.[123] One major reason for this is that these women deteriorate in coercive and institutional settings, lashing out and cutting themselves. The deterioration results in the perception by the mental health professionals and staff that they are even more dangerous to themselves, and because it seems counterproductive to discharge someone who is in worse condition than when she was admitted, the cycle of forced medication, seclusion, restraint, and escalatingly violent, assaultive, and angry behavior continues, to the detriment of the woman, the staff, and the unit. Often, a woman specifically asks for treatment related to her history of sexual abuse, which state hospitals generally refuse to give, either because they do not have trained staff or because they believe these issues are better confronted in the community.

Antidiscrimination Law

A number of federal statutes prohibit discrimination based on either physical or mental disability. The most important of these are the ADA[36] and Section 504 of the Rehabilitation Act of 1973.[34] These statutes forbid discrimination against "otherwise qualified" disabled persons. Both statutes require that people who would be qualified for employment or educational or other programs if they received "reasonable accommodations" must be provided with those accommodations. Accommodations are not reasonable if they would cause undue financial hardship or transform the fundamental nature of the job or program.

The ADA is relatively new, and there are few cases applying its provisions to women with borderline personality disorder. However, when women who have had borderline personality disorder diagnoses and conduct that points strongly to childhood sexual abuse have brought suits under the Rehabilitation Act, they have lost in ways that particularly underscore the legal dilemmas faced by women with this diagnosis.

The most famous of these cases is *Doe v. New York University Medical School*.[18] In that case, "Jane Doe" applied to New York University (NYU) Medical School, and she was one of 170 persons accepted out of 5,000 applicants. The application asked (probably illegally[u]) whether she had any "chronic or recurrent illnesses, emotional problems, or bodily defects."[18] She indicated that she did not. In fact, Doe had a history of cutting herself severely and numerous brief psychiatric hospitalizations, which were notably unsuccessful in resolving her emotional problems and apparently only exacerbated them.

Upon being asked about the scars on her arms during a required physical examination, Doe told an NYU doctor about "some of her problems." The doctor's immediate response was to tell her she should "undergo a psychiatric examination to determine whether she was fit to stay at the school."[18] Doe's reply was that "it's my body and what I do to it is my concern. If I want to go out and f— a cat, I can." She walked out without completing the examination.[18]

Soon after, Doe was required to undergo a battery of psychiatric interviews by Associate Dean Scotch. Although she had been doing satisfactorily in school, Dean Scotch asked her to withdraw on the basis of the interviews. She appealed to the dean of the medical school, who permitted her to· stay on the condition that she undergo psychiatric treatment.

Three months passed uneventfully until Doe had to see Dean Scotch to sort out a schedule problem. He was not in his office when she arrived for appointment, and she became distressed and angry:

> She left the office and attempted to calm herself, but to no avail. She returned and told Dean Scotch that she would have to revert to her past habits in order to cope with the situation. She retreated to a bathroom, where she bled herself with a catheter.[18]

After this episode, Doe was allowed to withdraw from medical school on the understanding that she could seek reinstatement. Her diagnosis was borderline personality disorder, which the court of appeals characterized in the following way:

> [Borderline personality disorder] is a serious condition. . . . A person suffering from it is likely to have it continue through most of his or her adult life, subject to modification only by treatment by well-trained therapists over a period of years and adoption of a lifestyle which avoids situations that subject the person to types of stress with which he or she cannot cope.[18]

Following her withdrawal from NYU Medical School, Doe worked at an advertising agency, received a master's in science from Harvard's School of Public Health, and worked in an extremely stressful position for the Department of Health, Education and Welfare, where she received awards for outstanding performance.

During this time she sought readmission to the medical school. She was denied readmission and she sued. After both the Office of Civil Rights and the district court judge found that she had been discriminated against, she was permitted to reenter NYU Medical School in the fall of 1981 while the Court of Appeals considered NYU's appeal on an expedited basis. She had not cut herself or been hospitalized since March 1976, but, as the district court noted, "based upon its acceptance of this diagnosis [borderline personality disorder], New York University has taken the position that there is nothing Jane Doe can do or prove (now, or in the future) that will convince them she is cured."[127] The district court, on the other hand, "finds the plaintiff's actual behavior and condition over the past five years to be more reliable criteria for predicting her future behavior."[127]

The court of appeals reversed, finding her not "otherwise qualified" to be a medical student. Although it did not erase her accomplishments, as the court erased Velma Hunt's, it minimized them, attributing her excellent record since leaving NYU to "the fact that the types of stress to which she has been subjected at the Harvard School of Public Health and as an HEW employee do not approximate the seriousness of those she would experience as a medical student and doctor."[18]

Rather than looking at Doe herself and her accomplishments, the Court of Appeals chose to listen to the psychiatric experts, many of whom testified that Doe could not possibly recover from her borderline personality disorder without more therapy than she had received, thus portraying her apparent recovery of the last five years as fragile and dooming her to likely recurrence. While the court noted that mental illness itself should not be seen as automatically rendering a person not otherwise qualified, it distinguished Doe's situation as one where "long-term treatment has been prescribed by competent psychiatrists and Doe has declined to accept such treatment."[18] This is particularly ironic in light of the fact that, by the time of the decision, Doe had received over 20 years of intermittent mental health treatment of all kinds, most of which had been completely unsuccessful. The fault for this was laid by the court squarely at Doe's door.

Like the mothers in the parental termination cases, few of whom had any history of abusing their children, there was no history of Doe's being unable to get along with fellow students, patients, or faculty members at NYU. Most of her violence was self-directed, with occasional assaults directed at mental health professionals, usually in the context of involuntary treatment. Her last assault on a mental health professional predated the court's decision by over seven years. Nevertheless, the court found that "NYU is of necessity concerned with the safety of other students, faculty, and patients to whom Doe would be exposed."[18]

The appeals court disagreed with the lower court's standard, which would have granted Doe admission if it appeared more likely than not that she could complete her medical training and serve successfully as a physician. The appeals court outlined its own standard for decision in the case, which predetermined the outcome:

> If she presents *any* appreciable risk [of harm to herself or others], this factor could properly be taken into account in deciding whether, among qualified applicants, it rendered her less qualified than others for the limited number of places available. In view of the seriousness of the harm inflicted in prior episodes, NYU is not required to give preference to her over other qualified applicants who do not pose any such appreciable risk at all.[18] (emphasis added)

This standard essentially makes it impossible for anyone with a diagnosis of borderline personality disorder, and especially anyone with a history of self-injurious behavior, ever to prevail in a civil rights case involving admission to graduate school.

The facts presented in the case suggest that Doe may well have had a history of sexual abuse. The violence she directed at herself usually came about in the context of confrontations with mental health professionals (and sometimes others) attempting to assert authority and control over her. If the experts and the court had understood the source and meaning of her behavior, the case would have looked completely different, both in terms of the determination of Doe's qualifications for medical school and in the discussion (which never occurred in either court) of what reasonable accommodations might be provided for her to enable her to succeed. Doe's cutting behavior could be explained in terms of its coping function by experts (the opinion notes that she herself explained it that way)[18] and perhaps might seem less bizarre, more explicable and predictable. The dangers of medical school for Doe would be seen not in terms of the stress, which was the focus of expert testimony and the court's opinion, but of the powerlessness of the medical student and the authoritarian nature of medical education. The medical school's insistence on therapy that Doe did not want might have been seen not only as counterproductive but as itself causing the very behavior the therapy was designed to address.

Instead, women in Doe's situation—a substantial number of professionally successful women who deteriorate badly when they interact with the mental health system, particularly involuntarily—are left with one of the most misguided legal decisions on record. The court has essentially imposed an impossible burden of proof on such a woman—she must prove that there is no appreciable risk that her difficulties will recur. This is impossible to prove, even with expert witnesses; Doe had expert witnesses (as is usual in cases involving diagnoses of borderline personality disorder, her witnesses either testified she no longer had borderline personality disorder or never had it).

The lesson of the appellate court in this case is a particularly searing one for women with histories of childhood sexual abuse: You cannot overcome your past. Nothing that Jane Doe could testify about herself or that she accomplished was given as much credence as the predictions of psychiatrists who met her for an hour. Rather than celebrating and praising her accomplishments as even more remarkable in the face of the pain and suffering that she obviously had survived, the court saw her as causing her own problems.

This is the crux of both the clinical and legal treatment received by women who are diagnosed with borderline personality disorder. They lose their children, their commitment hearings, their civil rights cases, and they are blamed for their own losses by the experts and courts that deprive them of the control, liberty, and connection they need to survive. Thus, law responds to them in a way that replicates their abuse. They are discredited as witnesses, confirming prophecies by their abusers that they would not be believed. They lose control as they did in childhood over their lives and bodies and privacy when they are institutionalized, medicated against their will with psychotropic medication (often by injection in the buttocks), and tied down in four-point re-straints. Their attempts to reconstitute a family are shattered by loss of custody and termination of parental rights, often for reasons having more to do with their diagnosis and antagonism toward caseworkers than their treatment of their children. The courts' perception of their illness, fueled by the testimony of "helping" professionals, overwhelms their achievement in civil rights cases.

IMPLICATIONS FOR MENTAL HEALTH POLICY AND SERVICES DELIVERY

The public health perspective has been invaluable in linking health problems with their sources and introducing preventive or ameliorative interventions. In seeking the source of disease and illness, public health research has sometimes traced the proliferation of disease to hospitals themselves. By tracing illness to certain conditions in the hospital, pub-lic health has assisted in making hospitals safer places for people to be treated and to recover from illness.

It is not too much to say that there is an epidemic of borderline per-sonality disorder. This diagnosis was included in the *Diagnostic and Sta-tistical Manual of Mental Disorders* for the first time in 1980, and it now makes up about 15 percent of inpatient diagnoses and 8 percent of out-patient diagnoses.[21] Although no studies have been done of mental ill-ness diagnoses in parental termination proceedings, it appears that a substantial number of women who lose their children in these cases have a diagnosis of borderline personality disorder.

One of the reasons for this borderline personality disorder epidemic may be that, like the hospitals of the 19th century, the state's mental health, legal, and foster care systems are themselves triggering or exac-erbating mechanisms for the condition we call borderline personality disorder. This may be for a variety of reasons. First, each of these sys-tems is undergirded by coercive procedures, which can take away from a woman what matters most to her: her liberty, her bodily integrity, her children, her choices. Second, each of these systems cloaks these actions with reassurances of benevolent intent contradictory to the reality that she experiences. In fact, the woman who is told she will be assisted and protected is rarely attended to in the ways that she wants, and she is ultimately powerless to prevent the most devastating outcomes. For women with a history of childhood sexual abuse, interactions with the state mental health, legal, and child welfare systems may so replicate the conditions of abuse as to literally drive them "crazy."

Like the hospitals of the 19th century, these systems appear utterly unconscious of their impact on the individuals they are required to evaluate, classify, and categorize. The legal system that determines whether an individual is mentally ill and dangerous to herself does not take into consideration that sudden detention by the police and involuntary transport to a psychiatric hospital for examination may have an impact on both mental illness and danger to self. Judges rarely, if ever, inquire whether a caseworker's negative report about a mother has more to do with power struggles between the caseworker and the mother than with the mother's ability to care for her children. State institutions employ male attendants who restrain women with histories of childhood sexual abuse in positions with their legs spread, with no consciousness of paradox.

Like the doctors, researchers, and public health workers of the past two centuries, we must work to make our places of treatment and justice safer for those they purport to serve. There are isolated examples of such work: the development of systems of therapy that seek to enhance power, control, and responsibility for clients with borderline personality disorder;[7] the testimony of expert witnesses explaining the effect of child protective proceedings and legal proceedings on a mother's mental health;[20] and the publication of this and other books. But presently the interaction of the legal and mental health systems in the lives of these women is far more damaging than helpful.

There is much to be done. The use of coercion—especially four-point restraints—on women with histories of sexual abuse should be minimized or eliminated. Judges should be educated about the effect of legal proceedings on women with histories of sexual abuse. Women are traumatized by depositions where strangers probe and explore sensitive and painful memories. A woman's lack of control over her life is underscored by forced appearance in court, where control over what she says and when she speaks is in the hands of lawyers (who may successfully object to what she has to say and silence her) and judges (who may rule that her testimony as a witness is irrelevant or out of order). This understanding has begun to develop in criminal and civil litigation involving children who are victims of sexual abuse. The focus on the impact of legal proceedings on the victim should also be given to women whose abusers were not identified, blamed, and prosecuted when the women were children.

It is tragically unlikely in this society that childhood sexual abuse can be eliminated, but the conditions under which its casualties are treated can be altered to support, rather than undermine and destroy, their struggle to survive. These are systemic issues, but each case terminating parental rights, civilly committing a woman, denying her disability benefits, or taking away custody of her child happens individually. A public health approach is needed to step back and examine the impact of the legal, mental health, and foster care systems on creating and exacerbating psychiatric disorder rather than healing or restoring or treating it.

ENDNOTES

a. The diagnostic criteria for borderline personality disorder are described in the fourth edition of the American Psychiatric Association's *Diagnostic and Statistical Manual of Mental Disorders* as follows:

A pervasive pattern of instability of personal relationships, self-image, and affects, and marked impulsivity beginning by early adulthood and present in a variety of contexts, as indicated by five (or more) of the following:

(1) frantic efforts to avoid real or imagined abandonment. *Note:* Do not include suicidal or self-mutilating behavior covered in Criterion 5.

(2) a pattern of intense and unstable personal relationships characterized by alternating between extremes of idealization and devaluation.

(3) identity disturbance: markedly and persistently unstable self-image or identity of self.

(4) impulsivity in at least two areas that are potentially self-damaging (e.g. spending, sex, substance abuse, reckless driving, binge eating). *Note:* Do not include suicidal or self-mutilating behavior covered in Criterion 5.

(5) recurrent suicidal behavior, gestures, or threats, or self-mutilating behavior.

(6) affective instability due to a marked reactivity of mood (e.g. intense episodic dysphoria, irritability, or anxiety usually lasting a few hours and rarely more than a few days).

(7) chronic feelings of emptiness.

(8) inappropriate, intense displays of anger or difficulty controlling anger (e.g. frequent displays of temper, constant anger, recurrent physical fights).

(9) transient, stress-related paranoid ideation or severe dissociative symptoms. (*Diagnostic and Statistical Manual of Mental Disorders,* fourth edition [*DSM-IV*] 301.83, p. 654)

In the discussion of reported case law involving women with diagnoses of borderline personality disorder, it should be noted that (as might be expected) the diagnosis was rarely the only one that the women had ever received. I made an effort, however, to ensure that the description of the woman's behavior that was seen as relevant by the court matched the *DSM-IV* and literature descriptions of behavior associated with borderline personality disorder and specifically behaviors associated with childhood sexual abuse. However, while many researchers have noted an association between a history of childhood sexual abuse and the diagnosis of borderline personality disorder (see notes 2-7, 11-13, and 17), it is questioned by some, for example, Zanarini MC, Williams AA, Lewis RE, et al.: Reported pathological childhood experiences associated with the development of borderline personality disorder. *American Journal of Psychiatry* 1997; 154:1101-1106.

b. Women with diagnoses of borderline personality disorder who self-injure, frequently report that they do so to relieve unbearable pain and help keep themselves alive, see, for example, *The Cutting Edge* (a newsletter for women who self-injure). The research literature bears this out. Cutting and self-injury have been recognized as an attempt at self-healing for many years. Karl Menninger posited in 1938 that it could reduce the risk of suicide (*Man Against Himself,* Harcourt, Brace and World, New York, 1938), and many therapists have echoed this point in different ways more recently. Marsha Linehan's dialectical behavior therapy is based on a construct of self-injury as "problem-solving behavior emitted to cope with or ameliorate psychic distress" that occurs "when the individual believes that an intolerable, inescapable life problem exists and that parasuicide (self-injury) is the only or best possible solution." Linehan M: Dialectical behavior therapy: A cognitive behavioral approach to parasuicide. *Journal of Personality Disorders* 1987; 1:328-333. Favazza, who had conducted one of the most thorough investigations of self-injury, has concluded that self-injury occurs "to correct or prevent a pathological, destabilizing condition that threatens the community, the individual, or both . . . deviant self-mutilation is best thought of as a purposeful, if morbid, act of self-help." Favazza A: Why patients mutilate themselves. *Hospital and Community Psychiatry* 1989; 40:137-145. Others who concur include: Leibenluft EL, Gardner DG, Cowdry RC: The inner experience of the borderline self-mutilator. *Journal of Personality Disorders* 1987; 1:317-324, and Rockland L: A supportive approach: Psychodynamically oriented supportive therapy—Treatment of borderline patients who self-mutilate. *Journal of Personality Disorders* 1987; 1:350-353.

c. For a remarkable analysis of this issue in the context of sexual harassment and battered women, see Mahoney M: Exit: Power and the idea of leaving in love, work, and the confirmation hearings. *Southern California Law Review* 1992; 65:1283-1319, and Mahoney M: Victimization or oppression? Women's lives, violence, and agency. In: Fineman M, Mykitiuk R (Eds.): *The Public Nature of Private Violence: The Discovery of Domestic Abuse.* New York: Routledge, 1994.

d. In fact, the expert in *In re McCormick*, 1992 Ohio App. LEXIS 4337 (August 30, 1992), testified that "people in the caring professions, such as nurses, frequently possess borderline personalities."

e. This is true on both the federal and state levels. Federally, the Protection and Advocacy for Mentally Ill Persons Act, 42 U.S.C. §10801 *et seq.* (West 1996) provides funds for states to establish protection and advocacy systems to investigate abuse of persons with mental illness who live in institutions and certain other locations; many states have similar laws. In addition, the Civil Rights of Institutionalized Persons Act (CRIPA) authorizes the Department of Justice to bring litigation to protect the civil rights of persons in institutions, including those in mental institutions, 42 U.S.C. §1997 (West 1996).

f. In some states such as New York and Florida, people with active cases of tuberculosis who refuse to submit to treatment can be hospitalized against their will as a quarantine measure. A diagnosis of mental illness is not constitutionally sufficient to involuntarily institutionalize a person, *Donaldson v. O'Connor*, 422 U.S. 563 (1975), and *Foucha v. Louisiana*, 405 U.S. 71 (1992). However, the additional requirements of "danger to self or others" can be met, as a practical matter, rather easily. The following facts were found legally sufficient, by themselves, to prove dangerousness to the Colorado Supreme Court: a woman who bought a gun "impulsively" (she said she bought the gun because she was raped three months earlier); showed the gun to strangers; overreacted to police officers (who showed up at night unannounced at her apartment and took her to a mental hospital); made a phone call to the governor claiming she had been forced to take medication and had been denied access to an attorney; telephoned her parents claiming the hospital had put poison or drugs in her food; and dressed inappropriately and responded inappropriately while watching television, *People v. Stevens*, 761 P.2d 768, 775 (Colorado 1988). The examining mental health professionals disagreed as to whether these facts made her dangerous to herself or others. The certifying psychologist found that since being unexpectedly forced into an institutional setting, she had "experienced rapid mood swings, fixation on revenge fantasies, denial of mental illness and need for treatment, and feelings of victimization." *id.* All agreed that she had not been aggressive since being hospitalized, even when assaulted herself. *id.*

g. There is considerable conflict in the courts over the degree to which experts can testify about a witness's credibility. Thus, most courts will exclude expert testimony that a particular witness is lying or telling the truth. The First Circuit recently permitted expert testimony regarding a defendant who claimed to be suffering from "pseudologia fantastica," an extreme form of pathological lying, *United States v. Shay*, 57 F.3d 126 (1st Cir. 1995). However, most courts will admit testimony regarding a witness's diagnosis or mental condition that might help the jury decide whether the witness is lying or telling the truth, see, for example, *State v. Sasnett*, 1996 Wisc. App. LEXIS 1046 (August 29, 1995) (in prosecution for rape of mentally retarded woman, therapist allowed to testify that complainant's mental retardation would not interfere with her memory and might even enhance it). This has been the basis for expert testimony regarding how victims of sexual abuse, particularly children, behave in the aftermath of the abuse.

h. Although no research or studies were found substantiating any connection between borderline personality disorder and deliberate falsification, there is a fair amount of anecdotal (and often highly affectively charged) reporting, see, for example, Snyder S: Pseudologia fantastica in the borderline patient. *American Journal of Psychiatry* 1986; 143:1287-1289. This correspondence is not, of course, equivalent to research or a controlled study.

i. Hunt "did not recall telling Dr. Traver that she had sex with her brothers. Sometimes she goes off into a 'twilight zone,' like she is not there—she could be daydreaming. . . . Respondent denies telling Dr. Traver she saw a flame of fire in her children's eyes or any of the other hallucinations to which Traver testified, saying she [presumably Dr. Traver] was exaggerating. If she did say it, she was in a twilight zone. She has headaches and stated a doctor told her she has a *split* personality." 633 N.E.2d 27,31.

j. Although the court does not make the connection, it seems possible that Hunt's kidney problems resulted from the physical abuse she suffered as a child.

k. The court also notes that the department had required Ms. Hunt to use birth control and she did not. 633 N.E.2d 27,32.

l. The court discounts this effort: "Despite an obvious need for her to make an effort to improve her ability to read and write, she undertook efforts in that direction only shortly before the hearings on the State's petition to terminate." It was only shortly before the petition to terminate that she managed to find a place to live.

m. After court decisions holding that mental illness alone cannot be a reason for terminating parental rights, for example, *Matter of J.L.B.*, 594 P.2d 1127 (Montana 1979), some states do not predicate termination of parental rights around a finding of mental illness, but do list mental illness or even a history of mental illness as a factor to be considered, Montana 41-3-609 (2). The extent to which the ADA requires that decisions regarding termination of parental rights be based on the parent's conduct, and prohibits the use of diagnoses as even partial proxies for parental unfitness, has yet to be litigated.

n. In states where parents are not entitled to reunification services at all, disabled parents cannot state a claim of discrimination under the Americans With Disabilities Act for failure to provide them with services appropriate to their disabilities, *Stone v. Davies County Division of Child and Family Services*, 656 N.E.2d 824 (Indiana App. 1995).

o. For example, in a case involving parents with mental retardation, the court noted that the agency had provided pictorial instructions, ensured that those instructions were posted on the refrigerator, and used visual aids in its instructions on basic hygiene and cooking, *Robinson v. State*, 896 P.2d 1298 (Washington App. 1995). These modifications were found to satisfy the requirements of the Americans With Disabilities Act.

p. The dissent notes that the mother's emotional problems and attempted suicide were associated with being forced by her ex-husband to abort a child conceived during their marriage, *Jones v. Jones*, 907 S.W.2d 745,754 (Arkansas App. 1995). The other factors that the court cited in approving the change of custody were that the husband offered a more stable home because he had married and had a new baby. There was uncontradicted evidence that the husband's relationship with his present wife antedated his divorce from his first wife; in fact, he married the labor nurse who attended delivery of the parties' child, 907 S.W.2d 745, 754 (Arkansas App. 1995).

q. In *Elkins v. Brown*, 8 Vet. App. 391, 1995, U.S. Vet. App. LEXIS 811 at *2 (November 7, 1995), a male service member who cut his arms with razor blades was "diagnosed with inadequate personality" and "discharged as a consequence of an air force psychiatrist's diagnosis of personality disorder."

r. Supplemental Security Income is a form of disability benefits given to blind, aged, and disabled individuals without sufficient work history to qualify for Social Security Disability Insurance (SSDI). The benefit amount is significantly lower than that given to people who qualify for SSDI.

s. Social Security Disability Insurance is given to disabled individuals who have sufficient work history to qualify for such benefits.

t. Interestingly, few published cases about involuntary commitment involve diagnoses of borderline personality disorder, especially women with the diagnosis. We learn of most cases involving involuntary commitment of women with borderline personality disorder through other kinds of cases, such as parental termination cases, for example, *In the Matter of Declaring V.B., et al. ,Youths in Need of Care*, 744 P.2d 1248 (Montana 1987) (mother with borderline personality disorder "admitted to Warm Springs State Hospital eleven times"), or discrimination cases, *Doe v. New York University*, 666 F.2d 761 (2nd Cir. 1981).

u. Although the Court of Appeals found that New York University "was entitled, in determining whether she was qualified, to be advised of and to take into account her mental impairment," *id.*, at 777, the Department of Education's Office of Civil Rights and the regulations governing Section 504 indicate that an institution of higher education cannot ask about disabilities or histories of disabilities on their applications, 34 C.F.R. 104.,42 (b) (4).

REFERENCES

1. American Psychiatric Association: *Diagnostic and Statistical Manual of Mental Disorders*. 4th ed. Washington, DC: American Psychiatric Association, 1994.
2. Widiger T, Weissman MA: Epidemiology of borderline personality disorder. *Hospital and Community Psychiatry* 1991; 42:1015-1021.
3. Wonderlich SA, Swift WJ: Borderline versus other personality disorders in the eating disorders: Clinical description. *International Journal of Eating Disorders* 1990; 9:629-638, citing to Herman J, Perry JC, van der Kolk B: Childhood trauma in borderline personality disorder. *American Journal of Psychiatry* 1989; 146:490-495.
4. Carrol J, Schaffer C, Spensley J, et al.: Family experiences of self-mutilating patients. *American Journal of Psychiatry* 1980; 137:852-853.
5. Zanarini MC (Ed.): *The Role of Sexual Abuse in the Etiology of Borderline Personality Disorder*. Washington, DC: American Psychiatric Press, 1996.
6. Bryer JB, Nelson BA, Miller JB, et al.: Childhood sexual and physical abuse as a factor in adult psychiatric illness. *American Journal of Psychiatry* 1987; 144:1426-1430.
7. Dawson D, MacMillan H: *Relationship Management of the Borderline Patient: From Understanding to Treatment*. New York: Brunner/Mazel, 1993.
8. *Brooks v. State*, 655 A.2d 1311, 1313-14 (Ct. Spec. App. Md. 1995) (criminal defendant suffered borderline personality disorder due to severe childhood sexual abuse).
9. *Corbett v. Morgenstern*, 934 F.Supp. 680, 684 (E.D. Pa. 1996).
10. *U.S. v. Prevatte*, 36 M.J. 1075 (C.M. App. 1993) (expert testifies that likely result of child's sexual abuse will be later development of borderline personality disorder or multiple personality disorder).
11. Briere J, Zaidi L: Sexual abuse histories and sequelae in female psychiatric emergency room patients. *American Journal of Psychiatry* 1989; 146:1602-1606.

12. Stone MH: A psychodynamic approach: Some thoughts on the dynamics and therapy of self-mutilating borderline patients. *Journal of Personality Disorders* 1987; 1:347-349.
13. Josephs L: Women and trauma: A contemporary psychodynamic approach to traumatization for patients in the OB/GYN psychological consultation clinic. *Bulletin of the Menninger Clinic* 1996; 60:22-38.
14. *Ford v. United States,* CA 84-1013, 1987 U.S. Dist. LEXIS 5971 at *22 (E.D. Pa. June 30, 1987).
15. Schwartz R, Cohen P, Hoffman N, et al.: Self-harm behaviors (carving): In female adolescent drug abusers. *Clinical Pediatrics* 1989; 28:340-346.
16. Kramer P: *Moments of Engagement.* New York: Norton, 1989.
17. Vaillant G: The beginning of wisdom is never calling a patient a borderline, or the clinical management of immature defenses in the treatment of individuals with personality disorders. *Journal of Psychotherapy and Research* 1992; 1:117-134.
18. *Doe v. New York University,* 666 F.2d 761 (2nd Cir. 1981).
19. Hubbard J, Saathoff G, Bernardo M, et al.: Recognizing borderline personality disorder in the family practice setting. *American Family Physician* 1995; 52:908-913.
20. *In re Kristin H.,* 46 Cal. App. 4th 1635, 1645 (Cal. App. 1996).
21. *In the Matter of M.B. and C.B.,* 570 N.E.2d 78,80-81 (Ind. App. 1991).
22. Stewart L: Testimony. In: Grobe J (Ed.): *Beyond Bedlam.* Cambridge, MA: Third Side Press, 1995.
23. *Tandi v. Henry,* 571 N.E.2d 1020 (Ill. App. 1991) (nurse).
24. *Jones v. Jones,* 907 S.W.2d 745, 752 (Ark. App. 1995) (registered nurse).
25. *California v. Brown,* 479 U.S. 538, 545 (1987) (O'Connor J., concurring).
26. *People v. Watters,* 595 N.E.2d 1369, 1375-76 (Ill. App. 1992).
27. 20 U.S.C. §1400 *et seq.* (West 1996) (Individuals With Disabilities in Education Act).
28. *Nunnally v. McCausland,* 966 F.2d 1 (1st Cir. 1993) (mental illness appropriate basis for tolling 30-day filing period set forth in Civil Service Reform Act).
29. *Moody v. Bayliner Marine Corp.,* 644 F.Supp 232 (E.D.N.C. 1987) (recognizing that mental incapacity may toll Title VII limitations period).
30. *Bassett v. Sterling Drug,* 578 F.Supp 1244 (S.D. Ohio 1984) (tolling ADEA limitations period if plaintiff mentally incompetent or institutionalized during filing period).
31. 42 U.S.C.A. §1437 (a) (b) (3) (West 1996) (Section 8 housing program).
32. The Supplemental Security Income for Aged, Blind and Disabled (SSI) is found at 42 U.S.C. §1382 (West 1996).
33. Title XIX of the Social Security Act, 42 U.S.C. §1396 (West 1996).
34. Section 504 of the Rehabilitation Act, 29 U.S.C. §794 (West 1996).
35. 42 U.S.C. §3604 (West 1996) (Fair Housing Act).
36. 42 U.S.C. §12101 *et seq.* (West 1996) (Americans With Disabilities Act).
37. *Jaffee v. Redmond,* 116 S. Ct. 1926, 135 L.Ed.2d 337 (1996). All states have some form of protection for communications between psychiatrists or psychotherapists and their patients, see, for example, Ala. Stat. 34-26-2 (1996); Cal. Evid. Code 1012 (Deering 1995); Conn. Gen. Stat. 52-146f (1994); Del. Rules of Evid. 503 (1995); O.C.G.A. 24-9-21 (1995).
38. *United States v. Hiss,* 88 F.Supp. 559-560 (S.D.N.Y. 1950).
39. *United States v. Moore,* 923 F.2d 910, 913 (1st Cir. 1991).
40. *United States v. Partin,* 493 F.2d 750, 762 (5th Cir. 1974).
41. *United States v. Lindstrom,* 698 F.2d 1154, 1160 (11th Cir. 1983).
42. Restatement of Torts (Second) 436a, Comment b (1965) ("Emotional disturbance may be too easily feigned").

43. Stefan S: *PTSD and Law: Variations Based on Gender and Etiology*. Paper presented at the annual conference of the American Psychiatric Association, New York City, May 5, 1996.
44. Levesque R Jr: Regulating the private relations of adults with mental disabilities: Old laws, new policies, hollow hopes. *Behavioral Sciences and the Law* 1996; 14:83-106.
45. Ala. 26-18-7 (a) (2) ("emotional or mental illness . . . of the parent of such duration or nature as to render the parent unable to care for the needs of the child").
46. Arizona, A.R.S §8-533 (B) (3).
47. Nebraska, §42-364 (7) (d) (1995).
48. Illinois, §40-1501-D-p (inability to discharge parental responsibilities supported by competent evidence from a psychiatrist or clinical psychologist of mental impairment, mental illness, or mental retardation [as defined by Illinois statute] and there is sufficient justification to believe that such inability to discharge parental responsibilities shall extend beyond a reasonable time period).
49. *In re Fant*, 335 N.W.2d 314, 315 (Neb. 1983).
50. *In re Maricopa County Juvenile Action No. JS-5209* 692 P.2d 1027, 1037 (Ariz. 1994).
51. Mont. Stat. §41-3-609.
52. Federal Rules of Evidence 608(a).
53. Nev. Stat. §50.085 (1995).
54. Wisc. Stat. §906.8 (1995).
55. Ok. Stat. Title 12 §2608 (1995).
56. *McClelland v. McClelland*, 595 N.E.2d 1131, 1137 (Ill. App. 1992).
57. *United States v. Jordan*, 24 M.J. 573, 575 (Navy-Marine Court of Military Review 1987) ("she [the witness] was impeached by . . . the testimony of a clinical psychologist that she had a severe borderline personality disorder and routinely distorted reality. If confronted with a traumatic event she was likely to project blame on someone else [footnote omitted to the effect that she had been "confronted" with traumatic events]. Revenge, such as making a false accusation against her former intimate partner, was consistent with her personality.").
58. *State v. Griggs*, 794 P.2d 1179 (Kan. App. 1990) ("fabrication of a prior claim by V.F. that she was forced to engage in sexual intercourse was consistent with her diagnosed condition of borderline personality disorder").
59. *S.V. v. R.V.*, 933 S.W.2d 1 (Tex. 1996).
60. *Goldberg v. Davis*, 602 N.E.2d 812 (Ill. 1992).
61. *Daniels v. Board of Registration in Medicine*, 636 N.E.2d 258, 264 (Mass. 1994).
62. *Johnson v. Johnson*, 471 N.W.2d 156, 163 (S.D.1991).
63. *People v. Walker*, 636 N.Y.S.2d 765 (New York Supreme Court 1996).
64. *State v. Munoz*, 546 N.W.2d 570 (Wisc. App. 1996).
65. *State v. Shiffra*, 499 N.W.2d 719, 723-24 (Wisc. App. 1993).
66. Gutheil T: Borderline personality disorder, boundary violations, and patient-therapist sex: Medicolegal pitfalls. *American Journal of Psychiatry* 1989; 146:592-602.
67. *Daubert v. Merrell-Dow*, 509 U.S. 579 (1993).
68. Reiser DE, Levenson H: Abuses of the borderline diagnosis: A clinical problem with teaching opportunities. *American Journal of Psychiatry* 1984; 141(12):1528-1532.
69. Gallop R, Lancee WJ, Garfinkel P: How nursing staff respond to the label "borderline personality disorder." *Hospital and Community Psychiatry* 1989; 40:815-819.
70. *Hoult v. Hoult*, 57 F.3d 1,7 (1st Cir. 1995).
71. *Santosky v. Kramer*, 455 U.S. 745, 753 (1982).
72. *In re B.M.*, 475 N.W.2d 909, 913 (Neb. 1992).

73. *In re J.P.*, 633 N.E.2d 27 (Ill. App. 1994).
74. *In re Hurlbert*, 465 N.W.2d 36 (Mich. App. 1990).
75. *In re McCormick*, 1992 Ohio App. LEXIS 4337 (August 28, 1992).
76. *In the Matter of Welfare of N.F.*, 1993 Minn. App. LEXIS 108 at *7 (Minn. App. February 2, 1993).
77. *Samantha Simms v. State of Florida*, 641 So.2d 957, 963, n.2 (Fla. App. 1994) (Jorgenson, J., dissenting).
78. *In re Misty Lee H.*, 529 A.2d 331 (Me. 1987).
79. *In re Christina A.*, 213 Cal. App.3d 1073 (1989).
80. *In re Donald LL*, 591 N.Y.S.2d 876 (N.Y. App. 1992).
81. *Matter of Guynn*, 437 S.E.2d 532 (N.C. App. 1993).
82. *R.M. v. Tippecanoe Dept. of Public Welfare*, 582 N.E.2d 417, 419 (Ind. App. 1991).
83. *Robinson v. State*, 896 P.2d 1298 (Wash. App. 1995).
84. *In the Interest of W.D.T.*, 785 S.W.2d 286, 290 (Mo. App. 1990).
85. See also *In re Alexander V.*, 613 A.2d 780 (Conn. 1992) ("[The evaluator] opined that the respondent would have difficulty remaining in one occupation or residence and that she did not keep stable personal relationships.").
86. *In re Pronger*, 517 N.E.2d 1076, 1078 (Ill. 1987).
87. *In re Jason M.*, 1991 Conn. Super. LEXIS 1604 (July 15, 1991).
88. Mahoney M: Victimization or oppression? Women's lives, violence and agency. In: Fineman M, Mykitiuk R (Eds.): *The Public Nature of Private Violence: The Discovery of Domestic Abuse*. New York: Routledge, 1994.
89. Ca. Welfare and Institutions Code §361.5 (b) (2).
90. *In re Angel B. et al.*, 659 A.2d 277 (Me. 1995).
91. *In the Interest of C.M.*, 526 N.W.2d 562 (Iowa App. 1994).
92. *New Mexico v. Penny J.*, 890 P.2d 389 (N.M. App. 1994).
93. *In the Interest of Torrance P.*, 522 N.W.2d 243 (Wisc. App. 1994) (holding that the Americans with Disabilities Act applied, but that any challenge to the procedures employed by the state agency would have to be brought separately from an individual parent's termination proceedings).
94. *Arkansas D.H.S. v. Clark*, 802 S.W.2d 461 (Ark. 1991). The Arkansas D.H.S. fought this order (amounting to $41.50 a month) all the way to the Arkansas Supreme Court.
95. Schneider C: Symposium: One hundred years of uniform state laws: Discretion, rules and law: Child custody and the UMDA's best-interest standard. *Michigan Law Review* 1991; 87:2215-2298.
96. *In re James J.*, 65 Cal. App.3d 254 (1976).
97. "Who gets child from Pensacola—murdering father or lesbian mother?" *Orlando Sentinel*, April 23, 1996.
98. This decision was reversed by the California Supreme Court, *In re Marriage of Carney*, 598 P.2d 36, 40-42 (Ca. 1979).
99. *Eisenberg v. Eisenberg*, 595 N.Y.S.2d 498, 499 (Supreme Ct., 2nd App. Div. 1993).
100. *In re Marriage of Patroske*, 888 S.W.2d 374, 383 (Mo. App. 1994).
101. *Evenson v. Evenson*, 538 N.W.2d 746, 748 (Neb. 1995).
102. *Jones v. Jones*, 907 S.W.2d 745, 750 (Ark. App. 1995).
103. 38 C.F.R. 4.127 (1994) ("Personality disorders will not be considered as disabilities under the term of the schedule.").
104. *Pleasant v. Pleasant*, 628 N.E.2d 633, 639 (Ill. App. 1993) (reversing lower court order that visitation must be supervised because mother was a lesbian and that mother be

involved in regular psychotherapy for her "borderline personality disorder" in order to have visitation).

105. *Leidel v. Madison County*, 891 F.2d 1542 (11th Cir. 1990).
106. *Palmore v. Sidoti*, 466 U.S. 429 (1984).
107. 38 C.F.R. 3.304 (1994).
108. See *YY v. Brown*, No. 94-1003, 1995 U.S. Vet. App. LEXIS 549 (U.S. Ct. Veterans Appeals July 7, 1995) at *2.
109. *Brooks v. Brown*, 1995 U.S. Vet. App. LEXIS 857 at *3 (November 14, 1995).
110. Veterans Administration Adj. Manual, M21-1, Part VI P 7.46(e)-(f) (December 1992).
111. 42 U.S.C. §1382c (a) (3) (B). The impairment must also be one either expected to result in death or expected to last for a continuous period of not less than 12 months. 42 U.S.C. §1382c (a) (3) (A).
112. 20 C.F.R. Part 404, Subpart P, App. 1, 12.08 (A) and (B).
113. *Williams v. Sullivan*, 1992 U.S. Dist. LEXIS 8286 (E.D.N.Y. May 26, 1992).
114. Mill L: A calculus for bias: How malingering females and dependent housewives fare in the Social Security disability system. *Harvard Women's Law Journal* 1993; 16:211-232.
115. *Ellingson v. Sullivan*, 1989 U.S. Dist. LEXIS 6952 (D.Ore. 1989).
116. See, for example, *Vanderford v. Heckler*, CA No. 84-2281-T (D. Mass. March 7, 1985) (Reversing determination that woman diagnosed with borderline personality disorder, who had 82 hospitalizations and emergency room visits in 13 years, was not disabled because in one calendar year she was not receiving any regular psychiatric treatment and visited emergency room only twice).
117. *Sarago v. Shalala*, 884 F.Supp. 100, 102 (W.D.N.Y. 1995).
118. *Smith v. Sullivan*, 776 F.Supp. 107 (E.D.N.Y. 1991).
119. *Donaldson v. O'Connor*, 422 U.S. 563 (1975).
120. *Foucha v. Louisiana*, 504 U.S. 71 (1992).
121. *State v. Paradis*, 455 A.2d 1070 (N.H. 1983).
122. *Jones v. State*, 482 So.2d.571 (Fla. App. 1986).
123. *In re Elizabeth M.*, 514 N.W.2d 424 (Wisc. App. 1993).
124. *Becky Moore v. Wyoming Medical Center*, 825 F.Supp. 1531, 1535 (D.Wyo. 1993).
125. *McCabe v. Lifeline Ambulance Service, Inc.*, 77 F.3d 540 (1st Cir. 1996). The appellate court reversed a district court finding that police had acted improperly.
126. Beck JC, van der Kolk B: Reports of childhood incest and current behavior of chronically hospitalized psychotic women. *American Journal of Psychiatry* 1987; 144:1474.
127. *Doe v. New York University Medical School*, No. 77-CIV-6285, 1931 U.S. Dist. LEXIS 14904 (S.D.N.Y. Oct. 2, 1981) (*slip op.*).

13

Abuse Histories, Severe Mental Illness, and the Cost of Care

Joy Perkins Newmann, M.S.W., Ph.D.
Dianne Greenley, M.S.W., J.D.
J. K. Sweeney, M.S.
Gillian Van Dien, M.S.

The past decade has witnessed a growing concern about the high rates of physical and sexual abuse in the lives of adults with serious mental illnesses. This concern is expressed, in large part, as a quality of care issue. That is, although studies show that 30 to 70 percent[1-6] of outpatients and 40 to 72 percent[4-13] of inpatients have histories of abuse, it is believed that few treatment providers are adequately trained to sensitively address the abuse histories of clients who enter their care.[14-17] Indeed, some critics of the mental health care system contend that abuse survivors are often revictimized by the care they receive, whether through a denial of the abuse history, inappropriate use of medications, excessive reliance on restrictive settings, or the inappropriate use of restraints to prevent self-destructive behaviors.[14-17]

Although such claims have been buttressed by individual case histories and/or anecdotal evidence,[15-17] few studies have investigated whether the course or quality of care for clients with histories of abuse is fundamentally different from that provided to clients with no abuse history. Moreover, there have been no attempts to investigate the cost implications of the different care trajectories presumed to be associated with histories of abuse. The purpose of the present study is to pursue such an inquiry. Specifically, we investigate the link between histories of abuse and the course and cost of care for 1,600 men and women, all of whom met criteria for a diagnosis of severe mental illness and were being served in one of ten systems of care in Wisconsin at the time of the study.

We begin with a review of the literature on the link between histories of abuse and the course and cost of care for adults with serious mental illnesses, which forms the basis for our hypotheses. We subsequently describe our sample and data and the methods of analysis, structural equation modeling techniques, which will be used to investigate our hypotheses. A central assumption underlying this study is that a failure to attend to histories of abuse as part of the routine assessment and treatment planning for adults with serious mental illnesses is a widespread and potentially costly practice. Moreover, it is a practice that disadvantages disproportionate numbers of women, because they are more likely than men to be victims of abuse. Thus, we conclude with a discussion of the policy implications of our findings with a special focus on the implications for women's mental health services.

HISTORIES OF ABUSE AND THE
COURSE AND COST OF CARE

Although a number of studies conducted in the past two decades have investigated the cost of care for persons with serious mental illnesses,[18-32] none has investigated the relationship between a history of sexual or physical abuse and cost of care in this population. There are, however, two distinct literatures that together form the basis for our hypotheses regarding the link between abuse histories and the course and cost of care. One focuses on the link between abuse histories and the course of care for adults with serious mental illnesses. The other focuses on the characteristics of clients or their patterns of use that drive up the cost of care for systems serving the seriously mentally ill. We review each of these literatures below.

Abuse Histories, Serious Mental Illness, and the Course of Care

A number of recent studies indicate that persons with abuse histories are not only more likely to end up in systems of care for adults with serious mental illness, but they are also more likely to present with a severe array of symptoms that increase the probability of (a) being treated with psychotropic medications, (b) being treated in emergency outpatient settings and/or hospitalized, and (c) having longer hospitalization stays than those with no abuse history.

For example, although community studies report rates of childhood sexual abuse ranging from 10 to 45 percent,[33-36] and childhood physical abuse ranging from 11 to 14 percent,[37] studies of rates of abuse among those consumers of mental health services who have a diagnosis of serious mental illness tend to be higher. Among six studies of severely mentally ill outpatient populations, histories of childhood sexual abuse ranging from 25 to 45 percent of the samples were reported.[1-6] Two of the studies reported rates of childhood physical abuse of 34 percent[4] and 31 percent.[5] Among five studies of inpatient populations, rates of childhood sexual abuse ranging from a low of 20 percent[11] to a high of 60 percent[7] have been reported with three studies reporting rates in the midrange of 40 percent.[8-10] Two of the inpatient studies reported rates of childhood physical abuse of 34.3 percent[9] and 38 percent.[11] Thus, we see, on average, a linear increase in rates of both physical abuse and sexual abuse as we move from community samples to treated samples of adults with serious mental illnesses, with the highest rates of all among the latter group who are in inpatient settings. Moreover, although few community studies investigate the co-occurrence of physical and sexual abuse, several studies of treated samples of adults with serious mental illness show disturbingly high rates of co-occurring forms of abuse. In one study of inpatients,[9] 59 percent of the subjects had been abused before their 16th birthday, almost half of whom had experienced both physical and sexual abuse. In a second study, also of inpatients, 43 percent had abuse histories, a quarter of whom had experienced both physical and sexual abuse.[11]

However, we must be cautious in generalizations we draw from these findings, since three of the six outpatient studies and five of the seven inpatient studies were exclusively of women, whose rates of reported abuse tend to be substantially higher than reported abuse rates for males in community studies.[38] Thus, it is unclear whether the appearance of a trend is an artifact of (a) the greater selection of women into these settings, or (b) something about the abuse experiences of women that may place them at greater risk for serious mental disorders or more likely to end up in treatment, as opposed to the criminal justice system, than their male counterparts.

If we turn to the handful of studies that compare the abuse experiences of men and women with serious mental disorders, there is some basis for assuming that abuse may be a more salient treatment issue for women than for men. Here we review five studies, four noted above, and a fifth, larger study of the abuse histories of 947 men and women consecutively admitted to inpatient care in a military hospital.[2,4,11,12,39] Three gender differences in abuse experiences are noted in these studies.

First, reported rates of childhood abuse are generally higher for women with serious mental illnesses than for men, regardless of type of abuse, although the difference is greatest for sexual abuse experiences. Two studies that provide a breakdown of rates of physical abuse by gender both show a 7 percent excess in rates for females compared with males.[4,39] However, five studies providing a breakdown of sexual abuse histories by gender show excess rates for females ranging from 17 to 37 percent.[2,4,11,12,39]

A second finding is that women with serious mental illnesses are more likely than men to have experienced co-occurring physical and sexual abuse during childhood.[39] Brown and Anderson propose that the higher risk of women to a combined history of physical and sexual abuse may be linked to their greater risk of being abused by a male family member as a child, particularly a family member with a history of alcohol abuse. Although this is the only study to provide a gender breakdown by co-occurring forms of abuse during childhood, it echoes a theme noted in three other studies of the substantially higher risk of abuse in families with a substance abusing parent, usually a father.[2,9,11]

Third, several studies report a pattern of revictimization during adulthood for many adults with serious mental illnesses who have experienced childhood abuse,[6,7,9] a pattern that may be more characteristic of the life trajectories of women than of men. For example, Lipschitz and associates[4] found that childhood sexual assaults, which were much more common for women than for men, were associated with an increased risk of adult assaults of both a physical and sexual nature. Childhood physical assaults, by contrast, were not related to adult victimization experiences. A similar finding was reported by Carmen and associates,[11] who observed that males were more frequently abused by parents during childhood and adolescence, while females were abused by parents, spouses, and strangers over a much longer period of time.

In sum, these findings suggest that although rates of abuse are generally higher among adults with serious mental illnesses receiving mental health care compared with adults living in the community, rate differentials may have been inflated due to the disproportionate number of studies that have focused exclusively on female outpatients or inpatients. What we can conclude is that abuse is a more common childhood experience among women with serious mental illnesses than among their male counterparts who enter systems of care. This is particularly true for histories of sexual abuse and for histories of co-occurring sexual and physical abuse. Moreover, women with serious mental illnesses who were victimized as children seem to be at higher risk than their male counterparts of being revictimized as adults.

An important question is, what evidence is there that a history of abuse is linked to different treatment experiences among adults with diagnoses of serious mental illness, particularly experiences that may contribute to a higher cost of care? Furthermore, what are the mechanisms or avenues through which different treatment experiences occur? Several studies have compared the symptom profiles and treatment experiences of adults with serious mental illnesses who have been abused as children with those who have not.[1-9,11] Interestingly, they provide a composite profile, much like the moving account Ann Jennings offers of her own daughter's mental anguish and multiple encounters with mental health care systems and providers over a 19-year period.[16]

A key characteristic of abuse survivors is that their diagnostic picture is often very complex, which is reflected in histories of having multiple diagnoses that have changed over time;[1,15,16] a higher probability of having both Axis I and Axis II diagnoses, the latter often including a diagnosis of borderline personality disorder;[1,9,10] and no clear or consistent pattern of an Axis I diagnosis.[10,11,13] However, several studies report that clients with abuse histories have significantly more symptoms than their nonabused counterparts, including more symptoms of sleep

services,[18-22] strategies for estimating the total costs associated with community treatment of persons with serious mental illness,[23] and the characteristics of persons who are heavy users of services or are high-cost clients.[43-48] A consistent finding in this body of work is that higher costs are primarily related to a greater use of inpatient treatment. Thus, programs that have been successful in maintaining clients in the community and reducing inpatient use are generally less costly than those having higher rates of inpatient use.[19,21,22,24,26]

Studies that have identified characteristics of clients who either are heavy users of mental health services[43-48] or are more likely to use services that are particularly costly, such as inpatient services,[19,28,29,31,32] suggest several consistent themes. One theme is that these are largely socially disconnected individuals who either have never married or are divorced or separated and have few family ties or other social resources.[20,26,28,29,43,46] A second theme is that most have less than a high school education, are unemployed, poor, and often homeless.[20,26,28,46]

Like abuse survivors, the clinical profile of heavy services/high-cost users is complex.[43,44] Many have diagnoses of schizophrenia[19,28] or other psychotic illnesses, usually complicated with physical illnesses,[44] substance abuse,[14,31,32,43,44] and personality disorders.[21,43,44,46] Moreover, in contrast to low-cost individuals, high-cost or heavy services users are less engaged in ongoing outpatient services, are characterized as treatment resistant,[19,44] and tend to rely on emergency psychiatric care when in crisis situations.[29]

Finally, although some studies suggest that males are overrepresented in the heavy user/high-cost users group,[26,28,31,32] other studies reveal an overrepresentation of women.[19,21,29,43,45] Geller's findings suggest that both men and women fall into the heavy user/high-cost group, although their pathways to emergency care may be different.[46] Although similar in social and economic circumstances, Geller found that the vast majority of women who were rapid cyclers into a state hospital had diagnoses of borderline personality disorders, while the men had diagnoses of schizophrenia. Moreover, while men were readmitted because of danger to others (35 percent), danger to self (40 percent), and inability to care for self (20 percent), the vast majority of women were readmitted because of danger to self (70 percent). Third, what led to readmission for the male patients was often noncompliance with drug regimen and a recurrence of psychotic symptoms. By contrast, most of the women were not on medications in the community, although many were abusing alcohol, suicidal, or were otherwise in crisis.

Summary and Hypotheses

One implication of the above literature review is that pathways to costly forms of mental health care, inpatient hospitalization in particular, may be different for men and women. Drawing on the above literatures, we offer three hypotheses regarding different pathways to higher cost of care for men and women:

> H1: Women with serious mental illnesses are more likely than men with serious mental illnesses to have experienced a history of severe abuse, particularly sexual abuse, but also co-occurring sexual and physical abuse.
>
> H2: Such abuse experiences are likely to increase the risk of being hospitalized in crisis situations and increase the risk of longer hospital stays, although they are unlikely to increase use of outpatient services.
>
> H3: Controlling for abuse-related costs, which will be significantly higher for women than for men, men will have significantly higher cost of care that is related to the use of inpatient services, although not mediated by exposure to reported abuse experiences.

METHOD

Sample

The data for the present study come from a large naturalistic study of adults with chronic mental illness who were served by one of 43 mental health organizations within ten systems of care spanning 16 counties in Wisconsin. The state is noted for its innovative treatment of adults with serious mental illnesses, and programs were selected that were considered to provide quality care, albeit through different models of care.

Clients eligible for inclusion in the study were those persons who were 18 years of age or older and who met Wisconsin's definition of chronic mental illness, outlined below:

"Chronic mental illness" means a mental illness which is severe in degree and persistent in duration, which causes a substantially diminished level of functioning in the primary aspects of daily living and an inability to cope with the ordinary demands of life, which may lead to an inability to maintain stable adjustment and independent functioning without long-term treatment and support and which may be of lifelong duration. (p. 345-a)[49]

A third criterion for inclusion is that all were identified as being the primary responsibility of one of the mental health organizations sampled in the study, referred to subsequently as the primary provider organization (PPO). Of the 2,528 eligible clients identified in the ten systems of care, 198 clients were not approached for consent for a variety of reasons (e.g., case managers thought they were too impaired to give informed consent). Consent was sought from the remaining 2,330, of whom 83 percent agreed to participate.

Data Sources

Each of the client's case managers completed a Client Assessment Questionnaire (CAQ), which was based on the National Institute of Mental Health's Uniform Client Data Instrument. It asks the key informant to provide a variety of information, including client's functioning, diagnosis, living situation, daily activities, and sociodemographic characteristics. Usable CAQs were completed for 1,571 clients, representing 67.4 percent of the clients from whom consent was sought and 81.2 percent of those clients who signed the consent form.

Although these data were cross-sectional in nature, they were eventually linked with three independent sources of data on the course, content, and cost of care over a period of one year. These sources included:

1. Data from the client's service provider, which detailed the specific types of services received by the client over the course of the year, the units of time, and the cost of services not covered by Medicaid;
2. All Medicaid claims files for those clients who were Medicaid-eligible for the same one-year period; and
3. Medicare reimbursement for eligible Medicaid clients.

Thus, the final data set is longitudinal by virtue of concatenating the four data sources.

Measures

In the concluding section of the CAQ, case managers were asked a series of questions about the client's life and functioning prior to entering the county's system of care and the case manager's particular program. These included questions about date of onset of illness, prior treatment history, and two questions about the client's abuse history: (1) Does the client have a history of being physically abused? (yes, no, don't know), and (2) Does the client have a history of being sexually abused? (yes, no, don't know). We constructed three categorical measures from these two items, PABUSE (coded "1" if a yes response to the physical abuse question, "0" if answered otherwise); SABUSE (coded "1" if a yes response to the sexual abuse question, "0" if answered otherwise), and DONTKNOW (coded "1" if either or both abuse histories were unknown, "0" if answered otherwise).

Case managers also provided information regarding the client's gender, age, medical assistance status, and most recent diagnosis as part of the CAQ. For the purposes of the present analysis, gender was coded 1 = female and 0 = male and will be referred to subsequently as GENDER. AGE is a continuous variable reflecting the actual age of each client. MAstatus is a categorical measure (coded 1 if client received Medicaid, otherwise 0), which reflects the client's eligibility for state Medicaid funds. Information on the services provided to clients by the various organizations and programs in their respective mental health systems was received from two independent sources. First, much of the data were provided by the individual systems on specific services used by each client over the course of the prior year. These were categorized into relevant service categories, such as counseling, medication checks, nursing home care, and vocational services, each associated with a time amount and specific cost of care. A second source of information was the Medicaid claims files for those clients who were Medicaid-eligible and who received reimbursable services during the index year. Data from both of the above sources were combined into a clients' services file, which was carefully checked to ensure against duplication of service information. These data were subsequently grouped into broader service categories, including (a) outpatient service hours, (b) inpatient days, (c) nursing home days, and (d) residential days over the course of the index year.

OUTPATIENT HOURS are the actual hours of services received over the index year for each client for the following outpatient services: case management, counseling, evaluation, day treatment, community support, alcohol and other drug use treatment, crisis care, medication checks, daily living skills, and transportation services. INPATIENT DAYS are the actual number of days of inpatient psychiatric care the client received over the index year. These estimates do not include days in nursing homes, for which we constructed a separate measure, NURSING HOME DAYS. Finally, we constructed a measure of RESIDENTIAL DAYS for each client for the index year, which includes days spent in supported housing arrangements, such as group homes or supervised apartment living. The total COST OF CARE for mental health services for each client for the index year was constructed by combining direct cost information from the county service providers with data from the state Medicaid file.

Sample Characteristics

We turn first to a general description of client characteristics, which is presented in Table 13.1. Slightly over half of the clients in the sample are males (51.2 percent), reflecting very closely the gender makeup of the state as a whole. The client's ages ranged from 18 to 92 years with an average of 44.7. The vast majority are non-Hispanic White, and 70 percent have a high school diploma, GED, or higher. Yet almost 60 percent were unemployed during the past year and close to 70 percent are Medicaid-eligible. Indeed, the majority of clients received Supplemental Security Income (SSI) (51.2 percent) or Social Security Disability Insurance (SSDI) (40.7 percent) during the prior year (not presented in table) and had gross monthly incomes of $630.00.

The material resource deficits experienced by this sample of clients is matched by deficits in interpersonal resources and relationships. Over 50 percent of the clients have never been married and of those who have, 24 percent are separated or divorced and another 5.7 percent are widowed. Thirty-five percent live alone, 10.5 percent live with their

TABLE 13.1 Sociodemographic Characteristics of Clients, by Gender

Characteristic	Female (n = 770)	Male (n = 801)	Total (N = 1,571)
Age (average years)	47.5	42.0	44.7****
Race (%)			
Non-Hispanic White	98.5	98.1	98.3
African American	0.4	1.0	0.7
Native American	0.4	0.3	0.3
Hispanic	0.1	0.5	0.3
Other	0.3	0.2	0.3
Education (%)			
Less than high school	31.5	28.9	30.2
High school	42.7	42.4	42.5
Post high school	18.1	21.4	19.8
College	7.7	7.3	7.5
Marital status (%)			
Never married	36.1	71.9	54.4****
Separated or divorced	32.5	15.7	24.0
Widowed	10.6	1.0	5.7
Married	20.8	11.3	16.0
Living status (%)			
Alone	36.1	34.6	35.3****
Family of origin	4.3	16.5	10.5
Family of procreation	29.1	13.5	21.1
With other adults (independently)	11.9	15.4	13.7
Supported living	17.5	18.6	18.1
Other	1.0	1.5	1.3
Region (%)			
Urban	69.2	74.9	72.1**
Rural	30.8	25.1	27.9
Employment status (%)			
Unemployed	63.6	53.8	58.6***
Employed part of year	15.6	21.6	18.7
Employed all year	20.9	24.5	22.7
Income (gross monthly)	$611.00	$650.00	$630.00*
Medicaid-eligible (%)	70.3	64.5	67.3*

NOTE: Ns with complete data on each contrast range from 1,419 (income) to 1,571.
*$p < .05$. **$p < .01$. ***$p < .001$. ****$p < .0001$ for gender comparisons.

family of origin, and another 21 percent live with their families of procreation. Another 13.7 percent live independently, but with unrelated
adults, while 18 percent live in supported housing or in inpatient settings. Finally, although the vast majority of clients live in urban areas,
these are predominantly small to large towns, rather than large metro-

politan centers, which accounts for the relatively low numbers of clients of color.

The statistical tests for gender comparisons show patterns that are reflected in the larger population as well. Although there is no significant difference in education or in racial background, women are significantly older than men in this sample. Moreover, they are more likely than the men to have married and to have experienced marital disruption, whether through separation, divorce, or widowhood. Furthermore, more women than men are currently married and living with their spouse and/or children. The vast majority of men, by contrast, have never married (71.9 percent of men vs. 36.1 percent of women). Moreover, if they live with family members, they are more likely to live with their family of origin (16.5 percent) than with their family of procreation (13.5 percent). Men are also significantly more likely than women to reside in urban, rather than rural, areas of the state.

Women's greater economic disadvantage within this population of individuals with serious mental illness is reflected both in their gross monthly incomes, which are significantly lower than men's, and in the high proportion of women (63.6 percent) compared with men (53.8 percent) who have been out of the labor market for at least the full year prior to the study. Indeed, fully 70 percent of the women are Medicaid-eligible compared with 64.5 percent of the men, which is another indication of the extent to which this population, and particularly women, are impoverished.

In Table 13.2 we present additional client characteristics, including their abuse histories, age of illness onset, most recent diagnoses, and course and cost of care over the index year. Again, the data are broken down by gender and a statistical test of the gender comparison has been performed, using either a t test or χ^2 statistic.

The abuse reports show several interesting findings. First, almost a third of the clients' abuse histories are unknown to their case managers. Those that are known show that women are significantly more likely to have histories of abuse than men. Approximately 23 percent of women and 8.5 percent of men are reported to have had physical abuse in their histories, and 21.2 percent of women and 3.6 percent of men have known histories of sexual abuse. Moreover, a notable percentage of clients, women in particular, have histories of both forms of abuse (13.5 percent vs. 2.5 percent). Thus, women's known abuse rates are substan-

TABLE 13.2 Abuse Histories, Diagnoses, and the Course and Cost of Care, by Gender

Characteristic	Female (n = 770)	Male (n = 801)	Total (N = 1571)
Abuse histories (%)			
Physical abuse, any	23.0	8.5	15.6****
Sexual abuse, any	21.2	3.6	12.2****
Both abuses	13.5	2.5	7.9****
No abuse	44.7	62.9	53.9****
Unknown	33.5	32.1	32.8
Age of illness onset	29.1	25.6	27.0****
Diagnosis (primary) (%)			
Schizophrenia	48.8	65.0	57.0****
Schizoaffective	13.2	9.0	11.1**
Bipolar depression	12.8	11.5	12.2
Unipolar depression	15.5	6.5	10.5****
Organic brain syndrome	1.3	1.5	1.4
Borderline personality disorder	3.7	0.1	1.9
Other	22.4	16.8	19.5****
Outpatient services (average hours per year)	180	188.0	184
Residential care (average days per year)	34.6	28.8	31.6
Inpatient care			
Average days in nursing home	4.85	5.19	5.02
Average days in psychiatric impatient	12.7	18.6	15.7*
Cost of care: Average cost of all care over past year	$6,610	$7,442	$6,987

NOTE: *N*s with complete data on each contrast range from 1,408 (residential days) to 1,571.
*$p < .05$. **$p < .01$. ***$p < .001$. ****$p < .0001$ for gender comparisons.

tially higher than men's, although both rates are much lower than reported in several studies of adults with serious mental illness.[1-11] This is most likely because the abuse information came from case managers, who were not required to assess for abuse histories and, thus, were likely to underestimate true rates of abuse for their clients.

We noted earlier that the average age of these clients is 44.7 years. As shown in Table 13.2, the average age of illness onset is 27 years of age. Thus, this client population has, on average, a 15-year history of illness, although we do not know much about the course of their illnesses. What we do know is that all presumably meet the state's criteria for a chronic mental illness. Within this broad diagnostic category, the vast majority of clients suffer from symptoms of schizophrenia (57 percent) or schizoaffective disorders (11 percent). Twelve percent are diagnosed as having a bipolar disorder, and 10.5 percent have major depressive disorders. Less than 2 percent have organic brain syndrome; another 2 percent are diagnosed as having borderline personality disorder. Other diagnostic categories account for the remaining 20 percent of the sample.

Gender differences in rates of the different disorders are largely specific to four diagnostic groups. That is, males are significantly more likely to have a diagnosis of schizophrenia than are females (65 percent vs. 49 percent). Females, by contrast, have significantly higher rates than males of schizoaffective disorders (13.2 percent vs. 9 percent), major depressive disorders (15.5 percent vs. 6.5 percent), and a group of disorders not specified (22.4 percent vs. 16.8 percent). They are also more likely to receive a diagnosis of borderline personality disorder (3.7 percent vs. 0.1 percent), although the differences are not significant due to the small numbers of persons in the sample with this diagnosis.

We turn now to the final section of the table that presents data on the course and cost of care. The average cost of care over the index year is somewhat higher for males ($7,442) than for females ($6,610), although these differences are not statistically significant. However, males do spend, on average, significantly more days in inpatient care (18.6 days vs. 12.7 days) than do females. In fact, there is no evidence that women receive services of any kind more frequently than do their male counterparts.

Plan of Analysis

In the analysis that follows, we used structural equation modeling to investigate the hypothesized links between gender, abuse histories, and the course and cost of care. Based on initial exploratory analyses, we chose to use separate measures of physical and sexual abuse, because they have different associations with other constructs in the model, despite their common co-occurrence for a number of participants. Thus, we will be examining each of their influences on the course and cost of care, independent of their common covariation in a portion of the sample.

The data screening and preparation were performed with PRELIS II,[50] with values imputed for missing data on RESIDENTIAL DAYS and NURSING HOME DAYS. Subsequently, a listwise deletion of data with missing values for any of the variables in the analyses yielded a final sample size of $N = 1,510$, representing 64.8 percent of clients from whom consent was sought and 78.1 percent of those who signed a consent form. A comparison of respondents and nonrespondents yielded no significant differences in the variables employed in the present analysis.

The analysis, which was performed with LISREL VIII,[51] proceeded in three steps. First, we estimated a model, Model 1, in which cost of care was regressed on abuse histories to determine if sexual abuse or physical abuse or both are associated with a significantly higher cost of care in contrast to those with no abuse history. A dummy variable was included for those whose histories are unknown to control for their costs without eliminating them from the analysis. In the second model, Model 2, we include gender, age, and Medicaid status to investigate the link between gender, abuse histories, and cost of care, controlling for age and Medicaid status. Finally, in Model 3, we added measures of course of care to the model to investigate hypothesized pathways to higher cost of care for men and women.

RESULTS

Model 1: Abuse Histories and Cost of Care

We begin our analysis with a test of the hypothesized link between abuse histories and cost of care. The model presented in Figure 13.1 shows the regression of cost of care on abuse histories of clients as reported by their case managers. We have included three measures of abuse in our model: physical abuse histories, sexual abuse histories, and abuse histories unknown. Thus, the coefficients for the model, which are presented in standardized form, represent a comparison of each type of abuse history with those with no abuse histories, which are the omitted category in the analysis.

This model reveals four noteworthy findings. First, clients with known sexual abuse histories have significantly higher service costs

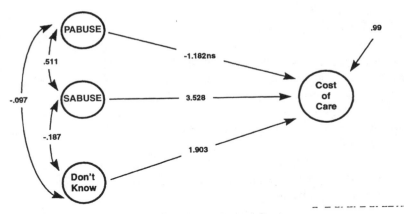

Figure 13.1. Model 1: Abuse Histories and Cost of Care
NOTE: $\chi^2 = 0$, $df = 0$, $p = 1.000$. PABUSE = yes response to physical abuse question; SABUSE = yes response to sexual abuse question.

over the course of the year than do clients with no history of abuse (the omitted category) by an average of $3,528.00 for the index year. Second, despite the fact that there is a strong positive association between having a history of both physical and sexual abuse (.511), physical abuse histories are not associated with a significantly higher cost of care. Indeed, if anything, physical abuse seems to suppress the cost of care, as shown by the negative, but nonsignificant, coefficient (–1.182 ns). By contrast, those whose abuse histories are unknown have significantly higher cost of care than those with no abuse history, averaging $1,903.00 for the index year. Finally, although we find support for the hypothesis that people with abuse histories have significantly higher mental health care costs than those who have no abuse histories, abuse histories account for only 1 percent of the variance in total cost of care.

To illustrate these associations in dollar terms, we display the average cost of care associated with each of the four groups of clients in Figure 13.2. These dollar amounts show rather dramatically the high average cost of care among clients with histories of sexual abuse ($9,701) compared with those with no known abuse history ($6,173). Moreover, they show a very similar, although less dramatic, pattern for those whose abuse histories are unknown, whose average cost of care was $8,076 for the index year. Interestingly, a history of physical abuse, de-

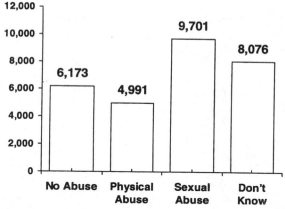

Figure 13.2. Abuse Histories and Cost of Care (in thousands of dollars)

spite the fact that it often accompanies sexual abuse, seems to have a suppressor effect on the cost of care. Indeed a statistical test of the differences in cost of care associated with physical and sexual abuse shows that the difference of $4,710 is statistically significant.

Why then, one might ask, do histories of abuse not account for more of the variance in cost of care, as shown in Model 1? The answer rests with the substantial variation in cost of care within the contrasting abuse categories. We turn now to Model 2, which incorporates other measures that may reduce some of the variability.

Model 2: Abuse Histories and Cost of Care, Controlling for Gender, Age, and Medicaid Status

In Model 2, presented in Figure 13.3, we show the link between abuse histories and cost of care, controlling for gender, age, and Medicaid status. We included the latter variable in the model because of its link to gender, as well as to cost of care, given that Medicaid benefits are an important source of money for services to adults with serious mental illness. We have also fixed all nonsignificant paths at zero.

First, the χ^2 (5, $N = 1,510$) = 8, $p = .13$, shows that the overall fit of the model to the data is very good. This is also shown by the adjusted goodness-of-fit index (AGFI) of .991. Thus, we can assume that paths fixed

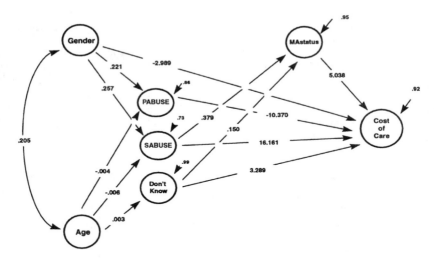

Figure 13.3. Model 2: Abuse Histories and Cost of Care, Controlling for
Gender, Age, and Medicaid Status
NOTE: $\chi^2 = 8$, $df = 5$, $p = .13$. PABUSE = yes response to physical abuse question; SABUSE = yes re-
sponse to sexual abuse question; MAstatus = Medicaid status.

at zero are plausible, as is the structure of the model. An important
question is: Has the relation between abuse histories and cost of care
been substantially altered with the addition of these variables to the
model? The answer is a qualified yes.

Clients with sexual abuse histories, as well as clients whose abuse
histories are unknown, have significantly higher costs of care than those
with no abuse history, replicating the finding in Model 1. However, in
this model, the relationships are even stronger than in the former and
are mediated through two paths of influence. First, we find that clients
with sexual abuse histories and unknown abuse histories are more
likely than those with no abuse history to be Medicaid-eligible, which,
in turn, is linked to a higher cost of care by an average of $5,038 for the
index year in contrast to those who are not Medicaid-eligible. Second,
independent of this path of influence, sexual abuse has a direct association with cost of care amounting to an average of $16,161 more for the
index year than those with no known abuse history. A similar, albeit
weaker association between abuse history and cost of care is shown for

those whose abuse history is unknown ($3,289). Thus, sexual abuse histories have both significant direct and indirect effects on cost of care, a cost trajectory pattern that is very similar to that found for clients whose abuse histories are unknown. Persons with histories of physical abuse, on the other hand, have significantly lower care costs than those with no known abuse by an average of $10,370 for the index year.

If one looks at the path of influence of both gender and age on cost of care, we can understand why the abuse coefficients are larger in Model 2 than in Model 1. We noted earlier that women in this sample of clients are significantly older than men, which accounts for the positive correlation between age and gender in the model (coded "1" for women and "0" for men). Although gender is positively related to having a reported history of physical or sexual abuse, age is not. In fact, older clients are significantly less likely than younger clients to have a reported history of physical or sexual abuse, but more likely to have abuse histories that are unknown.

A second important finding in this model is the direct path between gender and cost of care with the negative coefficient of −2.989 associated with it. What this coefficient tells us is that the cost of care for women is significantly lower than the cost of care for men by $2,989 for the index year, once we have controlled for the cost-inflating effects of sexual abuse histories for women. Thus, although we find no significant difference in the cost of care for men and women overall, these findings suggest support for our hypothesis that the pathways to higher mental health care costs for men and women may be different.

Model 3: Abuse Histories, Course, and Cost of Care, Controlling for Gender, Age, and Medicaid Status

We turn now to our final model, Model 3 presented in Figure 13.4, which includes four measures of what we referred to earlier as our course-of-care constructs: (1) number of days of inpatient care for the index year, (2) number of days of residential care for the same period, (3) number of days of nursing home care, and (4) number of outpatient hours over the course of the index year. Again, as with Model 2, we have fixed all nonsignificant paths; thus, all paths shown are significantly different from zero.

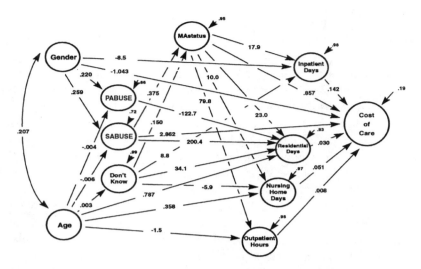

Figure 13.4. Model 3: Abuse Histories, Course, and Cost of Care, Controlling
for Gender, Age, and Medicaid Status
NOTE: χ^2 = 19, df = 17, p = .332. PABUSE = yes response to physical abuse question; SABUSE = yes
response to sexual abuse question; MAstatus = Medicaid status.

The overall goodness-of-fit statistics show that the model affords a
good fit to the data. This is shown both by the χ^2 (17, N = 1,571) = 19, p
= .322, and by the AGFI of .998. In short, we cannot reject the hypothesis
that this is the true model underlying the observed pattern of relations
among the observed data. Indeed, the addition of the course-of-care
measures in the model accounts for 81 percent of the variance in cost of
care, a 73 percent increase over the former model. Let us turn, then, to
the substantive findings.

Earlier we hypothesized that abuse experiences are likely to increase
the risk of being hospitalized in crisis situations and increase the risk of
longer hospital stays, although they are unlikely to increase use of, or
access to, outpatient services. Do we find support for this hypothesis?
The answer, again, is a qualified yes. That is, although histories of sexual
abuse are not directly linked either with outpatient hours or inpatient
days, there is an indirect association, which is largely mediated by the
path linking sexual abuse histories with Medicaid status (.375). Medicaid status, in turn, is associated with more inpatient days (17.9 days),

more residential days (23.0 days), more nursing home days (10.0 days), and more outpatient hours (almost 80 hours of outpatient care over the index year), as well as a higher average cost of care ($857) independent of costs associated with these four service measures.

A second path linking sexual abuse histories with a higher cost of care is through its association with residential treatment. That is, persons with histories of sexual abuse have, on average, 200 more days of residential care over the index year than persons with no known history of abuse, each day costing an average of $30. Finally, the direct path from sexual abuse histories to cost of care shows that persons with sexual abuse histories cost, on average, $2,862 per year that is over and above the two other indirect paths of association.

Indeed, if we combine these indirect and direct paths linking histories of sexual abuse with the course and cost of care, we find that clients with histories of sexual abuse use, on average, 6.7 more inpatient days, 3.8 more nursing home days, 209 more residential treatment setting days, and 30 more hours of outpatient care than do their nonabused counterparts, resulting in an average of $10,888 higher overall service costs for the index year. Thus, much of the relation between sexual abuse histories and cost of care is indirect (73.7 percent of the total effect) and mediated through the use of more restrictive, and costly, living arrangements.

Interestingly, clients whose abuse histories are unknown have cost-of-care trajectories that closely parallel those of clients with known histories of sexual abuse, with a few notable exceptions. First, the link between unknown abuse status and Medicaid status is much weaker, as shown by the path coefficient of .150. Second, although unknown abuse histories are associated with more days of residential care over the index year, the average number of days is much smaller (34.1) compared with persons with sexual abuse histories. Moreover, persons whose histories are unknown have on average 5.9 fewer days of nursing home care than their nonabused counterparts. In fact, the only association that is stronger for persons with unknown abuse histories, compared with those with sexual abuse histories, is that the former is associated with more inpatient days (8.8) compared with those with no known abuse experiences. Again, if we combine the direct and indirect paths of association with cost of care, we find that persons whose abuse histories are unknown have 11.5 more inpatient days, 37.6 more residential days, and

11.95 more outpatient hours than those with no known abuse experiences, which translates into an average higher cost of care of $2,759 for the index year.

Physical abuse histories, by contrast, seem to have precisely the opposite association with cost of care. That is, they are associated with significantly fewer days in residential settings over the course of the year (123 fewer days), which translates into $3,701 less over the index year compared to persons with no known history of abuse. Thus, despite its positive association with histories of sexual abuse, physical abuse seems to diminish clinical contact of all sorts, contrary to our initial hypothesis.

Although these findings suggest that women who are being served in public mental health programs are more likely than men to be placed in restrictive settings as part of their treatment, which is likely to drive up the cost of their care, we must qualify this claim in two ways. First, this effect is largely specific to those clients who have histories of sexual abuse, which includes disproportionate numbers of women, particularly younger women. Second, once we have controlled for this cost-inflating factor, women, in the aggregate, have significantly lower overall cost of care than do men. This is shown by two paths of influence in the model: (1) the path between gender and inpatient days (associated with a coefficient of –8.5) and (2) the path between gender and cost of care (associated with a coefficient of –1.043). These findings indicate that women, on average, have 8.5 fewer inpatient days than do men, and cost on average $1,043 less over the index year, once we have controlled for the impact of abuse histories on cost of care. Thus, although men and women do not differ in overall cost of care for mental health services, these findings suggest that pathways to higher cost of care are very different for men and women.

SUMMARY AND IMPLICATIONS FOR MENTAL HEALTH SERVICES

Over the past 25 years, significant advances have been made in developing community treatment systems that reduce hospitalization rates, thereby controlling costs for persons with schizophrenia and other serious mental illnesses. Case management programs, continuous treatment teams, day treatment, and residential alternatives have all been part of this effort.[18-21,24] This is certainly the case in the state where this study took place.[49] However, the results presented in these analyses indicate that the many services that have been developed for most persons with serious mental illness are not achieving the same outcomes for persons with serious mental illness who have a sexual abuse history.

We must, of course, acknowledge that we know little about the quality or kind of community-based care that clients with serious abuse histories are receiving within the systems of care included in the present study. Nor do we know whether clients with histories of abuse are receiving treatment that addresses their trauma experiences. Thus, an important area for further inquiry is to determine in what ways, if any, attempts are being made to address the special problems of trauma survivors within existing case management, residential, and inpatient programs.

Given the concentration of sexual abuse survivors in more restrictive living settings, it is particularly imperative that we ask: How relevant are existing treatment programs in these higher-cost settings to the special problems and needs of victims of abuse? Indeed, is the pattern of more days in restrictive settings for persons with histories of sexual abuse a function of longer stays, or more frequent entries and exits, in contrast to those with no abuse history? Finally, to what extent is a greater use of such settings for persons with abuse histories a consequence of the failure of community-based case management programs to address the special needs of abuse victims? Clearly, answers to such questions must be sought in an effort to bring down the cost, as well as improve the quality, of care.

Harris[52] has recommended modifications in community and residential treatment programs for women diagnosed with severe mental illness who also have histories of sexual abuse. These include changing the case manager's approach and relationship with the client, reevaluating the use of medications, helping clients develop ways of experiencing and controlling feelings, making efforts to develop and/or replace social networks, educating clients about sexual abuse trauma, and modifying social skills training programs. Treatment approaches that incorporate these elements need to be designed, implemented, and evaluated to determine if inpatient and residential use, and the resulting higher cost of care, can be reduced.

Clearly, an important first step in such efforts is the need for a careful assessment of the client's abuse history, as well as revictimization experiences that may be more salient and recent in the lives of adults with serious mental illnesses. It is striking that in this sample of clients within ten community treatment systems in a state with fairly well-developed community mental health services, a third of the clients' histories of physical or sexual abuse were unknown to their case managers. Given the seriousness of symptoms that can result from histories of abuse, and the growing body of evidence documenting that substantial numbers of adults with serious mental illnesses have had such histories, it is critically important that case managers and other mental health professionals include this information in their assessment procedures. Training in assessment for histories of physical and/or sexual abuse should be incorporated into the educational programs of case managers and clinicians at all program levels.

Such assessments must be conducted for all clients, young and old, male and female, so that stereotypes about who are usual victims of abuse do not determine the trauma assessment process. For example, in the present study, patterns of service use are similar for persons with a known history of sexual abuse and for persons whose abuse history is unknown. Both have higher use of residential and inpatient care than persons with no abuse history or a history of only physical abuse. This finding raises the possibility that many of the persons in the "don't know" category may have a history of sexual abuse. Moreover, since many of the "don't knows" are older women, it may be that case managers and others do not think of older women as being sexually abused or sexually active or simply feel it would be inappropriate to ask.

Another important finding of the study that has clear implications for the assessment process is the very different effect that physical and sexual abuse histories have on service use and cost of care. That is, although persons with histories of sexual abuse often have histories of physical abuse, physical abuse appears to suppress cost of care largely through diminishing clinical contacts of all kinds. For example, persons with histories of physical abuse have significantly fewer days of inpatient care and residential care than persons with histories of sexual abuse. Moreover, there was a general pattern of negative coefficients in the model linking physical abuse histories with utilization patterns, although all were not statistically significant.

These findings suggest that when designing services for persons who are abuse survivors, it is essential to explore all forms of abuse in the client's history. Indeed, one of the factors that may complicate the clinical picture for some sexual abuse survivors is a mixed history of both physical and sexual abuse. Persons with such histories may be more ambivalent about using services, as well as more unpredictable in their feelings and behaviors toward service providers, than persons with a sexual abuse history only or no abuse. Alternatively, persons who have a history of physical abuse, in the absence of other abuse experiences, may be particularly reticent to reach out for help or trust the help that is offered. These observations suggest that the particular configuration of services needed, or the way in which they are offered, may be quite different for persons with different kinds or combinations of abuse experiences.

As we move toward managed care for adults with serious mental illnesses, the higher use of inpatient care for persons with a history of sexual abuse is a finding that has important fiscal implications. Rather than simply restricting access to the hospital as a response, managed care programs should review the appropriateness of the assessment and treatment being provided to persons with histories of abuse. Our findings suggest that an assessment of physical and/or sexual abuse should be required prior to the commencement of treatment. If more appropriate community treatment is provided to persons who have such histories, inpatient use may be reduced without the need for arbitrary restrictions.

In conclusion, this study documents the increased cost of care for persons with serious mental illness who have a history of sexual abuse. Advocates, survivors, policymakers, treatment providers, and researchers must now join together to demand that treatment programs designed to meet the special needs of abuse survivors be developed, implemented, and evaluated. Failure to do so is costly in both human and financial resources and is a form of systematic discrimination against women that must be addressed.

REFERENCES

1. Briere JN, Zaidi LY: Sexual abuse histories and sequelae in female psychiatric emergency room patients. *American Journal of Psychiatry* 1989; 146(12):1602-1606.
2. Rose SM, Peabody CG, Stratigeas B: Undetected abuse among intensive case management clients. *Hospital and Community Psychiatry* 1991; 42(5):499-503.
3. Muenzenmaier K, Meyer I, Struening E, et al.: Childhood abuse and neglect among women outpatients with chronic mental illness. *Hospital and Community Psychiatry* 1993; 44(7):666-670.
4. Lipschitz DS, Kaplan ML, Sorkenn JB, et al.: Prevalence and characteristics of physical and sexual abuse among psychiatric outpatients. *Psychiatric Services* 1996; 47(2):189-191.
5. Ross CA, Anderson G, Clark P: Childhood abuse and the positive symptoms of schizophrenia. *Hospital and Community Psychiatry* 1994; 45(5):489-491.
6. Darves-Bornoz JM, Lemperiere T, Degiovanni A, et al.: Sexual victimization in women with schizophrenia and bipolar disorder. *Social Psychiatry and Psychiatric Epidemiology* 1995; 30:78-84.
7. Friedman S, Harrison G: Sexual histories, attitudes, and behavior of schizophrenic and "normal" women. *Archives of Sexual Behavior* 1984; 13(6):555-567.
8. Beck JC, van der Kolk B: Reports of childhood incest and current behavior of chronically hospitalized psychotic women. *American Journal of Psychiatry* 1987; 144(11):1474-1476.
9. Bryer JB, Nelson BA, Baker Miller J, Krol PA: Childhood sexual and physical abuse as factors in adult psychiatric illness. *American Journal of Psychiatry* 1987; 144(11):1426-1430.
10. Carlin AS, Ward NG: Subtypes of psychiatric inpatient women who have been sexually abused. *Journal of Nervous and Mental Disease* 1992; 180(6):392-397.
11. Carmen E, Rieker P, Mills T: Victims of violence and psychiatric illness. *American Journal of Psychiatry* 1984; 141(3):378-383.
12. Jacobson A, Herald C: The relevance of childhood sexual abuse to adult psychiatric inpatient care. *Hospital and Community Psychiatry* 1990; 41(2):154-158.
13. Henson CE, Colliver JA, Craine LS, et al.: Prevalence of a history of sexual abuse among female psychiatric patients in a state hospital system. *Hospital and Community Psychiatry* 1988; 39(3):300-304.
14. Rose SM, Peabody CG, Stratigeas B: Responding to hidden abuse: A role for social work in reforming mental health systems. *Social Work* 1991; 36(5):408-413.
15. Carmen EH: Inner-city community mental health: The interplay of abuse and race in chronically mentally ill women. In: Willie CV, Rieker PP, Kramer BM, Brown BS (Eds.): *Mental Health, Racism, and Sexism*. Pittsburgh, PA: University of Pittsburgh Press, 1995, pp. 217-236.
16. Jennings A: On being invisible in the mental health system. In: Levin BL, Blanch AK, Jennings A (Eds.): *Women's Mental Health Services: A Public Health Perspective*. Thousand Oaks, CA: Sage, 1998, pp. 326-347.
17. Herman J: *Trauma and Recovery*. New York: Harper Collins, 1992.
18. Weisbrod BA, Test MA, Stein LI: Alternative to mental hospital treatment: II. Economic benefit-cost analysis. *Archives of General Psychiatry* 1980; 37:400-405.

19. Quinlivan R, Hough R, Crowell A, et al.: Service utilization and cost of care for severely mentally ill clients in an intensive case management program. *Psychiatric Services* 1995; 46:365-371.

20. Jerrell JM, Hu T: Cost-effectiveness of intensive clinical and case management compared with an existing system of care. *Inquiry* 1989; 26:224-234.

21. Goldberg D: Cost-effectiveness studies in the treatment of schizophrenia: A review. *Schizophrenia Bulletin* 1991; 17:453-459.

22. Reed SK, Hennessy KD, Mitchell OS, et al.: A mental health capitation program: II. Cost-benefit analysis. *Hospital and Community Psychiatry* 1994; 45:1097-1103.

23. Wolff N, Helminiak TW, Diamond RJ: Estimated societal costs of assertive community mental health care. *Psychiatric Services* 1995; 46:898-906.

24. Dickey B, Binner PR, Leff S, et al.: Containing mental health treatment costs through program design: A Massachusetts study. *American Journal of Public Health* 1989; 79:863-867.

25. Ross CA, Dua V: Psychiatric health care costs of multiple personality disorder. *American Journal of Psychotherapy* 1993; 47:103-112.

26. Shern DL, Coen AS, Bradley L, et al.: The comprehensive costs of chronic mental illness: Estimates from two Colorado communities. In: *Proceedings of the National Association of State Mental Health Program Directors Research Institute National Conference on State Mental Health Service Systems Research*. Arlington, VA: National Association of State Mental Health Program Directors Research Institute, 1990, pp. 73-78.

27. Beecham J, Knapp M, Fenyo A: Cost, needs, and outcomes. *Schizophrenia Bulletin* 1991; 17:427-439.

28. Dickey B, McGuire TG, Cannon NL, et al.: Mental health cost models: Refinements & applications. *Medical Care* 1986; 24:857-866.

29. Smith ME, Loftus-Rueckheim P: Service utilization patterns as determinants of capitation rates. *Hospital and Community Psychiatry* 1993; 44:49-53.

30. Rubin J: Cost measure and cost data in mental health settings. *Hospital and Community Psychiatry* 1982; 33:750-754.

31. Kivlahan DR, Heiman JR, Wright RC, et al.: Treatment cost and rehospitalization rate in schizophrenic outpatients with a history of substance abuse. *Hospital and Community Psychiatry* 1991; 42:609-614.

32. Dickey B, Azeni H: Persons with dual diagnoses of substance abuse and major mental illness. *American Journal of Public Health* 1996; 86:973-977.

33. Finkelhor D: *Sexually Abused Children*. New York: Free Press, 1979.

34. Russell DEH. The incidence and prevalence of intra-familial and extra-familial sexual abuse of female children. *Child Abuse & Neglect* 1983; 7:133-146.

35. Siegel JM, Sorensen SB, Goldberg JM, et al. The prevalence of childhood sexual assault: Los Angeles Epidemiologic Catchment Area project. *American Journal of Epidemiology* 1987; 121:1141-1153.

36. Wyatt GE: The sexual abuse of African American and White American women in childhood. *Child Abuse & Neglect* 1985; 9:507-519.

37. Gelles RJ, Strauss MA: Is violence toward children increasing? A comparison of 1975 and 1985 national survey rates. *Journal of Interpersonal Violence* 1987; 2:212-222.

38. Briere J: *Child Abuse Trauma: Theory and Treatment of Lasting Effects*. Newbury Park, CA: Sage, 1992.

39. Brown GR, Anderson B: Psychiatric morbidity in adult inpatients with childhood histories of sexual and physical abuse. *American Journal of Psychiatry* 1991; 148(1):55-61.

40. Felitti VJ: Long-term medical consequences of incest, rape, and molestation. *Southern Medical Journal* 1991; 84(3):328-331.
41. Mitchell D, Gatson Grindel C, Laurenzano C: Sexual abuse assessment on admission by nursing staff in general hospital psychiatric settings. *Psychiatric Services* 1996; 47(2):159-164.
42. Eilenberg J, Thompson Fullilove M, Goldman RG, et al.: Quality and use of trauma histories obtained from psychiatric outpatients through mandated inquiry. *Psychiatric Services* 1996; 47(2):165-169.
43. Kent S, Fogarty M, Yellowlees P: A review of studies of heavy users of psychiatric services. *Psychiatric Services* 1995; 46:1247-1253.
44. Kent S, Fogarty M, Yellowlees P: Heavy utilization of inpatient and outpatient services in a public mental health service. *Psychiatric Services* 1995; 46:1254-1257.
45. Kent S, Yellowlees P: Psychiatric and social reasons for frequent rehospitalization. *Hospital and Community Psychiatry* 1994; 45:347-350.
46. Geller JL: In again, out again: Preliminary evaluation of a state hospital's worst recidivist. *Hospital and Community Psychiatry* 1986; 37:386-390.
47. Ellison JM, Blum NR, Barsky AJ, et al.: Frequent repeaters in a psychiatric emergency service. *Hospital and Community Psychiatry* 1989; 40:958-960.
48. Hadley TR, Culhane DP, McGurrin MC, et al.: Identifying and tracking "heavy users" of acute psychiatric inpatient services. *Administration and Policy in Mental Health* 1992; 19:279-290.
49. Wisconsin Department of Health and Human Services: *Wisconsin Mental Health Plan for Federal Fiscal Year, 1996*. Madison: Wisconsin Department of Health and Human Services, 1995.
50. Jöreskog KG, Sörbom D: *PRELIS II*. Mooresville, IN: Scientific Software, 1996.
51. Jöreskog KG, Sörbom D: *LISREL VIII*. Mooresville, IN: Scientific Software, 1996.
52. Harris M: Modifications in services delivery and treatment for women diagnosed with severe mental illness who are also survivors of sexual abuse trauma. In: Levin BL, Blanch AK, Jennings A (Eds.): *Women's Mental Health Services: A Public Health Perspective*. Thousand Oaks, CA: Sage, 1998, pp. 309-325.

14

Modifications in Services Delivery and Clinical Treatment for Women Diagnosed With Severe Mental Illness Who Are Also Survivors of Sexual Abuse Trauma

Maxine Harris, Ph.D.

Investigative reporting within the popular press has brought to light the incidence of childhood sexual abuse trauma, domestic violence, and sexual intimidation and harassment within the general population of women. More recently, scientific researchers have turned their attentions to discovering the rates of sexual abuse trauma in the lives of women diagnosed with serious mental illness.[1-3] Before clinicians and program planners begin making alterations in treatment protocols to address sexual abuse trauma in the lives of women with severe mental illness, two definitional issues must be addressed. First, what do we mean by sexual abuse trauma, and second, how do we define the population of women diagnosed with severe mental illness?

NOTE: This chapter appeared as an article in the *Journal of Mental Health Administration*, 1994, Vol. 21, No. 4, pp. 397-406.

Although distinctions can be made between sexual abuse trauma that occurs in childhood when cognitive and emotional schemata for understanding self and others are first forming, and abuse that occurs in adulthood as rape or domestic violence, many recent attempts to establish prevalence rates tend to aggregate sexual abuse that occurs in childhood with abuse that occurs later in adulthood.[4] This tendency to combine the two types of abuse may stem from the fact that women sexually abused in childhood are more likely to be victimized as adults resulting in substantial overlap between the two groups.[5] The tendency to group childhood and adult survivors of sexual trauma may also stem from a recognition that similar treatments apply regardless of when the trauma occurred.[6] For the purposes of this chapter, "sexual abuse trauma" will be used to refer to sexual assault experiences sustained during childhood and/or adulthood.

The designation "severe or chronic mental illness" also requires some clarification. It is generally accepted that such labeling does not refer exclusively to diagnosis, but rather that it takes into account both the duration of a person's psychiatric symptoms and the extent to which those symptoms impair level of functioning.[7] It is unclear, however, what role, if any, a history of sexual abuse trauma might play in a woman's being labeled as "severely" or "chronically" mentally ill. One study of female psychiatric inpatients suggests that those with a history of abuse are more likely than a nonabused cohort to have severe, psychotic-like symptoms; to be diagnosed as having borderline personality disorder; and to have suicidal symptoms.[8] It may well be, although it remains to be proven, that sexual abuse trauma is one route to patienthood for at least some women who come to be diagnosed as severely mentally ill.

While it is true that more research needs to be done before we fully understand the role that sexual abuse trauma plays in the lives of women diagnosed with severe mental illness, those studies that have been done reveal sufficient prevalence rates (from 34 percent in case management clients[3] to 51 percent in state hospital psychiatric patients[2]) to move clinicians and program planners to begin modifying treatment interventions to accommodate the special needs and vulnerabilities of trauma survivors. Treatment services for clients diagnosed with severe mental illness generally include case management, residential placement and supervision, inpatient hospitalization, medication management, network intervention, and social skills training. Each of these treatment or service interventions must be grounded in an understanding of the trauma experience and adapted to accommodate the vulnerabilities of the trauma survivor. The purpose of this chapter is to suggest a series of clinical and programmatic modifications in customary and usual treatment for persons diagnosed with severe mental illness that might render those treatments more suitable to women who have experienced sexual abuse trauma.

CASE MANAGEMENT

Case management is a systems and services intervention designed to coordinate, access, and often provide the full range of care that a person with severe mental illness needs to live in the community. Regardless of their theoretical orientation, case managers often share a willingness to be flexible and to bend the rules of traditional treatment, a sense of informality and collegiality that extends to both co-workers and clients, and a commitment to aggressive outreach.[9] Paradoxically, these very qualities, so important when engaging deinstitutionalized clients, may pose problems when working with trauma survivors. Trauma survivors are all too familiar with pseudo-intimate relationships in which traditional boundaries are violated and the will of the other is aggressively asserted "for their own good."

To avoid replicating the interpersonal dynamics of the abusive relationship, case managers must follow a set of guidelines that substitute structure and predictability for informality and flexibility:

1. Case managers should establish contracts with clients that spell out the obligations and responsibilities of both parties. The limits of the case management relationship should be articulated in these contracts; similarly, the terms under which the relationship will take place should be clarified;

2. Case managers should let clients know what they are going to do in advance of actually doing it. Even simple activities such as filling out a form should proceed with, "Now we are going to fill out this form; I will ask you 10 questions; the questions will all concern your medical

history." By walking the client through an interaction before it occurs, the case manager makes the encounter predictable and safe;

3. While case managers might do well to ask permission before they intervene with any client, they *must* ask permission when dealing with the survivors of sexual abuse trauma. Simple activities like making a home visit, riding in a car, or attending a recreational activity need to be agreed on in advance and need to proceed with the stated consent of the client. Such agreements not only demonstrate respect for the client's wishes but also give the client control over the interaction; and

4. Clients must have the right to say no to services. Case managers who are concerned with providing services to disenfranchised, "difficult" individuals sometimes forget that clients should always retain the right to reject services. When case managers foist services on unwilling clients, they risk creating an atmosphere in which a controlling adult asks a vulnerable child to do something that the child knows she does not want to do, in effect replicating the very dynamics of the trauma itself.

Because case management entails a relationship between two people in addition to being a services and treatment intervention,[10] case managers must be especially mindful of who they are when working with trauma survivors. One must be particularly cognizant of one's interpersonal style and how that style might be seen by a woman who has experienced abuse. Some variables that need to be considered are the following.

Degree of openness and friendliness. Because they have been abused in relationships that were supposed to be benign or positive, trauma survivors are naturally distrustful of new relationships. A case manager who is "too open" and "too friendly" may cause a client to ask somewhat suspiciously, "What does he/she want, anyway?"

Tendency toward being hierarchical and authoritarian. Since abusers use power to threaten and intimidate victims, clients are often wary of a case manager who is invested in "being in charge." For some clients, any relationship in which a power imbalance exists may be reminiscent of the abuse relationship.[4]

Degree to which one appears self-effacing and fragile. Because trauma survivors have an ambivalent, at best, relationship to their own "victim"-selves, they are often disdainful or even rageful toward case managers who appear too vulnerable. The client needs to believe that the case manager is strong enough to handle the powerful emotions that might arise in working together.

Gender. Because most abuse is perpetrated by men toward women, the gender of the case manager is a significant issue.[11] Male case managers tend to be feared as potential abusers. Clients may also try to seduce a male clinician, believing that all men are interested only in sex. Female case managers, on the other hand, may be seen as failed protectors and thereby become targets for rageful attacks. In general, it is wise to address issues of gender and the accompanying misperceptions early in the case management relationship. Also, case managers need to be aware of their own emotional reactions when working with trauma survivors. Both peer and individual supervision can be useful in helping case managers recognize and deal with their own feelings and responses.

RESIDENTIAL PLACEMENT AND SUPERVISION

At some point in their histories, most individuals who have severe and persistent mental illness receive assistance in securing and maintaining housing. Housing options range from structured group homes to independent yet supervised apartments, but they almost always include some support and supervision on the part of residential counselors or clinical case managers.[12] Because of economic and programmatic realities, however, residents in supervised housing experience a lack of privacy, control, and safety. Yet privacy, control, and safety are exactly what trauma survivors need if they are to succeed in residential placements. Moreover, concerns about privacy, control, and safety apply equally to independent and group home placements. Regrettably, even on-site supervision does not eliminate the element of dangerousness from some group homes.

Privacy. In most group homes and supported apartments, residents must share not only living, but also sleeping quarters. Boundaries are often blurred and a room that serves as a living or dining room by day may convert into a bedroom at night. Lack of secure, private sleeping space becomes especially problematic for a trauma survivor whose bedroom was violated by intruders in the past. It becomes difficult for a clinician to help a client develop emotional and psychological boundaries when her most fundamental physical boundaries are not secured.

Control. In residential programs, rules about when and where people sleep are determined and imposed by residential staff. If an individual is residing in a group home, for example, there will be specific times for sleeping, and individuals will be required to sleep in designated bedrooms on assigned beds. While this may seem like a relatively simple requirement, it can be problematic for the survivor of sexual abuse trauma who may have learned that the only safe time to sleep is during the day and that beds are unsafe places in which to sleep.

In most housing arrangements, residents do not have complete control over who is allowed to come into the home. While one may be able to control one's own visitors, in a shared apartment or a group home one may have no control over the visitors of one's roommates.

Safety. Because of the lack of affordable housing, most residential programs operate in marginal neighborhoods. It is difficult to feel safe where break-ins, rapes, and murders are a daily occurrence.

To provide clients with much needed privacy, control, and safety, residential planners must be mindful of the following guidelines:

1. Clients need private sleeping quarters. When economic realities prevent private bedrooms, room dividers and screens should be used to demarcate individual sleeping space. All residents should be helped to respect the privacy of roommates;

2. Residents should be allowed to maintain idiosyncratic sleeping patterns that feel safe to them. At the same time, they must be helped to respect group norms;

3. Rules about visitors and proper conduct within the home should be established to accommodate the needs of the most vulnerable house member. Whenever possible, needs for privacy should be considered and discussed when matching housemates;

4. Clients should be presented with a range of housing options and allowed to choose that which feels most safe;

5. Extra precautions such as door locks and window bars should be installed to help residents feel safe, even in those circumstances in which residential staff deem the precautions to be unnecessary; and

6. Whenever possible, planners should establish creative public/private partnerships to develop or subsidize more safe, affordable housing.

INPATIENT HOSPITALIZATION

Most adults diagnosed with severe mental illness will experience at least one inpatient stay over the course of their psychiatric treatment. Hospitalization is often indicated for the survivors of sexual abuse trauma who are suicidal, homicidal, psychotic, drug addicted, self-mutilating, or otherwise decompensating.[13] However, because many women with chronic mental illness have experienced sexual abuse or intimidation while being institutionalized, clinicians need to consider carefully how inpatient hospitalization will be used in the treatment of adult survivors of sexual abuse trauma who are diagnosed with severe mental illness.[14]

Before assuming that the hospital is a safe place, the clinician must understand the role that hospitals have played in the lives of individual survivors. In some cases, women were hospitalized and labeled as "crazy" when they first spoke of the abuse.[14] The hospital, rather than being a place of treatment, was an instrument of control and punishment. Many women who were hospitalized for long stays at public hospitals were abused while hospitalized.[14] The hospitalization thus became the site of more trauma.

When the need for inpatient and structured hospitalization does arise, clinicians need to carefully consider alternatives to traditional inpatient treatment as well as strategies for reframing inpatient treatment to render the hospitalization safe as well as therapeutic:

1. The alternative of using community-based and professionally staffed crisis beds should be considered. The need for a structured and safe environment is real; however, individuals can receive support and safe haven in environments other than hospitals;

2. When a hospitalization becomes necessary, it should, if possible, be voluntary and under the control of the patient herself. It is often useful to

establish contracts with individuals who both have chronic mental illness and are survivors of sexual abuse trauma, in which the client determines when and if a hospitalization will occur;

3. The rationale for an actual admission should be made explicit to the client as should the conditions for her release from the hospital. This explicit contracting makes the hospitalization a predictable experience rather than a frightening descent into a world over which the client has no control. Such contracting requires close coordination between the inpatient and outpatient treatment staffs; and

4. Clinicians should also reframe the hospitalization as being different from previous hospitalizations. Rather than meaning that the client is out of control and "crazy," this hospitalization means that the client is actually taking control of her life, asking for a safe space when she needs one, and demonstrating that she deserves to get the help that she requires.

MEDICATION MANAGEMENT

Most adults diagnosed with severe mental illness receive medications as part of their psychiatric treatment. Many receive several medications simultaneously. It is not uncommon to find a woman receiving antipsychotic, antidepressant, antianxiety, and possibly even antiseizure medication all at the same time. Regrettably, clinicians often medicate any sign of powerful affect in a client who has been labeled as "chronically mentally ill." Researchers have also found that there is a greater tendency to use psychotropic medications in adults who are survivors of abuse.[8]

Several factors may contribute to the manner and frequency with which psychotropic medications are prescribed. Some have suggested that the greater severity of symptoms has resulted in the increased use of medications.[8] It may also be possible that a lack of training and knowledge about sexual abuse trauma, coupled with exposure to media portrayals of trauma survivors as being out-of-control, has served to frighten practitioners into believing that they must medicate the powerful feelings of anger, sadness, and pain that accompany the exploration of a trauma history. Finally, medical practitioners historically have tended, in general, to "medicate away" the expression of powerful affect in female patients.[15]

Regardless of the reasons clients receive psychotropic medications, practitioners must be aware that otherwise helpful medications can contribute to the affective numbing so characteristic of many adult survivors of sexual abuse trauma. The ready use of medications to subdue or control feelings may also contribute to the client's naive beliefs that her feelings are bad and dangerous and should not be felt.

In light of a diagnostic reformulation that takes into account a trauma history, the medications of women diagnosed with severe mental illness who are the survivors of sexual abuse trauma need to be reevaluated. For some of these women, medications that address symptoms of anxiety and depression may be used to replace neuroleptic medications. Furthermore, it may be possible to use medications episodically and for a shorter duration rather than on a long-term, chronic basis. For other women, long-term antipsychosis medications may continue to be therapeutic. These evaluations will need to be made on an individual basis.

Recovery from sexual abuse trauma entails that the survivor feel powerful emotions of anger, pain, and sadness. Clients can, with the aid of clinical staff, experience their feelings and do so in ways that are safe and healthy. The relationship with a primary clinician or case manager creates a safe holding environment in which an adult survivor can begin to work through powerful feelings that have been locked away for a long time.

Both clinicians and clients must be trained to understand that starting to feel does not necessarily mean being overwhelmed by one's feelings. Clients can be taught to experience their feelings in small, manageable doses and can be given permission to shut down when feelings seem too powerful to control. As one client so aptly put it, "I can nibble at feelings rather than swallowing them whole."

Some of the expressive therapies used with women with nonchronic mental illness are appropriate for the chronic population with relatively little modification. Role plays, dance, movement and body work, anger and sadness rituals, and writing and drawing exercises are all viable techniques for work with women who are diagnosed with severe mental illness. These techniques are especially effective when the individual is also engaged in a close one-to-one relationship with a therapist or case manager in which the feelings can be worked through and further explored. By incorporating a variety of expressive therapies in treatment plans for clients who are trauma survivors, practitioners may find that they have to rely less on the use of psychotropic medications to control feelings and behaviors.

NETWORK INTERVENTIONS

The social support systems of adults diagnosed with severe mental illness are frequently impoverished. Research reveals that these networks contain fewer members and have scarcer resources than the networks of healthier adults of the same age.[16] Moreover, the reciprocity between individuals in relationships is often distorted with one member of the dyad doing most of the giving and the other member doing most of the taking. Because social support networks enhance one's ability to cope with crises and to function in general, interventions often focus on rehabilitating impoverished and diminished support networks.[17] These interventions seek to increase the size of the network or repair severed connections among network members. Clinicians often try to form an alliance with network members who can then assume some of the actual case management functions performed by mental health professionals.

Because trauma and abuse frequently occur in one's primary network, such interventions need to be modified when working with the survivors of sexual abuse trauma. First, clinicians must know the role that network members played in the abuse before routinely involving those network members in treatment. Clients should always have the option to refrain from contact with network members whom they deem to be dangerous and unsafe.

More difficult than honoring a client's request for no contact is the need to limit or modify contact when the network member is a past or current abuser and the client herself wants contact. Because their networks are so impoverished, these clients often desire to continue contact with network members who have been dangerous and abusive. In these cases, case managers need to find ways to permit contact to occur safely. Strategies similar to those used by child protective services with children whose abusive fathers have been removed from the home need to be adapted to working with adult survivors. It may be that contact should occur only, for example, when a disinterested and safe third person is also present.

Clinicians also need to be especially sensitive to the guilt and fear that a woman might feel if she is required to monitor and perhaps even report an abusive network member. Often abuse continues into the next generation, and a survivor of sexual abuse trauma may be witness to current abuse that is being perpetrated on her nieces, daughters, or granddaughters. Her own dilemma about whether to report a current abuser needs to be addressed within the clinical relationship. Issues of both loss and dangerousness must be considered.

Finally, case managers may need to focus on creating replacement networks for the survivors of sexual abuse trauma. New communities of women can join together to form replacement families.[18] Such efforts need to be encouraged and nurtured so that clients realize that distancing from an abusive network does not mean losing all social supports and human connections.

SOCIAL SKILLS TRAINING

Training in social and interpersonal skills is often based on the assumption that adults with severe mental illness do not have the interpersonal and practical skills needed to succeed in normal community living. The content of many social skills courses, known as modules, includes such behaviors as proper grooming, the use of leisure time, budgeting and money management, conversation initiation, and relationship building.

The first modification that clinicians must make in working with sexual abuse survivors in a social skills format is to understand the particular function that "apparent" skill deficits have served the abuse survivor. For example, many women consciously choose not to groom themselves because poor grooming protects them from further abuse and assault.[19] Other women who have been given money and gifts in exchange for sexual favors have difficulty managing money because, for them, taking money is shameful and reminiscent of acquiescing to sexual abuse. The difficulty these individuals have in managing their

help in accurately assessing dangerousness, respecting their own perceptions, and taking steps to make themselves safe.

Finally, decisions about sexuality need to address what it means to be seductive and flirtatious. Many women find themselves misreading the seductive behavior of others as well as being unclear about what nonverbal cues they themselves are giving. When sexuality has been confused, the whole idea of what it means to be seductive needs to be reexamined. Women need to be trained to attend to their own behavior as well as to learn what is normative behavior in intimate relationships.

Safety. Discussions of safety must address both physical and emotional safety and boundaries. Women need to be taught how to assess the actual dangers in their physical environment and how to take legitimate protective measures. For some women, this means avoiding certain neighborhoods at night; for others it may mean taking a self-defense course. All women must come to understand the limits on their abilities to avoid random physical violence.

Establishing emotional boundaries is especially difficult for trauma survivors. Women need to learn what rights they have in relationships, how to say no in a clear and direct way, and how to ask for what they need and want. For one whose most basic rights have been violated, it takes time and practice to begin to respect and to assert one's own needs and wishes in a relationship. A woman must be given support and encouragement that it is *always* right to take care of herself emotionally in a relationship.

Self-soothing. Women with serious mental illness need to be instructed in ways in which they can soothe themselves when they feel anxious, depressed, or frightened without using illegal substances, sexually acting out, or overmedicating themselves with prescription drugs. Techniques that help a woman to ground and center herself and to reestablish her own sense of who she is are especially important. It is also important for women to learn how to distract themselves from recurring thoughts and overwhelming feelings. Listening to music, meditating, watching television, or exercising often help a woman gain control over her own internal state. Women need to learn how to "talk themselves down," how to convince themselves that they have a right to live, and how to believe they can, in fact, get through the worst of times.

It is also important for women to know that certain standard defenses such as intellectual or compulsive activities are acceptable ways of modulating intense affect and anxiety. In the case of many, self-soothing begins by rereading notes or listening to tapes made by a therapist who instructs the woman in soothing "self-talk" to help her to cope with a difficult situation. All of these techniques come to be under the survivor's control and are understood as legitimate ways to manage one's anxiety and one's despair.

Regrettably, practitioners often believe that women diagnosed with serious mental illness do not have the same potential to soothe themselves that other men and women have, and consequently soothing often comes only via medication or hospitalization. If these women are to live successfully and independently in community environments, they need to learn ways to soothe themselves in the face of anxiety and depression.

Parenting. Although most women with serious mental illness do not raise their children full-time, many are mothers and have serious questions about how to be a good parent. If one has been raised in an abusive home where parenting was either neglectful or hurtful, one does not have a model of how to be a nurturing and constructive parent. Many women express fears over becoming abusive themselves and need to understand how to monitor their own behavior with children.

Several other issues that apply to motherhood and are especially salient for adult survivors of trauma include how to protect one's children without being overprotective, how to deal with one's envy over the safe childhood that one is providing for one's own children, and how to deal with the guilt one feels over not being able to raise one's children and guarantee their safety.

IMPLICATIONS FOR MENTAL HEALTH SERVICES DELIVERY

As clinicians and program planners begin to take into account the trauma histories of many women who have been diagnosed with severe mental illness, several modifications in services delivery must occur:

1. Assessment of current and childhood sexual abuse trauma must become part of the routine assessment of women diagnosed with serious mental illness.[5] Moreover, in addition to being performed at the time of intake, assessments might need to be conducted at several different times in an ongoing clinical relationship since some clients feel comfortable revealing a trauma history only after they have come to trust a service provider.

2. Clinical staff accustomed to working with persons diagnosed with severe mental illness must be trained to work with trauma survivors.

3. Existing treatment interventions for persons with serious mental illness must be revamped so as not to inadvertently retraumatize women who have suffered sexual abuse. In general, this means paying special attention to physical, psychological, and interpersonal boundaries.

4. Because trauma survivors often present with an array of symptoms (eating disorders, substance abuse histories, and psychiatric problems) that might well be treated by separate service delivery systems, overall coordination of an individual's treatment by a consistent and informed case manager is important.

While it may seem daunting to add yet another area of concern to the treatment of women who have serious mental illness, program planners would be remiss not to recognize the extent to which many women diagnosed with serious mental illness have suffered from sexual abuse trauma. An accurate assessment of the extent of trauma will allow clinicians to devise treatments that are truly relevant to the experiences of their clients. Current treatment approaches are adaptable for work with trauma survivors if clinicians take the necessary steps to accommodate the treatment program to a history of trauma.

REFERENCES

1. Beck JC, van der Kolk B: Reports of childhood incest and current behavior of chronically hospitalized psychotic women. *American Journal of Psychiatry* 1987; 144:1474-1476.

2. Craine LS, Henson CE, Colliver JA, et al.: Prevalence of a history of sexual abuse among female psychiatric patients in a state hospital system. *Hospital and Community Psychiatry* 1988; 39:300-304.

3. Rose SM, Peabody CG, Stratigeas B: Undetected abuse among intensive case management clients. *Hospital and Community Psychiatry* 1991; 42:499-503.

4. Jacobson A, Richardson B: Assault experiences of 100 psychiatric inpatients: Evidence of the need for routine inquiry. *American Journal of Psychiatry* 1987; 144:908-913.

5. Muenzenmaier K, Meyer I, Struening E, et al.: Childhood abuse and neglect among women outpatients with chronic mental illness. *Hospital and Community Psychiatry* 1993; 44:666-670.

6. Herman J: *Trauma and Recovery.* New York: Basic Books, 1993.

7. Bachrach LL: Defining chronic mental illness: A concept paper. *Hospital and Community Psychiatry* 1988; 39:383-388.

8. Bryer JB, Nelson BA, Miller JB, et al.: Childhood sexual and physical abuse as factors in adult psychiatric illness. *American Journal of Psychiatry* 1987; 144:1426-1430.

9. Harris M, Bergman HC (Eds.): *Case Management for Mentally Ill Patients.* Langhorne, PA: Harwood Academic, 1993.

10. Harris M, Bergman HC: Case management with the chronically mentally ill: A clinical perspective. *American Journal of Orthopsychiatry* 1987; 57:296-302.

11. Jacobson A, Herald C: The relevance of childhood sexual abuse to adult psychiatric inpatient care. *Hospital and Community Psychiatry* 1990; 41:154-158.

12. Bebout R, Harris M: In search of pumpkin shells: Residential programming for the homeless mentally ill. In: Lamb R, Bachrach LL, Kass FI (Eds.): *Treating the Homeless Mentally Ill.* Washington, DC: American Psychiatric Press, 1991.

13. Courtois CA: *Healing the Incest Wound.* New York: Norton, 1988.

14. Geller J, Harris M: *Women of the Asylum.* New York: Anchor, 1994.

15. Ehrenreich B, English D: *For Her Own Good.* New York: Doubleday, 1978.

16. Harris M, Bergman HC: Networking with young adult chronic patients. *Psychosocial Rehabilitation Journal* 1985; 8:28-35.

17. Harris M, Bergman HC, Bachrach L: Individualized network planning for young adult chronic patients. *Psychiatric Quarterly* 1986-1987; 58:51-56.

18. Bebout RR: Contextual case management: Restructuring the social support networks of seriously mentally ill adults. In: Harris M, Bergman HC (Eds.): *Case Management for Mentally Ill Patients.* Langhorne, PA: Harwood Academic, 1993, pp. 59-82.

19. Harris M: *Sisters of the Shadow.* Norman: Oklahoma University Press, 1991.

15

On Being Invisible in the Mental Health System

Ann Jennings, Ph.D.

This chapter brings into question one of the basic assumptions operating in the public mental health field today: that mental illness is biological or genetic in origin and is therefore treatable primarily by symptom control or management. A case study of my daughter Anna, a victim of early childhood sexual trauma, is used to demonstrate the need for inclusion in the field of an additional view of the etiology of mental illness. Forces supporting the emergence of a new trauma paradigm are highlighted.

ANNA'S STORY

From the age of 13 to her recent death at the age of 32, Anna was viewed and treated by the mental health system as "severely and chronically mentally ill." Communication about who she was, how she was perceived and treated, and how she responded took place through

NOTE: The reader is forewarned that to provide a realistic account of Anna's experience and her attempts to communicate it to others, explicit language and graphic descriptions of her behavior are included.

This chapter appeared as an article in the *Journal of Mental Health Administration*, 1994, Vol. 21, No. 4, pp. 374-387.

her mental health records. A review of 17 years of these records reveals her described in terms of diagnoses, medications, "symptoms," behaviors, and treatment approaches. She was consistently termed "noncompliant" or "treatment-resistant." Initially recorded childhood history was dropped from her later records. Her own insights into her condition were not noted.

When she was 22, Anna was re-evaluated after a suicide attempt. For a brief period, she was rediagnosed as suffering from acute depression and a form of post-traumatic stress disorder. This was the only time in her mental health career that Anna agreed with her diagnosis. She understood herself—not as a person with a "brain disease," but as a person who was profoundly hurt and traumatized by the "awful things" that had happened to her.

WHAT HAPPENED TO ANNA?

Anna was born in 1960, the third of five children, a beautiful, healthy baby with a wonderful disposition. At the age of about two and a half, she began to scream and cry inconsolably. At four, we took her to a child psychiatrist who found nothing wrong with her. When we placed her in nursery school, her problems seemed to lessen.

That Anna was being sexually abused and traumatized at the time is clear now, verified in later years by her own revelations and by the memories of others. Her memories of abuse by a male baby-sitter were vivid, detailed, and consistent in each telling over the years. They were further verified by persons close to the perpetrator and his family, one of whom witnessed the perpetrator years later in the act of abusing another child.

Anna described the experience of being forcibly restrained and sexually violated at the age of about three and a half: "He tied me up, put my hands over my head, blindfolded me with my little T-shirt, pulled my T-shirt over my head with nothing on below, opened my legs and was examining and putting things in me and all that . . . ugh. It hurt me. I would cry and he wouldn't stop. To do that when I was a little kid was like . . . uh, I don't know . . . it made me feel pretty bad. I remember after he did that I was walking toward the door out of the room and I was feeling like I was bad. And why not Sarah and Mary (her older and younger sisters) and why just me? And I had this feeling in me that I was bad, you know . . . a bad seed . . . and that I was the only one in the world."

Evidence that Anna was betrayed and sexually violated at an even earlier age by another perpetrator, a relative, came to light eventually through the revelations of a housekeeper whom Anna had confided in at the time. She had told this woman that a man "played with her where he wasn't supposed to" and that the man "hurted her." This abuse was kept secret for nearly 30 years.

Anna remembered trying to tell us, as a little child, what was happening, but there was no one to hear or respond. When she told me a man "fooled" with her, I assumed she meant a young neighborhood boy, and cautioned his parents. When we took her to a physician, she experienced the physical examination as yet another violation. "I remember the doctor you took me to when I told you. He did things to me that were disgusting (pointing to her genital area)."

The trauma Anna experienced was then compounded by the silence surrounding it. She tried to communicate with her rage, her screams, and her terror. She became the "difficult to handle" child. Her screaming and crying were frequently punished by spankings and confinement to her room. No one then could see or hear her truth; sexual abuse did not "exist" in our minds. When later, as a young girl, she withdrew within herself, somehow "different," and "apart" from her peers, we attributed it to her artistic talent or independent personality. We did not see or attend to the terror, dissociation, loneliness, and isolation expressed in her drawings, nor did we heed the hints of trouble expressed by her behaviors. Two grade school psychologists were alone among the professionals we encountered in sensing the turbulence underneath her silence. "Anna is confused about her sexual identity," one reported, "you must help her." The other wrote, "It would seem that Anna has suppressed or repressed traumatic incidents."

Chaos and parental conflict existed in Anna's family from the age of 11 to 13. Though her four brothers and sisters survived the multiple geographic moves, alternative lifestyles, disintegration of their parents' marriage, and episodic violence and alcoholism, Anna did not. She "broke" at the age of 13. A psychiatrist prescribed Haldol to "help her to sleep." She suffered a seizure in reaction, requiring emergency hospitalization. Thus was she introduced to the mental health system.

ANNA'S INVISIBILITY IN THE
MENTAL HEALTH SYSTEM

Anna was a client of the mental health system for 19 years, until age 32. For nearly 12 of those years, she was institutionalized in psychiatric hospitals. When in the community, she rotated in and out of acute psychiatric wards, psychiatric emergency rooms, crisis residential programs, and locked mental facilities. Principal diagnoses found in her charts included borderline personality with paranoid and schizo-typal features; paranoia; undersocialized conduct disorder aggressive type; and various types of schizophrenia including paranoid, undifferentiated, hebephrenic, and residual. Paranoid schizophrenia was her most prominent diagnosis. Chronic with acute exacerbation, subchronic, and chronic courses of schizophrenia were identified. Symptoms of anorexia, bulimia, and obsessive compulsive personality were also recorded. Treatments included family therapy; vitamin and nutritional therapy; insulin and electroconvulsive "therapy"; psychotherapy; behavioral therapy; art, music, and dance therapies; psychosocial rehabilitation; intensive case management; group therapy; and every conceivable psychopharmaceutical treatment including Clozaril. Ninety-five percent of the treatment approach to her was the use of psychotropic drugs. Though early on there were references to dissociation, her records contain no information about or attempts to elicit the existence of a history of early childhood trauma.

Anna was 22 when she learned, through conversation with other patients who had also been sexually assaulted as children, that she wasn't "the only one in the world." It was then that she was first able to describe to me the details of her abuse. This time, with awareness gained over the years, I was able to hear her.

Events finally became understandable. Sexual torture and betrayal explained her constant screaming as a toddler, her improvement in nursery school, and the re-emergence of her disturbance at puberty. It explained the tears in her paintings, the content of her "delusions," her image of herself as shameful, her self-destructiveness, her involvement in prostitution and sadistic relationships, her perception of the world as deliberately hurtful, her isolation, and her profound lack of trust. I thought, with relief and with hope, that now we knew why treatment had not helped. Here at last was a way to understand and help her heal.

The reaction of the mental health system was to ignore this information. When I or Anna would attempt to raise the subject, a look would come into the professionals' eyes, as if shades were being drawn. If notes were being taken, the pencil would stop moving. We were pushing on a dead button. This remained the case until she took her life, 10 years and 15 mental hospitals later.

There was one exception. When Anna was 25 years old, the chief psychologist on a back ward of a state hospital listened to her after a suicide attempt, and took what she told him seriously. He initiated a new treatment approach that addressed her experiences of sexual abuse. Antidepressant medication was prescribed, but psychotropic drugs were viewed as suppressing the thought processes and emotions she needed to feel fully and begin healing. Rather than relying on drugs as a solution to escalating stress, Anna was helped through these crises and taught how to deal with them. Art therapy was de-emphasized and art lessons were begun, building her artistic talent and increasing her self-esteem. Discussions began about what she needed so that she could leave the hospital and live in the community.

This situation was not to last. The state hospital was closed because of rampant and intractable abuse. Anna's treatment team disbanded. She returned to the system of public mental institutions and community mental health agencies, a world where she was—once again—invisible and undefended. In and out of the "protected environments" of mental health institutions, she repeatedly experienced coerced or manipulated sex, verbal and physical abuse, and rape. When she "broke," she became like a three- or four-year-old consumed by rage and terror. The thoughts, voices, and nightmares that tormented her were sexual and torturing in nature. Violent itches, twitching, stabbing pains, ice cold spots, and innumerable other somatic symptoms invaded her slight body.

Over her remaining years, in community agencies, acute psychiatric hospitalizations, medical and psychiatric emergency rooms, and the back wards of state mental institutions, she experienced night terrors and insomnia; fears of being taken over by outside forces and of "becoming someone else"; voices telling her she was evil, commanding her to be raped and punished; and eating disorders, dysmenorrhea, and amenorrhea. She painted self-portraits covered with tears, bodies in bondage without hands or arms, and images of multiple persons and sexual acts. She was plagued by intrusive thoughts of abusing her own child, of being tortured, of being "seen" naked by everybody, and of people "getting off sexually" on her torment.

She would often flash back to experiencing her childhood trauma, screaming in terror and pleading for help. On one such occasion, I went with her to a psychiatric emergency service. Calmed enough to answer questions, she stated her diagnosis to be post-traumatic stress disorder. The psychiatrist seemed to be recording this information on the form. When my daughter went over and looked at what she had written, she turned to me and said, "Mom, she wrote down 'schizophrenic.' "

She disclosed in words and behavior fragmented details of the awful things that had happened to her. Once while in restraints she screamed over and over again, "I'm just a sex object, I'm nothing but a sex object." She told her therapist of the "voices" inside her saying "I'm a very young person," "I want you to help me," and "The baby is crying." Once she called her therapist late at night, pleading for her to come to the hospital because "the baby wants to talk to you." Permission was denied by the psychiatrist in charge.

Believing herself to be "bad," "disgusting," and "worthless," as child sexual abuse victims often do,[1-10] she hurt, mutilated, and repeatedly revictimized herself. She put cigarettes out on her arms, legs, and genital area; bashed her head with her fists and against walls; cut deep scars in herself with torn-up cans; stuck hangers, pencils, and other sharp objects up her vagina; swallowed tacks and pushed pills into her ears; attempted to pull her eyes out; forced herself to vomit; dug her feces out so as to keep food out of her body; stabbed herself in the stomach with a sharp knife; and paid men to rape her.

Again and again, as victims of sexual assault often do,[1-11] Anna sought relief through suicide. She tried to kill herself many times—slashing her wrists, attempting to drown herself, taking drug overdoses, poisoning herself by spraying paint and rubbing dirt into self-inflicted wounds, slitting her throat with a too dull razor, and hanging herself from the pipes of a state hospital. She dared men to kill her—on one occasion by throwing her off a bridge and on another by stepping on her back to break it. Many times she would have succeeded had it not been for outside interventions or her own fears of dying or eternal damnation.

Many of the mental health professionals she encountered were highly skilled in their disciplines. Many genuinely cared for Anna; some grew to love her. But in spite of their caring, her experience with the mental health system was a continuing re-enactment of her original trauma. Her perception of herself as "bad," "defective," a "bad seed," or an evil influence on the world was reinforced by a focus on her pathologies, a view of her as having a diseased brain, heavy reliance on psychotropic drugs and forced control, and the silence surrounding her disclosures of abuse.

In the months prior to her death, Anna and I began to reconstruct her story. She completed over 200 pages of detailed memories of her childhood from birth to age 15. In her own words, including her writings and artwork, and the memories of her brothers, sisters, and others who had been close to her, she spoke her truth. "Mom," she said, "I'm gonna try not to live in these places, because I want to get my *life*—find some friends—get out some day. Maybe this book will help. Maybe someone will come along and understand me. And they won't just say 'drugs, drugs, drugs!' " She gave her doctor a draft of her book. He did not read it.

Four days after her 32nd birthday, after another haunted sleepless night, she hung herself, by her T-shirt, in the early morning bleakness of her room in a California State mental hospital. She was found by a team of three night staff who were on their way in to give her another shot of medication.

THE WALL OF SILENCE AND INVISIBILITY

The tragedy of Anna's life is daily replicated in the lives of many individuals viewed as "chronically and severely mentally ill." Unrecognized and untreated for their childhood trauma, they repeatedly cycle through the system's most expensive psychiatric emergency, acute inpatient, and long-term institutional services. Their disclosures of sexual abuse are discredited or ignored. As happened during their early childhood, they learn within the mental health system to keep silent.

Clinicians who acknowledge the prevalence of traumatic abuse and recognize its etiological and therapeutic significance are deeply frustrated at being denied the tools and support necessary to respond adequately. Sometimes, as Anna's psychologist did, these clinicians leave the mental health system entirely, deciding they can no longer practice with integrity within it.

A seemingly impenetrable wall of silence isolates the reality and impact of childhood sexual abuse from the consciousness of the public mental health system. No place exists within the system's formal information management structures to receive these data from clients. We do not elicit the information, nor do we record it. Yet to respond therapeutically without such knowledge is analogous to "treating a Vietnam veteran without knowing about Vietnam or what happened there."[12] Why, with childhood sexual abuse an open issue for discussion and treatment elsewhere, is it not addressed in the public mental health system?

A PARADIGMATIC EXPLANATION: THE INABILITY TO SEE

Although rehabilitative, psychotherapeutic, and self-help approaches operate within the system, the dominant paradigm within which these approaches are subsumed is clearly that of biological psychiatry. Thomas Kuhn, in his analysis of the history and development of the natural sciences,[13] brought the concept of "paradigm" into popular usage. He defined paradigms as "the conceptual networks through which scientists view the world." Data that agree with the scientists' conceptual network are seen with clarity and understanding. But unexpected, "anomalous" data that do not match the scientific paradigm are frequently "unseen," ignored, or distorted to fit existing theories.

In the field of mental health, a biologically based understanding of the nature of "mental illness" has for years been the dominant paradigm. It has determined the appropriate research questions and methodologies; the theories taught in universities and applied in the field;

the interventions, treatment approaches, and programs used; and the outcomes seen to indicate success.

Paradigmatically understood, the mental health system was constructed to view Anna and her "illness" solely through the conceptual lens of biological psychiatry. The source of her pain, early childhood sexual abuse trauma, was an anomaly—a contradiction to the paradigm, and as such, could not be seen through this lens. Her experience did not match the professional view of mental illness. It did not fit within the system's prevailing theoretical constructs. There was not adequate language available within the professions to articulate or label it. There were not reimbursement mechanisms to cover its "treatment." It was not addressed in curricula for professional training and education, nor was there support for research on the phenomena. There were no tools—treatment, rehabilitation, or self-help interventions—for responding to it. And there was no political support within the field for its inclusion. Screened through the single lens of the biological paradigm, Anna's experience could not be assimilated. It had to be "unseen," rejected, or distorted to fit within the parameters of the accepted conceptual framework.

As a result of this paradigmatic "blindness," conventionally accepted psychiatric practices and institutional environments repeatedly retraumatized Anna, re-enacting and exacerbating the pain and sequelae of her childhood experience. Table 15.1 illustrates that retraumatization.

The effect of this institutional retraumatization was to continually leave Anna "in a condition that fulfilled the prophecy of her pathology."[14] This was especially true in the use of psychotropic medication. Survivors of trauma tell us the capacity to think and to feel fully is essential for recovery. Psychotropic drugs continually robbed Anna of these capacities. Several years ago, she had been through a crisis period without medication. For days following, she asked for me to hold her. She talked softly about her feelings, crying gently, showing trust through touching and hugs. One day after her newly prescribed meds were beginning to take effect, she said to me with a flatter voice and her eyes again haunted, "Mom, the feeling of love is going away." As her feelings of rage, grief, and terror were suppressed, so were her feelings of love and laughter, caring and intimacy, isolating her again from herself and from others and preventing the possibility of healing.

(text continues on p. 338)

TABLE 15.1 Institutional Retraumatization

	Early Childhood Trauma Experience	Common Mental Health Institutional Practices
Unseen and unheard	Anna's child psychiatrist did not inquire or see signs of sexual trauma. Anna misdiagnosed.	Adult psychiatry does not inquire into, see signs of sexual trauma. Anna misdiagnosed.
	Anna's attempts to tell parents and other adults met with denial and silencing.	Reports of past and present abuse ignored, disbelieved, discredited. Interpreted as delusional. Silenced.
	Only two grade school psychologists saw trauma. Their insight ignored by parents.	Only two psychologists saw trauma as etiology. Their insight ignored by psychiatric system.
	Secrecy: Those who knew of abuse did not tell. Priority was to protect self, family relationships, reputations.	Institutional secretiveness replicates that of family. Priority is to protect institution, jobs, reputations. Patient abuse not reported up line. Public scrutiny not allowed.
	Perpetrator retaliation if abuse revealed.	Patient or staff reporting of abuse is retaliated against.
	Abuse occurred at preverbal age. No one saw the sexual trauma expressed in her childhood artwork.	No one saw the sexual trauma expressed in her adult artwork with the exception of one art therapist.
Trapped	Unable to escape perpetrators' abuse.	Unable to escape institutional abuse. Locked up.
	Dependent as child on family, caregivers.	Kept dependent. Denied education or skill development.
	Abuser stripped Anna, pulled T-shirt over her head.	Stripped of clothing when secluded or restrained, often by or in presence of male attendants.
	Stripped by abuser to "with nothing on below."	To inject with medication, patient's pants pulled down, exposing buttocks and thighs, often by male attendants.
	"Tied up," held down, arms and hands bound.	"Take down," "restraint." Arms and legs shackled to bed.

TABLE 15.1 Continued

	Early Childhood Trauma Experience	Common Mental Health Institutional Practices
	Abuser "blindfolded me with my little T-shirt."	Cloth would be thrown over Anna's face if she spit or screamed while strapped down in restraints.
	Abuser "opened my legs."	Forced four-point restraints in spread-eagle position.
	Abuser was "examining and putting things in me."	Medication injected into her body against her will.
	Boundaries violated. Exposed. No privacy.	No privacy from patients or staff. No boundaries.
Isolated	Taken by abuser to places hidden from others.	Forced, often by male attendants, into seclusion room.
	Isolated in her experience: "Why just me?"	Separated from community in locked facilities.
	"I thought I was the only one in the world."	No recognition of patients' sexual abuse experiences.
Blamed and shamed	"I had this feeling that I was bad . . . a bad seed."	Patients stigmatized as deficient, mentally ill, worthless. Abusive institutional practices and ugly environments convey low regard for patients, tear down self-worth.
	She became the "difficult to handle" child.	She became a "noncompliant," "treatment-resistant," difficult-to-handle patient.
	She was blamed, spanked, confined to her room for her anger, screams, and cries.	Her rage, terror, screams, and cries were often punished by medications, restraint, loss of "privileges," and seclusion.
Powerless	Perpetrator had absolute power/control over Anna.	Institutional staff had absolute power/control over Anna.
	Pleas to stop violation were ignored: "It hurt me. I would cry and he wouldn't stop."	Pleas and cries to stop abusive treatment, restraint, seclusion, overmedication, and so forth, commonly ignored.

	Expressions of intense feelings, especially anger directed at parents, were often suppressed.	Intense feelings, especially anger at those with more power (all staff), suppressed by medication, isolation, restraint.
Unprotected	Anna was defenseless against perpetrator abuse. Her attempts to tell went unheard. There was no safe place for her, even in her own home or room.	Mental patients defenseless against staff abuse. Reports disbelieved. No safeguards effectively protect patients. Personnel policies prevent dismissal of abusive staff.
Threatened	As a child, constant threat of being sexually violated.	As mental patient, constant threat of being stripped, thrown into seclusion, restrained, overmedicated.
Discredited	As a child, Anna's reports of sexual assault were unheard, minimized, or silenced.	As a mental patient, Anna's reports of adult sexual assault were not believed. Reports of child sexual abuse were ignored.
Crazy-making	Appropriate anger at sexual abuse seen as something wrong with Anna. Abuse continued, unseen.	Appropriate anger at abusive institutional practices judged pathological. Met with continuation of practices.
	Anna's fear from threat of being abused was not understood. Abuse continued, unseen.	Fear of abusive and threatening institutional behavior is labeled "paranoia" by the institution producing it.
	Sexual abuse unseen or silenced. Message: "You did not experience what you experienced."	Psychiatric denial of sexual abuse. Message to patient: "You did not experience what you experienced."
Betrayed	Anna violated by trusted caretakers and relatives.	Anna retraumatized by helping professionals/psychiatry.
	Disciplinary interventions were "for her own good."	Interventions presented as "for the good of the patient."
	Family relationships fragmented by separation, divorce. Anna had no one to trust and depend on.	Relationships of trust arbitrarily disrupted based on needs of system. No continuity of care or caregiver.

Medication can be helpful, if used cautiously, with the full understanding and consent of the patient. But without particular knowledge of trauma and of the kinds of medications that can alleviate symptoms and facilitate recovery from trauma, medications can cause incalculable damage. For Anna, the system's reliance on psychopharmaceutical treatment was a metaphor for her original trauma. As sexual assault had violated physical and psychological boundaries of self, forced neuroleptic drugs also intruded past her boundaries, invading, altering, and disabling her mind, body, and emotions. She once said to me, "I don't have a safe place inside myself."

THE EMERGING PARADIGM

Although the established paradigm may help to alleviate the suffering of those whose mental illness is strictly genetic or biological in nature, it is failing for a significant group whose histories contain sexual and/or physical trauma. Rising cognizance of this failure is one of several factors currently affecting the mental health field, indicating the possibility that a new paradigm, based on trauma, is emerging. The extraordinary resistance to such a paradigm is also indicative of its power and its eventual emergence.

RESISTANCE TO A TRAUMA PARADIGM

Paradigm shifts, though they mark the way to progress and opportunity, are always initially resisted. They cause change, disrupt the status quo, create tension and uncertainty, and involve more work.[15] Resistance to a sexual abuse trauma paradigm has existed for over 130 years, during which time the etiological role of childhood sexual violation in mental illness has been alternately discovered, then denied. In 1860, the prevalence and import of child sexual abuse was exposed by Amboise Tardieu,[16] in 1896 by Sigmund Freud,[17] in 1932 by Sandor Ferenczi,[18] and in 1962[19] and 1984[20] by C. Henry Kempe. Each exposure was met by the scientific community with distaste, rejection, or discreditation. Each revelation was countered with arguments that in essence blamed the victims and protected the perpetrators. Freud, faced with his colleagues' ridicule of and hostility to his discoveries, sacrificed his major insight into the etiology of mental illness and replaced his theory of trauma by the view that his patients had "fantasized" their early memories of rape and seduction.[16] Today, 100 years later, in spite of countless instances of documented abuse, this tradition of denial and victim-blame continues to thrive.

Psychiatrist Roland Summit refers to this denial as "nescience" or "deliberate, beatific ignorance." He proposes that "in our historic failure to grasp the importance of sexual abuse and our reluctance to embrace it now, we might acknowledge that we are not naively innocent. We seem to be willfully ignorant, nescient."[21]

At this point in history, however, multiple and divergent forces are confronting nescience with truth. Although these forces will continue to meet resistance, they appear to be forming a powerful movement that will help to protect children from adult violation and will promote acceptance of a trauma-based paradigm recognizing the pain of individuals like my daughter and offering them "the radical prospect of recovery."[21]

IMPLICATIONS FOR MENTAL HEALTH ADMINISTRATORS AND POLICYMAKERS

Mental health administrators and policymakers are in a unique position today to prevent the re-creation of tragedies such as my daughter Anna's. The tools and resources they need to do so can be found in the following forces supporting the emergence of the new trauma paradigm.

• Among the most significant forces for change are the victims themselves. For the first time in history, survivors of sexual trauma are speaking out—revealing their experiences of having been sexually violated as children, lobbying politically for services and legislative action, challenging societal denial and nescience, and keeping the reality of the sexual assault of children in the arena of public awareness. Growing numbers of these survivors are recipients of mental health services and former mental patients with post-traumatic stress and dissociative disorders. After years of hospitalization and misdiagnoses such as borderline personality disorder, major depression, and schizophrenia, they talk of how they could not have begun to heal had not someone recognized and responded therapeutically to their childhood experiences of abuse and torture. Finally, ex-patients in the mainstream consumer movement are beginning to reveal their experiences of sexual violation, the ways in which they felt retraumatized by treatment in psychiatric hospitals and institutions, and their ongoing struggle to heal from both childhood abuse and adult institutional revictimization.

• The number of studies, instruments, articles, books, and professional journals based on a trauma paradigm is multiplying, making visible the most hidden and most damaged victims of childhood sexual assault, and heightening awareness of such anomalies to the psychiatric paradigm. Research is revealing significantly higher prevalence rates of childhood sexual abuse among female psychiatric outpatients and inpatients (as high as 70 percent)[2,22] than is found in the general population. Many of these clients require emergency, acute inpatient care and long-term hospitalization services.[2-4, 11,21-48] Studies establish a history of childhood sexual trauma to have significant implications for diagnosis and treatment,[1,2,4,8,21,22,24,25,27-31,33,35,36,38,40,41,46-84] and the routine inquiry about childhood sexual abuse to be an essential component of emergency, acute inpatient and outpatient psychiatric protocols.[2,23,28,30,36,37,65,85-87] The growing pool of data indicates that when trauma is recognized and responded to in specific therapeutic interaction, possibilities of recovery exist even for those survivors of sexual abuse who are viewed as schizophrenic, depressive, or borderline.[21,31,55,70,78,79,83,88-95] Research findings showing inextricable connections between trauma, physiology, and the brain are now pointing the way to new relationships between these areas of data under a trauma paradigm.[96]

• Political support for a new trauma paradigm is growing as government-sanctioned committees are formed and local, state, and federal governing bodies pass legislation requiring mental health systems to address issues of physical and sexual abuse trauma in their clients. One such notable step is a 1993 congressional mandate directing the national Center for Mental Health Services (CMHS) to pay attention to women's issues. After surveying the field, CMHS established its priority focus to be on physical and sexual abuse in the lives of women with severe mental illness.

• New therapeutic approaches to sexual and other trauma in persons with serious mental illness are being used and developed outside of and on the fringes of the public mental health system. Examples can be found in the dissociative disorder units of private psychiatric hospitals; in the work of art therapists using imagery and play therapy with traumatized children; in the treatment of severely traumatized war veterans; in the specialized victims and offenders services now serving individuals with severe mental illness; in incest survivor self-help groups; in rape treatment centers; increasingly in the field of child psychiatry; and in the work of private therapists.

• Respected national and international professional associations focused on research and treatment of severely traumatized children and adults have formed over the past decade, and networks of professionals, advocates, and ex-patient survivors increasingly proliferate.

• Women's rights and mental health litigators are being asked to recognize the connection between sexual violence, "craziness," and the treatment of women in psychiatric institutions. These connections are seen to have consequences for rights to treatment, rights to refuse treatment, and forced medication and seclusion and restraint cases.[14]

• Finally, a powerful force for paradigmatic change at this time in history is the advent of health care reform, introducing managed care, capitation, and the need for public mental health organizations to compete in providing quality services to consumers in a cost-effective way. Incorrect diagnoses and treatment exacerbates the condition of traumatized patients, making them dependent on the system's most restrictive and expensive services. An analysis of 17 years of Anna's records shows that she was hospitalized a total of 4,124 days. The total cost for this hospitalization, figured at $640 a day, was $2,639,360! Not included in this analysis is the cost of social services, police, ambulance and legal/court services, conservator and patient advocacy services, residential treatment, psychiatric and therapist sessions, crisis services, day programs, and intensive case management estimated to be over $500,000 for a total cost of over $3,000,000. By comparison, intensive trauma-based psychotherapy, figured at $150 a session, two sessions a week, for 17 years, would have cost a total of $265,200. With studies showing prevalence rates as high as 81 percent[37] of hospitalized patients to have histories of sexual and/or physical trauma, the fiscal implications to exploring a trauma paradigm are obvious.

CONCLUSION

The ideas, practices, and standard operating procedures that got the public mental health field and its various agencies and institutions to where they are today will clearly not take them into the future. The rules have changed dramatically. Forces shaping a new paradigm include: health care reform and managed care; the need to compete and to deliver quality services in cost-effective ways; the emergence of political activism and public testimony on the part of ex-patient survivors of trauma; the proliferation of research and writing about sexual trauma and serious mental illness; the intense interest and debate around the import of sexual abuse for treatment; the developing legal interest in the system's retraumatization of sexually abused patients; the growth of private psychiatric hospital services for persons with dissociative disorders; and finally, the advances around the fringes of the public mental health field providing evidence that, when trauma is recognized and responded to therapeutically, actual recovery is possible for persons with histories of hospitalization and use of the most expensive services of the system. Resources for "re-tooling" the mental health system to effectively address trauma are to be found in the forces pushing the field to change. Institutions, agencies, and systems that ignore the opportunities presented by the new trauma paradigm do their clients an injustice.

REFERENCES

1. Briere J, Runtz M: Post sexual abuse trauma. In: Wyatt GE, Powell GJ (Eds.): *Lasting Effects of Child Sexual Abuse*. Newbury Park, CA: Sage, 1988, pp. 85-99.
2. Briere J, Zaidi LV: Sexual abuse histories and sequelae in female psychiatric emergency room patients. *American Journal of Psychiatry* 1989; 12:1602-1606.
3. Briere J, Evans D, Runtz M, et al.: Symptomatology in men who were molested as children: A comparison study. *American Journal of Orthopsychiatry* 1988; 58:457-461.
4. Brown GR, Anderson B: Psychiatric morbidity in adult inpatients with childhood histories of sexual and physical abuse. *American Journal of Psychiatry* 1991; 148:55-61.
5. Bulik CM, Sullivan PF, Rorty M: Childhood sexual abuse in women with bulimia. *Journal of Clinical Psychiatry* 1989; 50:460-464.
6. Coons PM, Bowman ES, Milstein V: Multiple personality disorder: A clinical investigation of 50 cases. *Journal of Nervous and Mental Disease* 1988; 176:519-527.
7. Garnefski N, Egmond M, Straatman A: The influence of early and recent life stress on severity of depression. *Acta Psychiatrica Scandinavica* 1990; 81:295-301.
8. Heins T, Gray A, Tennant M: Persisting hallucinations following childhood sexual abuse. *Australian and New Zealand Journal of Psychiatry* 1990; 24:561-565.
9. Rew L: Long-term effects of childhood sexual exploitation. *Issues in Mental Health Nursing* 1989; 10:229-244.
10. Riggs S, Alario AJ, McHorney C: Health risk behaviors and attempted suicide in adolescents who report prior maltreatment. *Journal of Pediatrics* 1990; 116:815-821.
11. Ross CA, Norton GR, Wozney K: Multiple personality disorder: An analysis of 236 cases. *Canadian Journal of Psychiatry. Revue Canadienne de Psychiatrie* 1989; 34:413-418.
12. Gise LH, Paddison P: Rape, sexual abuse, and its victims. *Psychiatric Clinics of North America* 1988; 11:629-648.
13. Kuhn TS: *The Structure of Scientific Revolutions*. Chicago: University of Chicago Press, 1972.
14. Stefan S: *The Protection Racket: Violence Against Women: Psychiatric Labelling and Law*. Miami, FL: University of Miami, 1993.
15. Barker JA: *Discovering the Future: The Business of Paradigms* (video). Charthouse Learning Corporation, 221 River Ridge Circle, Burnsville, MN 55337.
16. Masson JM: *The Assault on Truth: Freud's Suppression of the Seduction Theory*. New York: Farrar, Straus and Giroux, 1984.
17. Freud S: The aetiology of hysteria (1896). In: *The Standard Edition of the Complete Psychological Works of Sigmund Freud*. London: Hogarth Press and the Institute of Psychoanalysis, 1953-1974, pp. 191-221.
18. Ferenczi S: Confusion of tongues between adults and the child: The language of tenderness and the language of [sexual] passion. (1932) [Translation by Jeffrey M. Masson and Marianne Loring] In: Masson JM: *The Assault on Truth: Freud's Suppression of the Seduction Theory*. New York: Farrar, Straus and Giroux, 1984, Appendix C, pp. 283-295.
19. Kempe CH, Silverman FN, Steele BF, et al.: The battered-child syndrome. *Journal of the American Medical Association* 1962; 181:17-24.
20. Kempe RS, Kempe CH: *The Common Secret: Sexual Abuse of Children and Adolescents*. New York: Freeman, 1984.
21. Summit R: The centrality of victimization: Regaining the focal point of recovery for survivors of child sexual abuse. *Psychiatric Clinics of North America* 1989; 12:413-450.

66. Kinzl J, Biebl W, Hinterhuber H: The significance of incest experience for the development of psychiatric and psychosomatic diseases. *Nervenarzt* 1991; 62:565-569.

67. Kluft RP: *Childhood Antecedents of Multiple Personality.* Washington, DC: American Psychiatric Press, 1985.

68. MacFarlane K, Waterman J, Conerly S, et al.: *Sexual Abuse of Young Children.* New York: Guilford, 1986.

69. Paddison PL, Gise LH, Lebovits A, et al.: Sexual abuse and premenstrual syndrome: Comparison between a lower and higher socioeconomic group. *Psychosomatics* 1990; 31:265-272.

70. Patten SB, Gatz YK, Jones B, et al.: Post-traumatic stress disorder and the treatment of sexual abuse. *Social Work* 1989; 34:197-203.

71. Peters F: Children who are victims of sexual assault and the psychology of offenders. *American Journal of Psychotherapy* 1976; 30:398-432.

72. Pribor EF, Dinwiddie SH: Psychiatric correlates of incest in childhood. *American Journal of Psychiatry* 1992; 149:52-56.

73. Russell DEH: *The Secret Trauma: Incest in the Lives of Girls and Women.* New York: Basic Books, 1986.

74. Stein JA, Golding JM, Siegel JM, et al.: Long-term psychological sequelae of child sexual abuse: The Los Angeles Epidemiologic Catchment Area study. In: Wyatt GA, Powell GJ (Eds.): *Lasting Effects of Child Sexual Abuse.* Beverly Hills, CA: Sage, 1988, pp. 135-154.

75. Summit RC: Recognition and treatment of child sexual abuse. In: Hollingsworth C (Ed.): *Textbook of Pediatric Consultation-Liaison Psychiatry.* New York: Spectrum, 1983.

76. Summit RC: The child sexual abuse accommodation syndrome. *Child Abuse & Neglect* 1983; 7:177-193.

77. Summit RC: Critical issues in counseling. In: *Protecting Our Children: The Fight Against Molestation: A National Symposium.* Washington, DC: U.S. Department of Justice, 1984.

78. Summit RC: Hidden victims, hidden pain: Societal avoidance of child sexual abuse. In: Wyatt GA, Powell GJ (Eds.): *Lasting Effects of Child Sexual Abuse.* Beverly Hills, CA: Sage, 1988, pp. 39-60.

79. van der Kolk BA (Ed.): *Psychological Trauma.* Washington, DC: American Psychiatric Press, 1987.

80. van der Kolk BA (Ed.): *Post-Traumatic Stress Disorder: Psychological and Biological Sequelae.* Washington, DC: American Psychiatric Press, 1984.

81. Whitman BY, Munkel W: Multiple personality disorder: A risk indictor, diagnostic marker and psychiatric outcome for severe child abuse. *Clinical Pediatrics* 1991; 30:422-428.

82. Whitwell D: The significance of childhood sexual abuse for adult psychiatry. *British Journal of Hospital Medicine* 1990; 43:346-352.

83. Wyatt GA, Powell GJ (Eds.): *Lasting Effects of Child Sexual Abuse.* Newbury Park, CA: Sage, 1988.

84. Young WC, Sachs RG, Braun BG, et al.: Patients reporting ritual abuse in childhood: A clinical syndrome: Report of 37 cases. *Child Abuse & Neglect* 1991; 15:181-189.

85. Ross CA, Miller SD, Reaagor P, et al.: Structured interview data on 102 cases of multiple personality disorder from four centers. *American Journal of Psychiatry* 1990; 147:596-601.

86. Goodwin J, Attiass R, McCarty T, et al.: Effects on psychiatric inpatients of routine questioning about childhood sexual abuse. *Victimology,* in press.

87. Jacobson A, Koehler J, Jones-Brown C: The failure of routine assessment to detect histories of assault experienced by psychiatric patients. *Hospital and Community Psychiatry* 1987; 38:386-389.

88. Goodwin JM, Talwar N: Group psychotherapy for victims of incest. *Psychiatric Clinics of North America* 1989; 2:279-293.

89. Goodwin JM: Applying to adult incest victims what we have learned from victimized children. In: Kluft R (Ed.): *Incest-Related Syndromes of Adult Psychopathology.* Washington, DC: American Psychiatric Press, 1990, pp. 55-74.

90. Herman JL: *Trauma and Recovery: The Aftermath of Violence—From Domestic Abuse to Political Terror.* New York: Basic Books, 1992.

91. Putnam FW: The treatment of multiple personality: State of the art. In: Braun BG (Ed.): *Treatment of Multiple Personality Disorder.* Washington, DC: American Psychiatric Press, 1986.

92. Putnam FW: *Diagnosis and Treatment of Multiple Personality Disorder.* New York: Guilford, 1989.

93. Ross CA: *Multiple Personality Disorder: Diagnosis, Clinical Features and Treatment.* New York: Wiley, 1989.

94. Wilbur CB: Treatment of multiple personality. *Psychiatric Annals* 1984; 14:2-31.

95. Wilbur CB: The effect of child abuse on the psyche. In: Kluft RP (Ed.): *Childhood Antecedents of Multiple Personality.* Washington, DC: American Psychiatric Press, 1985, pp. 22-35.

96. van der Kolk BA: The body keeps the score: Memory and the evolving psychobiology of post-traumatic stress. *Harvard Review of Psychiatry* 1994; 1:253-265.

16

From Chaos to Sanctuary

*Trauma-Based Treatment for Women
in a State Hospital System*

Lyndra J. Bills, M.D.
Sandra L. Bloom, M.D.

In 1993, I (LJB) was appointed medical director of a chronic, extremely violent, women's unit in a state hospital, in a rural, mid-Atlantic region. I accepted the position because of the challenge it presented. I had been trained as a resident and fellow in the relatively new field of psychotraumatology, the study of how psychological trauma, particularly early childhood trauma, affects adult functioning. The level of reported violence, particularly self-harming behavior, that was an endemic part of this environment convinced me that there must be a high level of previously unrecognized and unresolved traumatic experience in the backgrounds of these patients, a finding that has been recognized in previous research.[1] If this was the case, then perhaps the level of chronicity and violence could be decreased. To bring about such a change, it would be necessary to introduce two separate, but mutually compatible, theoretical systems to the inpatient unit: a trauma-based approach combined with the systematized use of a therapeutic milieu, previously articulated as the Sanctuary Model© of inpatient treatment.[2,3] This chapter summarizes the process of converting a deteriorated, chaotic, violent, and alienated culture into a community milieu with established nonviolent norms and the resultant changes in patient behavior and outcome.

BACKGROUND

As I entered the system, the hospital had been and was continuing to undergo significant change. The state hospital was the major employer for a very small town. Some of the local families could claim four generations working at the hospital. Like so many other mental health facilities in these times of economic decline for the mental health system, the hospital was in the midst of rapid downsizing with attendant staff layoffs and a dramatic switch from public to private management. Nursing staff members and other ancillary staff provided most of the patient care. There were only two psychiatrists for 250 patients. Several other physicians, who had no formal psychiatric training, supplemented the medical care, although they were expected to function in that role to the best of their ability.

Several years prior to my employment, there had been several patient deaths that were, at least in part, attributed to deficiencies in patient care. State officials had responded by instituting a patient advocacy system that answered directly to the state and not to the local hospital authorities. Intended as a solution to problems of deficient patient care, the advocacy system had somehow gone astray and the potential for abuse of patients by staff had made a pendulum swing in the direction of increased potential for abuse of staff by patients. The patient advocates were perceived as wielding an unusual amount of power, and staff members had reportedly been fired, without a chance for appeal, in the face of confronting a patient about violence. Allegedly, one of the male advocates had been accused of violence toward patients in the past and was rumored to have a personal history of domestic violence. I had no opportunity to search out the veracity of these incidents, but I did observe that the staff was extremely hesitant to establish any rules for the unit that could serve to curb the violence. They attributed their reluctance to fear of the patient advocates. They believed that if they were to set limits on patient behavior, it could cost them their jobs.

EVALUATION PHASE

My first day on the unit will always stand out vividly in my memory. I was freshly out of my residency and eager to start my new job. This particular unit was noted to be the most difficult and least desirable post in the hospital. I had deliberately chosen to assume leadership of the unit because I believed that there was a potential to make significant changes. I had also been impressed with the cohesion and humor of the staff already present on the unit.

But the first few moments of that first day forced me to question my decision. As I opened the door, I looked down a long, dimly lit, drab hallway. I stopped at the sound of women's screams filling the air. As I stared down the long corridor, a chair flew across the hallway and crashed to the floor, and then a large, disheveled woman came up behind a staff member and began to pound the nurse on the head. Several other staff members rushed up, grabbed the patient's arms, and began to talk to her. Only later did I learn that this was routine behavior for that patient. During the brief period of calm that ensued, I became more aware of the current situation on the unit. There were four rooms with staff posted on chairs outside because those four patients required one-to-one supervision for 24 hours per day, and one room with two staff posted outside because their patient required two-to-one supervision for 24 hours per day. Even with this close contact, however, the staff would rarely talk to the patients to whom they were assigned, but each 15 minutes they would carefully note the status of the patient on the clipboard that accompanied them throughout their long and tedious shifts. When they were not assigned to this kind of supervisory duty, the staff members would gratefully retreat behind a raised Plexiglas wall at the nursing station, which separated the staff from the patients. The nurses were clear that the job they had been instructed to do was to observe, record, and report. Talking to the patients, engaging in a therapeutic dialogue, was considered beyond their abilities. The nursing staff did not necessarily always follow this dictate, but it was clear that if they wished to do so, such a policy would be backed up by the normative expectations of the institution.

In my first days and weeks on the unit, I spent a great deal of time watching, listening, and learning. I attended many shift change reports and nurses' unit meetings, and I paid close attention to the everyday functioning and underlying norms of the unit milieu. There were two nurses and four to six psychiatric aides on every shift. There were no social workers, psychologists, or other unit-based support. Although the hospital had some strong therapeutic programming, including art therapy, recreational therapy, work programs, and psychoeducational programming, our patients were not considered to be safe enough to participate in these activities. The most basic needs or desires of the patients imposed what structure there was on the unit—the desire to eat, to smoke, or to have a pass. Usually, the patient was able to attain these privileges by simply nagging a staff member until she gave in to the request, as long as there were no immediate safety concerns. Patients were neither expected nor required to attend programming or to engage in treatment in any way. The barriers to any kind of therapeutic progress were immense.

My impressions of the first day were reinforced with every passing day. Violence was normative behavior. On the average, there were 100 reported violent episodes per month, which included violence to self, others, and accidents. But this did not take into account the hundreds of other violent incidents and threats that did not get reported, since only the most severe incidents were worth the trouble of filling out the inevitable and time-consuming paperwork. Susan was a 32-year-old patient who had been physically and sexually abused as a child, first by her family and then in numerous foster homes. She expressed her chronic feelings of distress and despair through self-harm. In one day alone, she stole staples from the nursing station and put them in her eye and then crushed tiny pieces of glass and put them in the other eye. She managed to extract the light bulb in her room out of its socket, smashed it, and with the pieces of glass, sliced up her arms. Geraldine was 22 and mildly retarded. She was an incest victim and had a child at age 12, by her father. She was put into foster care at the time, but placed back in the home with her abuser at age 18, and was sent to the state hospital at age 19, after her self-harming behavior had escalated to an unmanageable degree. At one point, the state had put her in a placement with eight staff members assigned to her to try to prevent self-harm, costing about $125,000 per year. Even with that regimen, her self-harming behavior could not be stopped. She repeatedly cut herself so severely that the wounds required plastic surgery. She also had frequent gynecological problems. Five times in one day, she placed objects into her vagina—the top of an aluminum soda can, a large square earring, broken glass, a pencil, and batteries. Neither she nor any of the staff appreciated this behavior as a symbolic re-enactment of her incest.

Everyone abhorred the violence, but felt helpless to do anything to stop it. No real effort was made to understand the factors that may have provoked the violence. It was as if "violence" was an active entity that ran the unit. The patients routinely lashed out violently at each other, sometimes provoked by an insult or a despised behavior, other times apparently provoked by nothing. The patients were frequently and un-remittingly violent toward staff, who resorted to the use of seclusion and restraint as their only defense against serious harm. Even in those early days, it was apparent to me that the patients were engaged in some kind of bizarre re-enactment behavior that was satisfied only by the use of strait jackets and solitary confinement.

One of the most accurate demonstrations of this was Michelle, 25 years old, very tall and obese, who had a serious substance abuse prob-lem and was hospitalized after an overdose and repeated episodes of self-mutilation. Her father was an alcoholic and unhappily married to Michelle's mother, and Michelle became a pawn in their routine marital battles. He would kill her pets in front of her as a way of exerting control and was physically violent toward her. On the unit, as Michelle's de-structive behavior escalated, the staff would begin to threaten conse-quences and their threats led to a further escalation. The staff would call an emergency code, and male staff members ran to the unit to provide assistance. Michelle would be roughly hauled into the seclusion room and tied down with restraints. She had become close to one of the nurs-ing staff who was involved in one such code. She felt betrayed by this staff member and subsequently cut off all interactions with the staff. She reported the incident to the patient advocates, who then confronted the staff. Until we all sat down together to debrief, no one had any insight into the fact that Michelle and the staff had become involved in a dra-matic re-enactment of her childhood experiences with her father. This resolved the problem and ended Michelle's use of restraint.

A less successful example was Ruth. Everyone in the town knew Ruth, who had been a beautiful young woman from a not so beautiful family. It was rumored that she had been sexually abused, but Ruth would not provide me with any family history. She had been raped as an adult and then supported herself as a prostitute in the town, but at some point, she had turned to violence and ended up hospitalized. She had been put on many drugs, but nothing controlled the violence. By the time I met her, she had already been in the hospital for more than 10 years and of those years had spent 4 continuous years in seclusion because of her repeated violence. She was hugely obese and only her history spoke of her former beauty. She engaged in a great deal of inappropriate sexual behavior with humans and even with animals. The best that the changed milieu could offer her was a less provocative environment and for her, no use of seclusion and restraint.

The level of self-mutilation was terrifying. One of the environmental reasons for this behavior rapidly became obvious. Being taken to the emergency room for suturing of self-inflicted wounds was one of the only times that a patient could count on the undivided attention of another human being. Throughout the drive to the local emergency room and the visit to the hospital, a patient would have a staff member entirely to herself, in close proximity and surrounded by strangers. This provided an increased likelihood that the staff member and the patient would actually carry on a conversation. Even though the emergency room staff would often disparage the patient with comments about her "manipulative," "needy," or "problem" behavior, the attention and change from the extreme monotony of everyday life was well worth the effort.

I was certainly not immune to the effects of this violent climate. I was hit in the head, thrown down steps, and repeatedly threatened. The patient who was on constant two-to-one supervision was a young woman diagnosed with dissociative identity disorder who was so volatile that she was allowed to get air outside only while cloaked in a strait jacket behind an enclosed and walled courtyard. On one occasion, she managed to climb her way up the bars of a window, punched out the window through the heavy mesh screen, and was preparing to slice her wrist with a long shard of glass when I spotted what she was doing. I climbed up behind her, grabbed her around the waist and yanked until we both fell about six feet to the ground, at which point I sat on top of her, held both her hands out, and tried to control my own impulse toward violence until help finally came. That night, and for many nights afterward, my own sleep was plagued by nightmares and, like other victims of violence, I became hypervigilant and on edge.

It took many days to go through every patient chart to perform a careful review of each case. There were 24 women on the unit, all involuntarily committed. One quarter of them had been hospitalized for six months to four years, and another one quarter had been in the hospital for more than 10 years. The charts were so voluminous that one patient's chart alone required two shopping carts to haul the paperwork onto the unit for my review. Their average age was 38. Fifty percent of the patients had a high school degree or equivalency and two had master's degrees. Three quarters were diagnosed with schizophrenia, 10 percent with mood disorders, 10 percent with personality disorders, and 5 percent with dissociative disorders. Many of them had not seen a psychiatrist or been re-evaluated in many years. I rediagnosed 60 percent of those carrying a schizophrenic diagnosis and of these, 50 percent met criteria for post-traumatic stress disorder (PTSD) or a dissociative disorder.

PLANNING PHASE: THE SANCTUARY MODEL©

After carefully evaluating the milieu from a cognitive and experiential point of view, I was ready to make some serious changes. But I needed some guidelines and some teaching materials to assist me in the process of transformation. I knew that I would need some support for this task. I sought consultation from two experienced clinicians who had helped me in the past. I spoke with them on the phone as often as I needed to help provide an objective viewpoint and a perspective outside of the system. Tinnin had been my fellowship supervisor and a proponent of a specific different treatment approach that focused on traumatic memory-processing procedures. From him I had learned the importance of finishing the trauma story or narrative using special techniques like trauma art, video dialogue, and recursive video therapy.

Bloom and her colleagues had created a specialized treatment program for adult survivors of childhood trauma and abuse in a general hospital setting. She had discovered, consistent with other research data,[1,4,5] that a substantial proportion of her general psychiatric population had a childhood history of extreme and traumatic experiences that had been neglected as contributory causes to their adult symptomatic picture. Once her treatment team revised their protocols to reflect an understanding of how childhood trauma and unresolved post-traumatic stress symptoms affect adult pathology, formerly resistant patients became treatable. The changes that this team made did not require fancy techniques or expensive equipment. Instead, change occurred at the level of system norms, a change in the way the treatment team approached the patient, understood and explained the problems, and altered their expectations of behavior for themselves and their patients. They based these changes on a series of shared assumptions rooted in a relatively new knowledge base about the effects of profound trauma[3,6-8] and a shared practice rooted in the decades-old methodology of the therapeutic community.[9-12] The trauma-based assumptions became the normative basis for understanding psychopathology and developing treatment strategies and the community practice became the platform for promulgating those norms and organizing interventions. In the next section, I have provided a summarized contrast of the two models. For the sake of clarity, I have focused on the extremes of the two positions. The traditional model is drawn from my own experiences, that of my colleagues, and several references.[13-16]

TRAUMA-BASED ASSUMPTIONS VERSUS TRADITIONAL/MEDICAL MODEL

Traditional/Medical Model

1. Patients are perceived to be too weak, impaired, or dysfunctional in comparison to normal people. They may have "nervous breakdowns" because of an inability to handle stress. The nervous breakdown is the basic failure of the patient as a person.

2. The focus of evaluation and treatment revolves around symptom description. In other words, there is little consideration for why someone is having the particular problem or symptoms.

3. The organization is hierarchical and revolves around the physician. There is a less involved approach, and less acceptance for non-physician involvement to patient treatment.

4. The patient is kept as a "child" in treatment, that is, helpless, powerless, and weak as compared to the physician parent.

5. The treatment environment is viewed as a "holding tank" for severe and/or chronic disorders.

6. The focus is on the individual with little attention to the group or community as a whole.

7. There is minimal regard for emotional safety because the problems are viewed as being more "biological" in nature.

8. The treatment is primarily short-term and behavioral with little input from the patient.

9. Even when emotional expression would be therapeutic, it would not be encouraged by the staff in hopes that the patient would more quickly return to premorbid level of function.

10. The primary mode of treatment is biological, with an emphasis on very brief medication management visits. There is very little individual therapy, with less skilled clinicians providing this form of treatment.

11. Medication is a primary treatment modality, but is used often as a restraint. There is little emphasis or understanding of the interactions and relationships between medication and psychotherapy.

12. Physicians are more and more isolated, often struggling with difficult transference and countertransference issues alone. There is little consideration for the overall well-being of staff. Physicians often get pulled in the direction of using their resources to do emergency coverage, consultation, and so forth. Thus, they are less involved in collaborative patient treatment.

13. The view of the family is more likely to support the patient as the "problem." There is little focus on family therapy or a systems view of the patients' presentation.

14. There is little linking between the treatment modalities and locations of treatment, that is, inpatient, outpatient, and so on. There is often no communication between the inpatient clinicians and the outpatient providers.

15. Returns to the hospital are considered the patients' failure. The patient is reminded of what he or she did that was "bad" leading up to the hospitalization.

16. Patients are not expected to get better or get beyond their "illness" or problem. They are reminded of the chronicity of mental illness and that their role should be one of acceptance. There is no room for a combination of serious mental illness and the potential for going beyond or overcoming tragedy.

17. The traditional model does not accept trauma/childhood abuse as a reasonable explanation for any type of problem.

Trauma-Based Model

1. Patients begin life with normal potentials for growth and development, given certain constitutional and genetic predispositions, and then become traumatized. "Post-traumatic stress reactions are essentially the reactions of normal people to abnormal stress."

2. When people are traumatized in early life, the effects of trauma interfere with normal physical, psychological, social, and moral development.

3. Trauma has biological, psychological, social, and moral effects that spread horizontally and vertically, across and down through the generations.

4. Many symptoms and syndromes are manifestations of adaptations, originally useful as coping skills that have now become maladaptive or less adaptive than originally intended.

5. Many victims of trauma suffer chronic PTSD and may manifest any combination of the symptoms of PTSD.

6. Victims of trauma become trapped in time, their inner experience fragmented. They are caught in the repetitive re-experiencing of the trauma that has been dissociated and remains unintegrated into their overall functioning.

7. Dissociation and repression are core defenses against overwhelming affect and are present, to a varying extent, in all survivors of trauma.

8. Although the human capacity for fantasy elaboration and imaginative creation are well-established, memories of traumatic experiences must be assumed to have at least a core of basis in reality.

9. Stressful events are more seriously traumatic when there is an accompanying helplessness and lack of control.

10. Traumatic experience and disrupted attachments combine to produce defects in the regulation and modulation of affect, of emotional experience. Human beings require other human beings to resonate with their emotions and to help contain feelings that are overwhelming.

11. People who are repeatedly traumatized develop "learned helplessness," a condition that has serious biochemical implications.

12. Trauma survivors often discover that various addictive behaviors restore at least a temporary sense of control over intrusive phenomena.

13. Survivors may also become addicted to their own stress responses and, as a result, compulsively expose themselves to high levels of stress and further traumatization.

14. Many trauma survivors develop secondary psychiatric symptomatology and do not connect their symptoms with previous trauma. They become guilt-ridden and depressed, and they exhibit low self-esteem and feelings of hopelessness and helplessness.

15. Trauma victims have difficulty with the appropriate management of aggression. Many survivors identify with the aggressor and become victimizers themselves. A vicious cycle of transgenerational victimization often ensues.

16. The more severe the stressor, the more prolonged the exposure to the stressor, the earlier the age, the more impaired the social support system, and the greater the degree of exposure to or involvement in previous trauma, the greater the likelihood of post-traumatic pathology.

17. Attachment is a basic human need from cradle to grave. Enhanced attachment to abusing objects is seen in all studied species, including humans.

18. Childhood abuse leads to disrupted attachment behavior, inability to modulate arousal and aggression toward self and others, impaired cognitive functioning, and impaired capacity to form stable relationships.

19. Although it may require lifelong processing, recovery from traumatic experience is possible. Over the course of recovery, survivors may temporarily need safe retreats within which important therapeutic goals can be formulated and treatment can be organized.

20. We are all interconnected and interdependent, for good or for ill. Safety must be constantly created and maintained by everyone in the community as a shared responsibility.

21. The whole is greater than the sum of the parts.

INTERVENTION PHASE: CREATING A COMMUNITY

Armed with a cognitive framework for beginning to organize change, I began my intervention by freely vocalizing the way I felt about the violence on the unit. I directed the staff to begin daily community meetings that would engage all of the patients in face-to-face encounters with each other, the staff, and myself. At these meetings, I spoke about the devastating effect that the unit violence was having on all of us. I shared my own experience and feelings about the conditions and urged other staff members to do the same.[17,18] Using violence as the central focus, I gradually trained the staff and the patients in the basic rules of the therapeutic milieu.

All therapeutic milieu environments rest on several assumptions: (1) Patient should be responsible for much of their own treatment, (2) the running of the unit should be more democratic than authoritarian, (3) patients are capable of helping each other, (4) treatment is to be voluntary whenever possible and restraint kept to a minimum, and (5) psychological methods of treatment are seen as preferable to physical methods of control. The most striking characteristic of the therapeutic milieu is that the community itself—and all the individuals who constitute it—are expected to be the most powerful influence on treatment.[3] These concepts were largely new to the staff and certainly new to the patients. There were many questions about how any of these ideas could be instituted with such a violent and unpredictable population. But I remained convinced that much could be done if we were jointly able to change the existing norms of the institution. In my analysis of the situation, I had come to recognize that violence was not only condoned, but encouraged by the normative structure of the unit and by the lack of an alternative model.[19]

And I was going to guarantee that there was, in fact, an alternative option. I met with the medical director and actively participated in the medical staff administration. I verbalized the enormity of the violence problem and the barriers to change, namely, the advocacy system. I also met fairly regularly with my department chair to express how overwhelming my situation was to me. He regularly stated that I was the perfect person for this job, and verbally patted me on the head.

In the Sanctuary Model,© progress in treatment can be expected only if safety has been established. Creating a safe environment free from physical and verbal violence is absolutely necessary before any other kind of progress can be made, and this nonviolent environment can be created and maintained only through the joint effort of the entire community. I educated the staff about the Sanctuary Model, and I wrote a beginning set of unit rules that were extremely definitive about the insistence on nonviolence. These rules are outlined in Figure 16.1. I repeatedly iterated my goals for the community to the staff and to the patients. Every episode of violence presented a renewed opportunity for the simple restatement of this changed norm. Instead of ignoring the episode, I would respond to it. I would use whatever method it took to get the violence under control and then altered the established pattern by insisting on reviewing what led up to the violence, how the pattern could have been altered, and alternative forms of coping with the same emotion.

1. Violence in general will not be tolerated on our unit. This includes verbal and physical violence, aggression, and abuse of other patients, staff, or property.
2. Treatment is an opportunity for you to work on your problems. Your program schedule is the most important thing you will be doing and is a requirement for all patients. We have a "No Class—No Pass" policy.
3. All patients should go to all meals unless specifically ordered not to by the physician.
4. Community meetings are an opportunity for patients to express concerns to each other and staff. It is also an opportunity to learn more about how to communicate and how to interact with each other.
5. All patients should observe quiet time after 11:00 p.m. (Staff may confiscate items like radios if the quiet time is not respected.)
6. The use of the phone is a privilege for everyone. Phone use is limited to 10 minutes per call. If you are unable to use the phone properly, then staff may ask you to get off the phone.
7. Patients are not allowed to come into staff offices unless requested by staff.
8. Patients who are on a level 3 or above will have pass time off the unit depending on their level of function.
9. During the weekdays, especially, treatment is top priority; therefore, no visitors are allowed before supper without treatment team approval.

Figure 16.1. Unit Rules

The use of mechanical restraint and seclusion provided frequent illustrations of the violence-begets-violence cycle. As I helped the staff and patients develop a methodology for reviewing episodes of violence,[2,17,18] it became increasingly easy to establish the patterns of re-enactment that were involved in the use of restraints. The patients were able to articulate how helpless, trapped, and revictimized they felt when the staff response to their violence began. They would often regress, dissociate, and begin experiencing flashbacks and increased autonomic arousal, often followed later by terrifying nightmares. They would perceive the staff as abusive. Likewise, the staff felt uncomfortable about having to resort to violence to curb violence, but had never before expressed their feelings and perceptions to the patients. Gradually, with repeated debriefings after every episode of seclusion and restraint, both the patients and the staff began to recognize what events in the

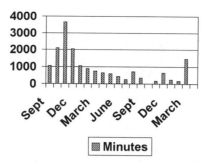

Figure 16.2. Number of Minutes Used for Seclusion/Restraint Per Month, September 1993 to March 1994

environment tended to trigger these episodes and how these triggers related to unresolved traumatic experiences from the past. As the violent episodes began to be contextualized and understood, it became possible for the staff and patient community to begin to experiment with other kinds of interventions that preceded and often prevented the violent outburst. Figure 16.2 reflects changes in seclusion/restraint episodes per month, over time. There was an obvious decrease in the level of violence felt on the unit within about 10 months, and certainly noticeable within a year.

I dealt with the issue of self-harm by addressing it head-on. In the trauma-based approach, self-mutilation is understood as an addictive and compulsive behavior that originates in attempts to self-soothe and then often takes on secondary meanings. Once it is understood as perpetration against the self, an internalized form of identification with the aggressor, the behavior becomes more accessible to treatment. I portrayed self-harm as no different from any other form of violence and an abuse of the entire community (as presented in Figure 16.3). I made the patients responsible for helping each other reduce the level of violence by helping to protect the safety of the unit and each other, rather than by encouraging or trying to ignore the violence. Since repeated self-mutilative behavior was one other way the patients had of seeking out extra staff attention, I decided that we needed to take away the secondary reinforcement for the behavior at the same time as we were understanding and explaining it using a trauma-based approach. In service of this, I insisted that the patients were to apply bandages and antibiotics

It shall be the policy of this unit to quickly establish a safe, constructive treatment plan with those individuals who, by history or current behavior, are self-mutilating or otherwise a danger to their own or to others' physical or emotional well-being and comfort. Furthermore, efforts to re-establish control over such behavior will be constructive, using the least amount of physical restraint necessary to ensure the individual's and the community's continued safety.

Procedure:
1. All admitted patients and/or transferred patients with a known history of self-harm or self-mutilative behavior will be advised of the unit policy regarding such behavior at the time of admission. The patient will be asked to make a written contract regarding his/her understanding of the policy (noted below).
    a. It is the responsibility of the admitting nurse to ensure that the patient reads and/or understands the self-harm behavior policy.
    b. The self-harm behavior policy will be an intervention for self-harm in the patients' treatment plan and the policy/contract will be placed in the permanent medical chart.
2. All patients with a history of self-mutilation will be involved in the following treatment:
    a. Referral and evaluation to Dialectic Behavior Therapy.
    b. Referral and evaluation for a post-traumatic disorder or dissociative disorder.
    c. Patients will be given a Trauma Profile upon admission or at any time self-mutilation is identified as a problem.
    d. Referral and evaluation for Anger Management.
3. If, despite the efforts to prevent such activity, there is evidence of self-mutilative behavior occurring or having occurred, efforts will be taken to ensure that there is adequate opportunity for treatment and observation.

Figure 16.3. Self-Harm Behavior Policy

to their own self-inflicted wounds and they had to fill out their own incident reports. As the unit became calmer, more hospital staff were willing to provide treatment, one psychologist[20] trained in Linehan's approach[21] and a good behaviorist, helped me to develop some self-harm protocols that were put into place. As the staff-to-patient inter-actions multiplied, patients were able to get attention from staff mem-

---

Self-Destructive Protocol
  1. There will be an immediate drop of at least one level for 24 hours.
  2. All sharps and items with potential for self-harm will be prohibited for 24 hours.
  3. There will be no group attendance or work program attendance for 24 hours, exclusive of community meeting, individual therapy, and Dialectic Behavior Therapy.
  4. Written assignments will be given and supervised by the patient's primary contact and/or nursing staff.
     These include the following:
     a. Self-Abuse Scale
     b. Refocusing Assignment
     c. Incident report
     d. Self-check time sheets (interval determined by patient and staff)
  5. Free time will be spent in the day room or at the nursing station.
  6. Visitation will be restricted to the immediate family for a period of 24 hours following the self-mutilative behavior.
  7. Meals will be eaten on the unit for 24 hours.

_____   _____
Patient Signature   Staff Signature

_____
Date

Figure 16.3. Continued

bers through healthy behavior, rather than having to depend on getting a meager amount of attention through self-harming behavior. As less staff time was consumed in one-to-one and two-to-one supervision, more time was available for positive patient contact.

The larger hospital environment noted these changes, of course. I educated the administration and medical staff about the trauma-based approach and my intention to reduce violence on the unit. The patient advocates initially posed some problems because they objected to any restriction of patients and my policies required that there be negative consequences for violent behavior, including the loss of privileges. I regularly accompanied my nursing staff to meetings with the patient advocates. The routine established by the advocates involved a sort of threatening interrogation of nursing staff about the ways they had "wrongly" or "badly" managed patients. To me, this was the same problem at a different level. Staff members did not feel safe. I tried not to be partisan in my approach. I also asked for advocacy help to improve services and the quality of patient care. I expressed to them my conviction that their role had become unfocused and, at times, they were interfering with the betterment of patient care by obstructing policies that were designed to help patients stop antisocial and self-destructive behavior. As a result, my communication with many of the advocates improved. I had to become increasingly firm in my insistence that these changes were necessary and nonnegotiable, but there were still occasions on which I found it necessary to accompany unit nurses when they were summoned by the advocates about my approach and policies. My presence clearly tended to have a muting effect on the proceedings.

When the violence had been reduced, therapy could really begin. Individual and group therapies were initiated and changes in the patients began to be noted. Morale improved for the staff and for the patients. But continuous and active leadership was necessary for these changes to remain in place.

RESULTS

The unit violence began to decrease, as can be seen in Figures 16.4, 16.5, and 16.6. For the first three months, the average number of violent episodes was about 100 per month. After that, the levels of violence began to decrease. In May 1994, a hospital move occurred and one result was that the unit was changed from all-female unit to a mixed unit. The addition of men to the unit appeared to affect the environment positively with a decrease in the average rate from 63 to 24 incidents per month. In August 1994, I went on vacation, and I left in November 1994; increases in violence can be seen at these points as well. These increases probably represented the effects of loss of leadership in a milieu that was still reconstituting itself and continued to require the strong norming

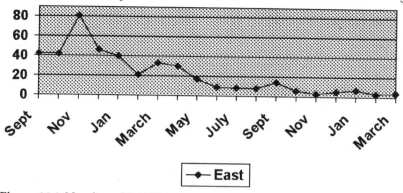

Figure 16.4. Number of Self-Harm Episodes Per Month, September 1993 to March 1994

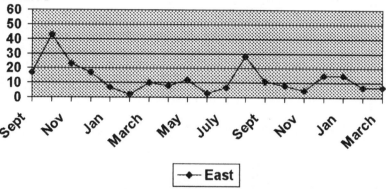

Figure 16.5. Number of Aggressive Episodes Per Month, September 1993 to March 1994

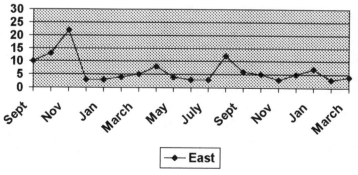

Figure 16.6. Number of Accident Episodes Per Month, September 1993 to March 1994

function that leaders must provide. A striking salute to the effectiveness of the trauma-based approach was the month of October 1994 in which no seclusion or restraint was used. This was a first in the history of the institution.

An important administrative consideration for any institution is the cost of violence. Employee time was lost as a result of being bitten, hit, splashed with hot coffee, and kicked. The average was about 20 hours per month at the peak of the violence, but in one month alone there were 74.5 hours of employee time lost from work.

As expected, many of the patients who had been considered untreatable and chronically mentally ill responded to a more intensive, trauma-based therapeutic milieu. By 1996, two years after I had left, one of the original patients had died, but only two others remained in the hospital. All the rest had been discharged. The dissociative identity disorder patient who had consumed so many months of two-to-one supervision was released from the hospital shortly after I left, 30 months after her admission; she had not self-harmed or been suicidal, nor had she been rehospitalized, during a subsequent 18-months follow-up period.

IMPLICATIONS FOR MENTAL
HEALTH SERVICES DELIVERY

Unfortunately, the constraints of the environment prevented me from engaging in any formal research on the unit, so my account must remain largely anecdotal. However, the dramatic alteration in violence patterns over such a comparatively short period certainly speaks to the possibility for change that does not require large reservoirs of capital or increases in personnel. It did require leadership, commitment, vision, and desire. Drawing on the time-proven tenets of the therapeutic milieu and the newer insights of the trauma field, we were able to accomplish a striking change in a setting that ostensibly was resistant to any improvement. As resources diminish and victims of interpersonal violence multiply, the mental health system must be prepared to use innovative, community-based approaches in an effort to help victims heal.

REFERENCES

1. Saxe GB, van der Kolk BA, Hall K, et al.: Dissociative disorders in psychiatric inpatients. *American Journal of Psychiatry* 1993; 1507:1037-1042.

2. Bloom SL: The sanctuary model: Developing generic inpatient programs for the treatment of psychological trauma. In: Williams MB, Somer JF (Eds.): *Handbook of Post-Traumatic Therapy: A Practical Guide for Intervention, Treatment, and Research.* New York: Greenwood, 1994, pp. 474-491.

3. Bloom SL: *Creating Sanctuary: Towards the Evolution of Sane Communities.* New York: Routledge, 1997.

4. Jacobson A, Herald C: The relevance of childhood sexual abuse to adult psychiatric inpatient care. *Hospital and Community Psychiatry* 1990; 41:154-156.

5. Jacobson A, Richardson B: Assault experiences of 100 psychiatric inpatients: Evidence of the need for routine inquiry. *American Journal of Psychiatry* 1987; 144:7.

6. Herman JL: *Trauma and Recovery.* New York: Basic Books, 1992.

7. van der Kolk BA: *Psychological Trauma.* Washington, DC: American Psychiatric Press, 1987.

8. van der Kolk BA, McFarlane AC, Weisaeth L (Eds.): *Traumatic Stress: The Effects of Overwhelming Experience on Mind, Body, and Society.* New York: Guilford, 1996.

9. Gunderson JG: Defining the therapeutic process in psychiatric milieus. *Psychiatry* 1978; 41:327-335.

10. Jones M: *The Therapeutic Community: A New Treatment Model in Psychiatry.* New York: Basic Books, 1953.

11. Jones M: *Beyond the Therapeutic Community: Social Learning and Social Psychiatry.* New Haven, CT: Yale University Press, 1968.

12. Wilmer H: Defining and understanding the therapeutic community. *Hospital and Community Psychiatry* 1981; 32:95-99.

13. Goffman E: *Asylums.* New York: Doubleday, 1961.

14. Greenblatt M, Levinson DJ, Williams RH (Eds.): *The Patient and the Mental Hospital: Contributions of Research in the Science of Social Behavior.* Glencoe, IL: Free Press, 1957.

15. Stanton AH, Schwartz MS: *The Mental Hospital: A Study of Institutional Participation in Psychiatric Illness and Treatment.* New York: Basic Books, 1954.

16. Wilmer H: *Social Psychiatry in Action: A Therapeutic Community.* Springfield, IL: Charles C Thomas, 1958.

17. Flannery RB, Fulton P, Tausch J, et al.: A program to help staff cope with psychological sequelae of assaults by patients. *Hospital and Community Psychiatry* 1991; 429:935-938.

18. Flannery RB, Hanson MA, Penk W: Risk factors for psychiatric inpatient assaults on staff. *Journal of Mental Health Administration* 1994; 211:24-31.

19. Katz P, Kirkland F: Violence and social structure on mental hospital wards. *Psychiatry* 1990; 53:262-277.

20. Bell T: Personal communication, 1993.

21. Linehan MM: *Cognitive-Behavioral Treatment of Borderline Personality Disorder.* New York: Guilford, 1993.

17

Specific Needs of Women Diagnosed With Mental Illnesses in U.S. Jails

Bonita M. Veysey, Ph.D.

The number of detainees in U.S. jails is exploding. From 1985 to 1995, this population rose from 265,010 to 509,828, an increase of 192 percent.[1] Women represent a growing proportion of these populations. In 1985, women represented 8.0 percent of adult jail inmates, a total of 19,077 women. In 1990, this percentage had increased to 9.2 percent and in 1995, 10.2 percent of jail detainees were female, a total of 52,136 women and a 273 percent increase since 1985.[1] Jail administrators are being more often challenged to find appropriate ways to provide safe pretrial and post-adjudication detention that is on a par with male detainees' correctional, treatment, and services opportunities to meet both constitutional and humane standards.

In a previous study of mental health services in U.S. jails, many jails were found that provided state-of-the-art and creative programming—for men.[2] However, even in these exceptional jails, rarely were comparable services provided for the female detainees. Women are typically underserved in correctional settings in all types of jail programming.[3] When women do receive services, such as mental health or substance abuse, the services tend to be based on models designed for the male population and simply applied to women. To achieve parity, jail programming must (1) provide women with access to the same medical, mental health, substance abuse, and other services that are available to men; and (2) where significant gender differences exist or when providing services to meet needs that are unique to women, these services should be modified or expanded to address the specific needs of women.

CHARACTERISTICS OF WOMEN IN U.S. JAILS

The increase in the number of women in U.S. jails is due in large part to changes in criminal justice policy, particularly the "war on drugs" and "getting tough on crime" policies. These policies mean that more women are being incarcerated for all crimes, especially crimes involving drugs.[4,5] Due to mandatory sentencing laws, the courts have less discretion in incarceration and term-length decisions. Because of these facts, a study of women in California prisons concluded that "the 'war on drugs' has become a war on women."[6]

While both the popular and news media have attempted to link the growing female offender population with the emergence of a new, more violent female criminal, current evidence does not support this conclusion. Female arrestees are being booked into U.S. jails predominantly for drug charges or nonviolent crimes that are often economic crimes committed to support drug habits. This fact alone accounts for most of the increase in the size of the population and does not represent a fundamental shift toward a new population of violent female offenders.[5,7]

Table 17.1 displays some key characteristics of male and female jail detainees. As can be seen, men and women in U.S. jails are similar in terms of age and race/ethnicity. The median age of both men and women in jail is 28. Slightly less than 40 percent of male and female detainees are White non-Hispanic, a little over 40 percent are Black non-Hispanic, about 16 percent were Hispanic, and less than 3 percent belonged to other racial and ethnic groups, such as Native Americans, Pacific Islanders, and Asian Americans. In comparison to men, however, a greater proportion of women have been married at some time (51.1 percent vs. 42.3 percent) and have completed high school or more (50.6 percent vs. 45.8 percent). In comparison to men, a smaller percentage of women were charged with violent crimes and a greater proportion with property and drug offenses.[8] Only 13 percent of women, compared with 24 percent of men, were arrested for violent crimes.

TABLE 17.1 Characteristics of Jail Detainees, by Gender

Variable	Female	Male
Median age	28	28
Race/ethnicity (%)		
White	37.8	38.7
Black	43.4	41.5
Hispanic	16.3	17.5
Other	2.5	2.3
Never married (%)	48.9	57.5
High school or more (%)	50.6	45.8
Arrest charge (%)		
Violent	13.2	23.5
Property	31.9	29.9
Drug offense	33.6	21.9
Other	21.2	24.7

SOURCE: Maguire K, Pastore AL: *Sourcebook of Criminal Justice Statistics—1993*. NCJ-148211. Washington, DC: U.S. Department of Justice, 1994.

Conversely, 34 percent of women were arrested for drug charges, while only 22 percent of men were arrested for the same kinds of crimes. This information continues to support the fact that women are increasingly being arrested and prosecuted for drug-related crimes. This also means that women are increasingly entering the criminal justice system with serious medical and mental health problems that are associated with drug use.

The association between the growth of the number of women in the criminal justice system with poverty and drug use is disturbing, particularly in an era of decreasing resources. Today, women have less access to public subsidies, including housing, health care, and financial entitlements. The change in national policies toward welfare and health care is anticipated to have a negative impact on this very group of people. In addition, these women face increasing discrimination due to their multiple statuses as offenders, mental health service users, substance abusers, and being predominantly people of color in poverty.

MENTAL HEALTH STATUS OF FEMALE JAIL DETAINEES

Many women are entering the criminal justice system diagnosed with serious mental illnesses. In addition to presenting symptoms related to serious mental illnesses, many women also enter jails with issues that complicate mental health problems and produce additional stress that affects a woman's mental health. A majority of women booked into jails have one or more of the following: substance abuse/dependence, serious physical illness, pregnancy and/or primary responsibility for minor children, history of adult or childhood physical or sexual abuse, self-esteem issues, and vocational and educational needs. These factors are not unknown among male populations, but they are much more prevalent among women. In addition, jails are typically designed and administered for a male population without regard to differences between the genders,[5] particularly differences in dangerousness and interpersonal interactional styles. This rigidly structured and controlled environment can create unnecessary stress for women, many of whom do not require high-security precautions.

Prevalence Estimates of Serious Mental Illnesses

Although women represent only a small percentage of jail inmates, studies show that they are more likely than incarcerated men to be diagnosed with serious mental illnesses.[9,10] In a prevalence study of mental illnesses among male and female admissions to a large urban jail, Teplin[9,11] found that 8.9 percent of males and 18.5 percent of females had diagnosable serious mental illnesses (see Table 17.2). Acute conditions of serious mental illnesses were found in 6.1 percent of men and 15.0 percent of women being booked into the jail. Compared with male detainees, women had fairly comparable rates of acute schizophrenia and bipolar disorder (1.8 percent females vs. 3.0 percent males diagnosed with schizophrenia, 2.2 percent vs. 1.1 percent bipolar-manic episode). However, 13.7 percent of female admissions to jail were diagnosed with a current episode of major depression, while only 3.4 percent of men were diagnosed with this disorder. In addition, a notable 22.3 percent of women in jail were diagnosed with post-traumatic stress disorder (PTSD), an additional 6.5 percent with dysthymia, and approximately 3.5 percent with anxiety and panic disorders.

The diagnosis of PTSD is noteworthy in the context of women in correctional settings, both because it reflects a common experience of many women—namely, repeated, severe, and/or long-term physical

TABLE 17.2 Lifetime Prevalence and Current Incidence of Mental Illnesses Among Jail Detainees, by Gender (in percentages)

Diagnosis	Current		Lifetime	
	Female	Male	Female	Male
Any severe disorder	15.0	6.1	18.5	8.9
Schizophrenia	1.8	3.0	2.5	3.8
Bipolar-manic	2.2	1.2	2.6	2.2
Major depression	13.7	3.4	16.9	5.1
Post-traumatic stress disorder	22.3	na	33.5	na
Dysthymia	6.5	na	9.6	8.5
Anxiety and panic disorders	3.5	11.6	4.0	21.0

SOURCE: Teplin LA: Psychiatric and substance abuse disorders among male urban jail detainees. *American Journal of Public Health* 1994; 84:290-293. Teplin LA, Abram KM, McClelland GM: Prevalence of psychiatric disorders among incarcerated women. *Archives of General Psychiatry* 1996; 53:505-512.

and sexual abuse—and because it has implications for service providers, corrections staff, and administrators. Women diagnosed with PTSD may exhibit a number of symptoms, including hypervigilance, startle reflex, phobias, auditory and visual flashbacks to incidents of abuse, and uncontrollable anger or rage. They may have problems that are directly associated with incidents of abuse, specifically interacting with authority figures or men in general (i.e., persons who remind them of the perpetrator of violence), being physically restrained or locked up, and being unclothed. Clearly, women with histories of physical or sexual abuse may experience extreme difficulties in jail settings.

Corrections and health care staff are often trained to recognize the symptoms of psychotic disorders and suicide risk. However, many of the psychiatric and emotional problems that women have are not so easily identified. Because corrections staff act as the gatekeepers to psychiatric evaluations, there is a significant risk that women who have serious mental health problems may not be identified and, therefore, not have access to mental health treatment during their confinement in jail. More important, some psychiatric disorders such as PTSD and anxiety disorders, if not specifically acknowledged and attended to within the jail, are likely to increase the risk that women will become management problems for security staff and may inappropriately use expensive medical and psychiatric services they would otherwise not require.

Because women represent a small proportion of jail populations, many facilities do not provide a full range of mental health services or appropriate housing options for female detainees. Furthermore, the mental health services that are offered are often based on the needs of men, including the criteria used in screening and psychiatric evaluations, the use of psychotropic medications, and specialized housing.

In addition to symptoms related to serious mental illnesses, many female detainees have substantial emotional difficulties related to separation from children, guilt and shame, conditions of confinement, and self-esteem. If these issues are addressed, women are more likely to be willing to engage in treatment services, cooperate in their adjudication process, and be less difficult to supervise.

Prevalence of Co-Occurring Substance Abuse

A majority of women diagnosed with mental illnesses in jails have current substance abuse problems. The National Institute of Justice's Drug Use Forecasting program indicates that 67 percent of female arrestees test positive for drugs.[12] Table 17.3 indicates that, compared with men, women arrestees are much more likely to abuse cocaine and opiates, while male arrestees are more likely to test positive for marijuana use. Lifetime prevalence rates of alcohol abuse/dependence and drug abuse/dependence disorders also reveal that female detainees are more likely than male detainees to be diagnosed with drug disorders. As indicated in Table 17.3, 70.2 percent of female admissions had diagnosable substance use disorders, 63.5 percent with drug abuse.[9] Among males, 61.3 percent were diagnosed with substance abuse disorders, 32.4 percent with drug abuse.[11] The rates of substance abuse are even higher for persons diagnosed with mental illnesses. Among jail detainees with serious mental illnesses, 74.9 percent of women and 72.0 percent of men have co-occurring substance abuse disorders.

Substance abuse treatment services have traditionally been designed by and for men.[4,13] However, men and women who abuse substances differ in important ways. When compared with men, women are more likely to be poor,[4,13-16] are more likely to be involved with a partner who also abuses drugs,[13,14] have lower self-esteem,[13] differ and

TABLE 17.3 Substance Abuse Among Arrestees and Jail Detainees, by Gender (in percentages)

Substance Abuse	Female	Male
Arrestees		
Any drug	67	66
Marijuana	17	30
Cocaine	50	41
Opioids	8	6
Jail detainees		
Substance abuse/dependence	70.2	61.3
Drug abuse/dependence	63.5	32.4
Alcohol abuse/dependence	32.3	51.1

SOURCE: National Institute of Justice: *Drug Use Forecasting: 1994 Annual Report on Adult and Juvenile Arrestees*. Washington, DC: U.S. Department of Justice, 1995. Teplin LA: Psychiatric and substance abuse disorders among male urban jail detainees. *American Journal of Public Health* 1994; 84:290-293.

exhibit more severe physiological effects,[4] and are more likely to be victims/survivors of violence as adults and as children.[14]

Histories of Childhood and Adult Physical and Sexual Abuse

Histories of physical and sexual abuse are common among incarcerated women. The Michigan Women's Commission[13] found that 50 percent of female Michigan jail detainees had been victims of physical or sexual abuse at some point in their lives. An American Correctional Association study[17] revealed that over half of adult female offenders had been victims of physical abuse and 36 percent had been sexually abused.

A review of histories of violence among female recipients of psychiatric inpatient and outpatient services revealed that 35 to 51 percent of women had histories of childhood physical abuse, 20 to 54 percent with childhood sexual abuse, 42 to 64 percent with adult physical abuse and 21 to 38 percent with adult sexual assault.[18] More than 70 percent of women with drug or alcohol abuse problems were victims of violence, including domestic assault by adult partners, rape, and incest.[19]

Women with histories of abuse may be diagnosed with a serious mental illness. The high prevalence rate of childhood abuse among female psychiatric inpatients (51 percent) seems to indicate that childhood trauma is a contributing, if not causal, factor to the diagnosis of a serious mental illness later in life. The factors associated with childhood sexual abuse among women diagnosed with mental illnesses are as follows: early age of onset, more sexual delusions, symptoms of depression and suicidality, and psychotic symptoms. They are also more likely to be diagnosed with borderline personality disorder and have higher rates of substance abuse and serious medical problems.[20,21]

Clearly, behavioral reactions to childhood physical and sexual abuse, including self-injury, flashbacks, instability in relationships, phobias, anger, and rage, may be misunderstood as symptoms of mental illnesses, such as schizophrenia or depression. Proper diagnosis of these symptoms has practical implications for medication and treatment. The treatment for multiple personality disorder or PTSD is significantly different than the treatment for schizophrenia, for example. While medication and treatment strategies differ depending on the diagnosis, it is important that jails do not create a two-tiered system of mental health care. Services must be available to all who need and want them and be provided with equal care, concern, and attention to the recipient.

During incarceration, women diagnosed with mental illnesses who have histories of violence are a particularly vulnerable group. Jails are designed to control the potential for violence. The jail is a highly coercive environment that is based on strict adherence to authority. It is also predominantly male, both detainees and staff. This kind of environment is extremely threatening to women with histories of abuse. The response to this perceived threat may be withdrawal, fighting back or extreme outbursts, and/or worsening of psychiatric symptoms or physical health problems.

Health Care Needs

The most pressing health problems among incarcerated women are HIV, AIDS, tuberculosis, hepatitis, and sexually transmitted diseases. According to the Centers for Disease Control and Prevention (CDC), HIV infection is increasing disproportionately among women. In the general population, HIV infection has a higher prevalence among males, African Americans, Hispanics, and persons of low socioeconomic status, with intravenous (IV) drug use being the predominant exposure source.[3] Among correctional populations, female admissions to U.S.

prison and jail systems are significantly more likely to be HIV seropositive than male admissions. Women are typically underserved in correctional settings. In the case of the HIV epidemic, this is alarming. Female jail detainees are more likely than men to be IV drug users and have greater family responsibilities.[3] In addition, many women enter the system pregnant or postpartum. This means that the health crisis extends beyond the woman to include her family.

Tuberculosis and other infectious diseases are a growing problem for correctional facilities. Not only do the populations in U.S. jails have a higher prevalence of these diseases, but the crowded conditions and poor ventilation of many facilities increase the risk of transmission.

Due to the high prevalence of sexually transmitted diseases, pregnancy, and postpartum conditions, good obstetric-gynecological (OB-GYN) care is critical. While jails are first and foremost detention facilities, the medical needs of these detainees incur a constitutional mandate to provide health care. In addition, it is good public health policy to intervene in public health crises in jails, where medical treatment can be carefully monitored during custody.

Pregnancy and Child Care

In 1991, 67 percent of women in prisons had one or more children under 18,[22] and approximately one quarter of all women who enter prison are pregnant or postpartum.[23] Estimates for jail populations are likely to be even higher, since most individuals spend a considerable amount of time in jail prior to sentencing and transfer to a prison facility. As noted above, women in jails bring with them serious mental health, substance abuse, and medical problems. Infants born to addicted mothers have a higher mortality rate than infants born to nonaddicted mothers.[23] In addition, medical and mental health conditions may present complicating factors in pregnancy that require careful prenatal care. Medications prescribed for psychiatric conditions must be carefully reviewed to ensure the health of both the mother and the developing fetus, particularly during the first trimester.

The responsibility for minor children creates additional stress for women in jail. Approximately 70 percent of incarcerated women lived with their minor children prior to being incarcerated and most expressed an intent to parent after release.[22] Women have a great concern about where and with whom their children are living. In about one third of the cases of incarcerated women with children, child protective services and other social services agencies are involved in the out-of-home placement of their children.[24] In addition, many women are in the formal process of losing custody of their children. These stresses, plus the limited access to children during visiting hours, make incarceration an extremely difficult time for parents.

SERVICES PARITY

The 14th Amendment of the U.S. Constitution, the "due process" clause, assures "nor shall any State deprive any person of life, liberty, or property, without due process of law, nor deny to any person within its jurisdiction the equal protection of the laws." This is the clause that is typically used in case law decisions regarding conditions of pretrial detention. Case law decisions, such as *Estelle v. Gamble,* established the right to minimal medical care and subsequently to other essential treatment. Similar arguments have been made for sentenced jail and prison inmates under the 8th Amendment's "cruel and unusual punishment" clause. To the extent that these constitutional mandates exist for male detainees, they also exist for female detainees.

Parity in correctional programming for female detainees means that services and programming available to male detainees are available to women in the facility, except when those services and programs can be shown to be male-specific. For example, arguments have been made that shock incarceration or "boot camps" are not appropriate for women. A sentence to a boot camp is typically made in lieu of a jail or prison term and is designed to reduce the amount of time an offender spends incarcerated. If this program is available only to men, and women have no equivalent, female offenders will serve longer terms in jail or prison. In this instance, female offenders are not accorded equal protection under the law. For parity to exist under these circumstances, equivalent programming should be made available.

Equivalent mental health and other correctional services for female detainees means that women should have the same range of services and opportunity to use those services with the same criteria and conditions for participation applied to their use. For true parity to exist in jail mental health programming, women must (1) have access to the same mental health services as men, and (2) the services must be tailored to women's unique needs. Many jails provide specialized mental health housing and services for male detainees, but not for their female population. In this case, administrators believe that it is not cost-effective to provide separate housing for women diagnosed with mental illnesses and, therefore, have adapted other procedures to accomplish the same ends, including transferring women who exhibit less severe symptoms to inpatient settings and overmedicating women to reduce behavioral symptoms so that they can remain in general population. These adaptations to procedure do not provide equal treatment.

In addition, some consideration must be given to where services are physically located, when the services may be used, and who they are designed to serve. Typically, female housing units are physically separated from the male units. Commonly, jail programming and services are located within the male housing area. This means that women must pass through or close to the male housing. When this happens, the women are often harassed by the male detainees. Administrators attempt to reduce contact to protect female detainees from harassment and assault and to reduce the risk of illicit activities, both of which compromise security. Many jails have solved this problem by bringing all services to the female housing units. The unintended consequence is that services are truncated, both in the breadth of services and the time available for specific activities.

Of critical importance in jail mental health and other programming is the question, "For whom are the services designed?" Most clinical interventions are based on the assumption that men and women will respond similarly to treatment given similar clinical characteristics.

However, there is a growing acknowledgment within the medical, psychiatric, and substance abuse treatment communities that women's psychosocial development, experiential characteristics, and physiology are sufficiently different from men to require that treatment interventions be designed specifically for them. This is especially true of psychiatric medications. Many medications have been tested only on men. Even in drug trials where women have participated as subjects, women of childbearing years are excluded. Careful consideration should be given to what medications are selected and how they affect the women for whom they are prescribed.

Given the growing population of female jail detainees and their unique characteristics, it has become increasingly necessary for jail administrators to begin developing appropriate, gender-specific services for women. This is not an option. It is a constitutional duty. In addition, providing appropriate services and programming to female detainees makes sense from a management perspective. Without these services, women can be disruptive and may, in fact, be more likely to use expensive medical and mental health services.

WOMEN-SPECIFIC JAIL MENTAL HEALTH SERVICES

Jails are first and foremost correctional institutions and should remain as such.[25] Jails that provide comprehensive mental health treatment services are at risk of becoming the treatment facility of choice in communities with dwindling community-based mental health resources. At the same time, jails incur a substantial constitutional mandate to provide minimum medical and psychiatric services to all detainees who need such services. Two basic principles guide the minimum requirements: (1) Persons in detention should not leave the facility in worse condition than when they arrived, and (2) persons should not be punished for being identified as having a need (i.e., the identification of a mental illness should not affect access to other services or length of time spent in jail). Jail mental health services are typically focused on identification, crisis management, and short-term treatment. Adaptations to typical services and resources to improve services delivery to female detainees are discussed below.

Screening, Assessment, and Evaluation

Screening, assessment, and evaluation is a three-stage process by which jails identify persons in need of psychiatric care. The *initial screen* is conducted by a corrections officer at booking. The purpose of this screen is to flag persons in need of a more detailed mental health evaluation and to identify persons at risk for suicide. Officers are not trained clinicians and are not expected to make decisions regarding treatment. The booking officer's job is to refer all individuals who, because of their responses to specific questions or by their appearance or behavior, appear to be at risk.

A *mental health assessment* is often a second step toward providing treatment. This can be done by a mental health worker or by medical staff within the context of a medical history. Both the booking screen and the medical exam are done on all individuals who are booked into the jail and assigned housing. The mental health assessment is conducted only on persons flagged by the booking screen or by the medical department. At the final stage, persons assessed as needing psychiatric services are referred for a full *psychiatric evaluation.* Psychiatric evaluations are conducted by a psychiatrist and often result in the prescription of medication.

Screening, assessment, and evaluation are critical points in the services delivery system for the provision of appropriate services to female offenders because information uncovered at these points affect classification decisions and whether women will receive mental health and other treatment services. Screening instruments used by booking officers should include a minimum set of questions related to symptoms of affective and psychotic disorders, history of mental health treatment, current use of prescribed psychotropic medication, and risk of suicide. For these screens to encompass the characteristics of women diagnosed with mental illnesses, questions should also ask about (1) symptoms of depression, (2) whether the woman was recently injured, and (3) whether she has minor children and, if so, whether they are currently being cared for.

In addition to more detailed information regarding the areas noted above, the medical and mental health assessments and the psychiatric evaluation are points where information about physical and sexual abuse should be gathered. This requires that medical and mental health staff receive training in assessing women with histories of abuse. This information is critical for the identification of the correct diagnosis and the development of appropriate mental health, health care, and substance abuse treatment plans.

Classification and Housing

Structurally, jails are designed to control the potential for violence. Their primary mandate is to hold individuals in a secure environment and prevent physical injury to either staff or detainees. Single-cell tiers and pods, highly regimented schedules, lack of privacy, and an expectation of an unquestioning response to authority are characteristics of correctional facilities designed to maximize control and reduce opportunities for breaches in security (e.g., escapes, riots and violent incidents, use of contraband). This structure, in fact, functions well for men who tend to be socialized to hierarchical authority. However, women tend to rely more heavily on flat structures of interpersonal relationships and desire more privacy. In addition, women do not pose the same threats to jail security as men. Jail facilities may, in fact, create an additional unintended burden on female detainees.

Classification refers to the process by which individuals booked into the jail are assigned housing. Appropriate classification takes into account seriousness of offense and risk of violence, special needs such as medical or mental health problems, gender and age, and adjudication status. Most jails assign different security levels within their facility and have different kinds of housing, including general population, medical (where persons diagnosed with acute mental illnesses or suicide risk may be placed), and administrative segregation. Some jails also provide specialized housing such as mental health units for persons with stable conditions, substance abuse therapeutic communities, trustee housing, and juvenile units.

In many jails, there is only one classification status for women—female. Because women comprise such a small proportion of the jail population, many facilities tend to group all women together, regardless of security risk or needs. However, women diagnosed with mental illnesses in jail have the right to the same protections as their male counterparts. Because many jails do not provide special housing for women diagnosed with mental illnesses, many facilities transfer female detainees with moderate symptoms to psychiatric facilities, where a male detainee with similar characteristics would remain in the jail. While this appears to be more humane, it has serious consequences. First, a transfer out of the jail for evaluation or inpatient treatment interrupts, and may significantly delay, the adjudication process, thus extending the period of confinement. Second, the inpatient facility may not be within the locality. This means that the woman may not be able to see family and other support persons easily, if at all. Also, some persons diagnosed with chronic mental health conditions resist transfers to inpatient settings, preferring the jail to a psychiatric facility. Jails must provide the same kinds of housing options to both men and women. They must also apply the same standards and procedures to both men and women when transferring detainees to psychiatric facilities.

Eighty-seven percent of female offenders are arrested for nonviolent crimes. For the most part, women do not require high-security supervision. Given this fact and the widespread prevalence of histories of abuse, several adaptions to housing and staffing may be suggested:

1. Staff must be trained in managing women in a nonaggressive and nonthreatening manner, realizing that women have been victimized predominantly by men and abandoned by their female protectors;
2. Housing units, particularly in jails with podular designs and direct supervision, should consider cell doors that are not locked; and
3. Jails should consider ways to normalize the jail environment, including more time out of the cells for the detainees to interact socially and more protections for personal privacy, such as shower curtains and doors on bathroom stalls.

Medication and Psychiatric Follow-Up Services

Medication and medication monitoring of women are major issues for jail psychiatry. Women are diagnosed at a much higher rate with unipolar depression. However, some jails do not allow the prescription of certain antidepressants, because of their potential for abuse. Despite indications or previous treatment, some women cannot receive the medication of choice due to standing policies. On the other hand, these policies exist for good reason. Women and men with significant addictive disorders may request antidepressants as a substitute for their drug of choice. Each individual case must be reviewed carefully prior to the prescription of medication, and at regular intervals thereafter, to assure that the medications are appropriate to the need.

Overprescription of medication is as problematic as underprescription. Because women's housing is limited and because women are not as easily managed as men in general, there is a tendency to overprescribe medications for the sole purpose of tranquilizing the detainee. From the jail's perspective, this is a reasonable policy, because it enhances the jail's security. From a human rights perspective, it is an unjustified use of chemical restraints and violates constitutional rights. In addition, the medication may interfere with the detainee's ability to participate in her adjudication process.

Crisis Intervention and Suicide Precautions

Women diagnosed with mental illnesses in jail do not typically exhibit the same symptoms as men. Nor should the crisis intervention responses be the same. Clinicians must be trained to identify suicide risk in women and how to appropriately intervene in mental health crises without retraumatizing a woman who typically has been repeatedly traumatized.

The policies and procedures governing the use of physical and chemical restraints should be carefully reviewed for their application on all female detainees, both those with diagnoses of mental illness and those without. Because histories of abuse are so prevalent among women in jail, these procedures should be developed for all women. Some mental health systems are beginning to review these issues in response to a growing awareness of the damage that these procedures have on individuals' physical and emotional well-being. This is critically important when managing women with significant histories of physical and sexual abuse.

If staff of jail psychiatric services expect to have a continuing relationship with a female detainee, it may be helpful to understand what actions or events cause distress and what interventions staff can use that will help to calm the detainee. It is also helpful to tell women diagnosed with mental illnesses who might require restraint what procedures are used in the facility early on in their confinement.

Other Mental Health Treatment

In jails where other kinds of mental health treatment are available, several considerations for women should be addressed. Single-gender groups are critically important. Women who have been victims of abuse do not function well in mixed-gender treatment groups. In addition, women who have experienced physical or sexual abuse as well as women diagnosed with mental illnesses appear to benefit from peer-support groups. Given the prohibitive costs of professional services and the benefit of peer support, jails may want to consider using community resources to supplement core psychiatric services.

Case Management and Discharge Planning

Most jails do not provide case management or discharge planning services. Arguably, release planning can be the most important service a jail can provide to reduce the probability of return. For all persons with special needs, both male and female, linkages to community services, particularly if the linkage is more than a telephone appointment, can make a significant difference in engagement in community-based services.

While most jails acknowledge this important service, the manner by which individuals are processed limits a jail's ability to develop effective linkages. Most important, it is critical to understand that release decisions are made from the court. Except when inmates serve specific sentences, jails do not typically know when someone will be released, whether it is pretrial or upon sentencing.

Beginning discharge planning early in confinement is important. Upon release, women in general, and women diagnosed with mental illnesses in particular, will require more community services, including housing for the women and their children, mental health and substance abuse services, social services and entitlements, and health care and vocational services. In the case of female detainees, discharge planning involves not only services for the individual released from jail but a web of services for single-parent families.

Because release from jail is complicated by the re-integration of a woman into multiple contexts—her family, significant relationships, and community—and requires a lifestyle change in all domains of her life if she is to remain free, lead time is important. Women recently released often express being overwhelmed by all the demands. To whatever extent possible, issues around release should be addressed early and often in mental health and substance abuse counseling. In addition, slow re-integration through halfway houses or other residential facilities is helpful.

IMPLICATIONS FOR MENTAL HEALTH SERVICES DELIVERY: APPROPRIATELY RESPONDING TO WOMEN'S SPECIAL NEEDS

To address the special needs of women diagnosed with mental illnesses in correctional settings, comprehensive and integrated strategies are necessary. To provide leadership in this area, specific attention should be given to the following areas.

Parity of mental health services. One of the major issues regarding women's mental health in correctional settings is the lack of services. The state of mental health services in U.S. jails is poor, but for women, it is worse. Because women represent such a low percentage of correctional populations, they often do not have access to the same mental health or other services that are available to men. In addition, when they do exist, rarely do mental health services give attention to the special needs of women. But before specialized programs can be developed, basic services must be available to all women who need them. This requires a commitment on the part of the jail administration. More important, this requires the allocation of resources, including staffing, space, and money.

Targeted screening/evaluation procedures and instruments. Currently, no screening and assessment tools exist that are designed specifically for women. A critical first step in the process of treatment is proper diagnosis and treatment planning. In corrections, woman-specific tools must be developed that support appropriate classification of women and can identify issues that complicate treatment and supervision, including histories of abuse, medical problems, and child care issues.

Furthermore, because major mental illnesses, such as major affective disorders, schizophrenia, and dissociative disorders precipitated by childhood trauma, and symptoms associated with PTSD have different courses and may involve different treatment interventions, screening and evaluation tools for women who have been diagnosed with a mental illness must be highly specific and sensitive. However, if the facility has no flexibility in treatment provision, jail staff must carefully consider the risks associated with identifying a woman as "mentally ill" with the benefits of more complete information.

Special crisis intervention procedures. Because so many women in jail, with and without diagnoses of mental illnesses, have experienced physical and/or sexual abuse, protocols for crisis intervention should be developed for use with all women in crisis. Jails may want to consider the use of advance directives and investigate noninvasive, nonthreatening de-escalation techniques for general use.

Peer support and counseling programs. Because some psychiatric interventions are coercive (e.g., seclusion and restraint, involuntary medication, locked rooms, and paternalistic treatment and infantilization of patients), the more so when delivered in jails, they may be resisted or rejected. Peer-counseling programs show great promise in helping women to address both mental health problems and the violent events in their lives. These programs are not designed to replace standard mental health treatment, and may, in fact, function best when coordinated with existing services. Peer-support programs also offer an opportunity to connect the woman with her community prior to release. Transition from jail to the community is often one of the most difficult steps for women to take. Continuity is critical. Many peer support programs (i.e., 12-step substance abuse programs, AIDS awareness, Double Trouble) have community groups.

Parenting programs. Research indicates that adult survivors of child abuse often repeat the behaviors of their parents with their own children. Furthermore, substance abuse is strongly associated with child abuse. To the degree that women in correctional settings are both victims of violence and perpetrators of violence, they are also at a higher risk of abusing their own children. Parenting programs directed at education, empowerment, and practical skills hold promise to break the cycle of violence in families.

Integrated services. Clearly, women in correctional settings are likely to face multiple issues, including substance abuse, mental illnesses or emotional difficulties, parenting, and dangerous or violent home environments. Integrating services, whether it is in the jail or transition to the community, holds the most promise in assisting women to remain safely in the community.

Training programs for security, mental health, and substance abuse professionals. Issues specific to women are not well-known. Even when the administration supports woman-specific programming, direct line staff do not always understand the need and therefore do not act in accordance with the program procedures. Training is necessary not only for criminal justice personnel, but also for mental health, medical, and substance abuse workers. Misdiagnosis, the medicalization of social problems, and sexist attitudes contribute to the continuing abuse of women in jail.

Outcome measures. How do we know when we are making progress? In regard to woman-specific services, this is an especially cogent question. Attention must be given to the development of appropriate outcome measures for treatment interventions designed to affect women diagnosed with mental illnesses in jails. Where most programs are designed for men, so too are most outcome measures. It is not that these indicators are not applicable; rather, they are insufficient. Attention must be given to outcomes that acknowledge the wide variation in women's life experiences, adaptive styles, and modes of recovery. Measures should be developed through a joint effort by mental health professionals, researchers, and the women using services. While this is a generic issue, it is equally valid in the assessment and evaluation of mental health programs in correctional settings.

U.S. jails vary enormously in size and resources. Not all facilities are large enough to provide a full array of mental health services and housing options on-site. However, all jails are required to provide *access* to necessary services. Small jails access psychiatric care typically by contracting with community providers. To ensure that the rights of women held in jails are protected, administrators and services providers should carefully review the services options and protocols applied to women to guarantee that (1) they have access to basic psychiatric care, (2) they have the same access as men in the same facility to other housing and support services, and (3) the services provided are modified to address woman-specific treatment issues and needs, where necessary.

REFERENCES

1. Gilliard DK, Beck AJ: Prison and jail inmates, 1995. *Bureau of Justice Statistics Bulletin.* NCJ-161132. Washington, DC: U.S. Department of Justice, 1996.
2. Morris SM, Steadman HJ, Veysey BM: Mental health services in American jails: A survey of innovative practices. *Criminal Justice and Behavior* 1997; 24:3-19.
3. Hammett TM, Daugherty AL: *1990 Update: AIDS in Correctional Facilities.* Washington, DC: U.S. Department of Justice, 1991.
4. Policy Research Incorporated: *Practical Approaches in the Treatment of Women Who Abuse Alcohol and Other Drugs.* DHHS Pub. No. (SMA) 94-3006. Rockville, MD: Center for Substance Abuse Treatment, 1994.
5. Chesney-Lind M: Rethinking women's imprisonment: A critical examination of trends in female incarceration. In: Price BR, Sokoloff NJ (Eds.): *The Criminal Justice System and Women: Offenders, Victims, and Workers.* New York: McGraw-Hill, 1995, pp. 105-117.
6. Bloom B, Chesney-Lind M, Owen B: *Women in California Prisons: Hidden Victims of the War on Drugs.* San Francisco: Center on Juvenile and Criminal Justice, 1994.
7. Steffensmeier D: Trends in female crime: It's still a man's world. In: Price BR, Sokoloff NJ (Eds.): *The Criminal Justice System and Women: Offenders, Victims, and Workers.* New York: McGraw-Hill, 1995, pp. 89-104.
8. Maguire K, Pastore AL: *Sourcebook of Criminal Justice Statistics—1993.* NCJ-148211. Washington, DC: U.S. Department of Justice, 1994.
9. Teplin LA: Psychiatric and substance abuse disorders among male urban jail detainees. *American Journal of Public Health* 1994; 84:290-293.
10. Rice ME, Harris GT: Treatment for prisoners with mental disorder. In: Steadman HJ, Cocozza JJ (Eds.): *Mental Illness in America's Prisons.* Seattle, WA: National Coalition for the Mentally Ill in the Criminal Justice System, 1993, pp. 91-113.
11. Teplin LA, Abram KM, McClelland GM: Prevalence of psychiatric disorders among incarcerated women. *Archives of General Psychiatry* 1996; 53:505-512.
12. National Institute of Justice: *Drug Use Forecasting: 1994 Annual Report on Adult and Juvenile Arrestees.* Washington, DC: U.S. Department of Justice, 1995.
13. Holden P, Rann J, Van Drasek L: *Unheard Voices: A Report on Women in Michigan County Jails.* Lansing: Michigan Women's Commission, 1993.
14. Finkelstein N, Duncan SA, Derman L, et al.: *Getting Sober, Getting Well.* Cambridge, MA: Women's Alcoholism Program of CASPAR, 1990.
15. Matteo S: The risk of multiple addictions: Guidelines for assessing a woman's alcohol and drug use. *Western Journal of Medicine* 1988; 149:742.
16. Moise R, Kovach J, Reed B, et al.: A comparison of Black and White women entering drug abuse treatment programs. *International Journal of the Addictions* 1982; 17:46-47.
17. Task Force on the Female Offender: *What Does the Future Hold?* Alexandria, VA: American Correctional Association, 1990.
18. Goodman LA, Dutton MA, Harris M: Episodically homeless women with severe mental illness: Prevalence of physical and sexual assault. *American Journal of Orthopsychiatry* 1995; 65:468-478.
19. National Council on Alcoholism and Drug Dependence. *NCADD Fact Sheet: Alcoholism, Other Drug Addictions and Related Problems Among Women.* New York: National Council on Alcoholism and Drug Dependence, 1990.

20. Brown GR, Anderson B: Psychiatric comorbidity in adult inpatients with childhood histories of sexual and physical abuse. *American Journal of Psychiatry* 1991; 148:55-61.

21. Bryer JB, Nelson BA, Miller JB, et al.: Childhood sexual and physical abuse as factors in adult psychiatric illness. *American Journal of Psychiatry* 1987; 144:1426-1430.

22. Snell TL: *Correctional Populations in the United States, 1991.* NCJ-142729. Washington, DC: U.S. Department of Justice, 1993.

23. Leukefeld C: *Planning for Alcohol and Other Drug Abuse Treatment for Adults in the Criminal Justice System.* DHHS Pub. No. (SMA) 95-3039. Rockville, MD: Center for Substance Abuse Treatment, 1995.

24. Smith B: Special needs of women in the criminal justice system. Center for substance abuse treatment. *TIE Communique* 1993; Spring:31-32.

25. Steadman HJ, McCarty DW, Morrissey JP: *The Mentally Ill in Jail: Planning for Essential Services.* New York: Guilford, 1989.

18

Risk Factors and Resilience

Mental Health Needs and Services Use of Older Women

Deborah K. Padgett, Ph.D.
Barbara J. Burns, Ph.D.
Lois A. Grau, Ph.D.

The mental health needs of older women are of increasing significance given demographic projections of explosive growth in the over-65 age group, of which women are a clear majority. However, relevant bodies of literature from the fields of gerontology, geropsychiatry, and mental health have shown a notable lack of attention to this topic.[1,2] With few exceptions,[3-6] the intersection of old age, female gender, and mental health remains relatively unexplored.

This chapter will seek to fill this gap in knowledge by reviewing what is known about the mental health needs of older women and their use of mental health services in community and institutional settings. Particular attention will be paid to discussing how gender and age may affect accurate and effective diagnosis and treatment of mental disorders as well as gender- and age-related barriers to the use of mental health services.

Any discussion of the mental health status of older women must address resilience as well as risk factors. That is, a balanced picture must

NOTE: We would like to thank Ryan Wagner, Ph.D., for assistance in data analysis, Ms. Kathy Miller for her work on table preparation, and Ms. Yelena Gubskaya for typing the many references.

discuss "success stories" of female aging as well as the risks associated with the "double jeopardy" of growing old in a society where being old and female entails one of the most devalued statuses available in American society.[3,7,8] In this context, many older women are not simply surviving, but are thriving in old age.

Contrary to stereotypical notions of aging as a time of inevitable decline and disability, recent research has produced a convincing picture of increasing robustness among America's elderly population. Analyses of the National Long Term Care Surveys from 1982 to 1994 show continuous declines in rates of chronic diseases such as hypertension, arthritis, and emphysema as well as work-related disability.[9] Steady declines in disability are traceable to public health improvements affecting the earlier lives of recent cohorts of elderly persons; improved self-care, such as reduced rates of smoking and increased exercise; and recent medical advances in hip replacement, cataract surgeries, and treatment of heart disease, stroke, and hypertension.[9]

These reports of vitality and resilience in old age belie traditional stereotypes of aging.[10] At the same time, broad population trends pointing to healthier aging do not mean that all older women are faring equally well. The task remains to identify gender-related risk factors associated with mental health problems and access to mental health services in the older years. As the older population grows dramatically in numbers, the problems and prospects for successful aging become a "women's issue."

ESTIMATING THE NEED FOR MENTAL HEALTH SERVICES AMONG OLDER WOMEN

Despite recent evidence of improved health of older men and women, the converging effects of ageism and sexism—termed "double jeopardy"[3,11,12]—place many older women at risk of mental disorders and inadequate or inappropriate treatment. Risks associated with double jeopardy include disproportionate economic losses,[12,13] a greater likelihood of widowhood and of living alone, societal devaluation, and the stress of taking care of spouses and/or aging parents.[3,14,15] For example, while widowhood is objectively the same life event for men and women, its consequences disproportionately affect older women since they live longer. Thus, while older men are more likely to remarry, older women are less likely to have the support of a spouse.[15] Problems of younger women—domestic violence, sexual abuse, and rape—may plague older women as well.[16]

While women benefit from greater longevity, they face the threat of chronic physical disability and institutionalization (albeit in later years in more recent cohorts). Moreover, they are more likely than men to face the stress of caregiving and widowhood and to suffer from related depression.[17] Estimates of rates of caregiving-related depression range from 14 percent[18] to 78 percent.[19] By comparison, men are more likely to have caregiving spouses or children and less likely to face widowhood.[17] At the same time, older men (particularly white men) have some of the highest rates of suicide of any age/gender subgroups.[20] Those who do survive to old age suffer more from acute, life-threatening illnesses than from chronic disability.[21]

Certain factors affect estimates of the need for mental health services of older women. First, older adults in general are more likely than younger adults to suffer from organic mental disorders (i.e., dementias). This has important implications for appropriate diagnosis and treatment as well as services delivery planning for elderly persons.[22] Second, estimates of need for mental health treatment can vary widely depending on the diagnostic criteria employed. This variation particularly affects estimates targeting older women since very few screening and diagnostic instruments are age- and gender-neutral.[23] For example, estimates based on *Diagnostic and Statistical Manual of Mental Disorders* (*DSM*) diagnoses tend to underreport the extent of psychiatric symptomatology among elderly persons since they neglect subclinical states such as distress.[22,24] Given the greater prevalence of distress among women,[14] diagnosis-based case finding may underreport the true extent of their psychological problems. The insensitivity of many depression scales to male-associated symptoms of depression may lead to underreporting for men as well.[25]

Third, older adults are more likely than their younger counterparts to suffer from comorbid physical and mental illnesses.[26-28] Estimates of need may neglect comorbid psychiatric disorders that accompany physical illness, an issue particularly affecting older women.[21]

Finally, the majority of psychiatric disorders are detected and treated de facto in the general medical sector.[29] This pattern of care is pronounced among elderly persons in general[30-33] and older women in particular.[14,33]

With these caveats in mind, we can proceed to review extant epidemiologic data. For example, the Epidemiologic Catchment Area (ECA) surveys in the early 1980s, sponsored by the National Institute of Mental Health (NIMH), provided clear evidence that older persons manifest a lower prevalence of mental disorders compared with those under age 65.[1,34] However, there is considerable age-by-sex diversity in the over-65 group. Table 18.1 shows both the rates of diagnoses and of mental health services use from the ECA data broken down by sex and age.

As shown in Table 18.1, women over age 75 have the highest rates of any mental disorder; these rates drop considerably when cognitive impairment is excluded but still remain higher than those for men. For men, disparities between the young-old and old-old are minimal except for diagnoses excluding cognitive impairment where men over 75 manifest much lower rates than their 65- to 74-year-old counterparts. Thus, a pattern emerges of greater prevalence of mental health problems of older women compared with older men, even when cognitive impairment is excluded. While the proportion of over-65 persons in need of mental health services is not large, the levels of *unmet* need are substantial.

Unfortunately, more recent national epidemiologic data are not available. The NIMH-sponsored epidemiologic study of the 1990s—the National Co-Morbidity Survey (NCS)—had an upper age limit of 54 years.[35] Major community surveys of the older population such as the EPESE (Established Populations for Epidemiologic Studies of the Elderly)[36] fail to assess mental disorders beyond use of a screening scale for depressive symptoms.

Compared with community rates, estimates of the prevalence of mental illness among institutionalized elderly persons residing in nursing homes are much higher,[37] as high as 65 percent.[38] Since women comprise the overwhelming majority of nursing home residents, these high rates underscore the need to consider older women's mental health needs in institutional as well as community settings.

TABLE 18.1 Prevalence of Mental Disorder and Use of Mental Health Services, by Sex and Age (over 65): Epidemiologic Catchment Area (ECA) Data[a] (in percentages)

	Diagnosis			Service Use		
	Any DIS[b] (6 mo.) Diagnosis	Any DIS Excluding Cognitive Impairment	Any DIS Excluding Phobia	Any Mental Health Use[c]	General Medical Mental Health Use	Specialty Mental Health Use
Men						
65-74	11.93	8.78	7.96	8.78	5.56	3.22
75+	10.04	5.44	8.03	8.53	5.81	2.72
Women						
65-74	13.16	11.65	5.27	13.37	11.13	2.24
75+	15.45	9.36	9.61	6.35	6.35	0

a. Rates represent all five ECA sites combined and were adjusted for differential probabilities of selection and weighted to reflect 1980 Census distributions for age, sex, and race as appropriate to the sample area.

b. Diagnostic Interview Schedule.

c. Either general medical or specialty mental health use.

USE OF AMBULATORY MENTAL HEALTH SERVICES BY OLDER WOMEN

There are a few sources of national data on mental health service use by older men and women during the 1980s. These include the ECA data, the National Medical Expenditure Survey (NMES),[39] and the Blue Cross/Blue Shield Federal Employee Program (FEP) studies.[40] Of these three sources of utilization data, only the ECA data provide measures of mental health needs as well as service use.[34]

As shown in Table 18.1, rates of mental health service use from the ECA data demonstrate that women over 75 have the lowest rates of any mental health service use despite higher rates of disorder. Furthermore, none of the women over age 75 received specialty mental health services. In contrast, there were few age differences in service use among men—the 65- to 74-year-olds resembled their over-75 male counterparts. While unmet need is disproportionately high for all older persons in the ECA surveys,[34] women over 75 appear to have the highest levels of unmet need.

Table 18.2 presents age and sex differences in use of various types of mental health services from the 1987 NMES. As shown, the utilization rates for any type of mental health visit were lowest for the over-65 age group of adults—3.1 percent for men and 5.5 percent for women. For use of mental health services in the specialty sector only, the rates were .9 percent for men and 1.2 percent for women over age 65. On the other hand, rates of use of psychotropic medications (with or without a mental health visit) were highest for those over age 65—7.5 percent for men and 14.8 percent for women.[41] The latter rate for older women far exceeds any other type of mental health service use for any of the age-by-sex groups.

These findings raise concerns about appropriate use of psychotropic medications among older persons in general (older women in particular) and about the general absence of a knowledgeable mental health professional supervising use of these drugs.[42] Concerns have been expressed about inappropriate use of psychotropic drugs in the primary care sector[43] and in institutional care.[44] A study by Burns and Kamerow[45] found that 30 percent of psychotropic drug prescriptions for elderly persons in nursing homes were inappropriate due to a lack of a psychiatric diagnosis or notation of symptoms warranting use of psychotropic drugs.

Compared with younger adults, all older persons who are eligible for Social Security have some type of health insurance from Medicare, Medicaid, and/or private sources. However, mental health coverage tends to be limited. Medicare limits lifetime mental health benefits to 190 days in a private psychiatric hospital and limits stays per episode to 90 days. Outpatient mental health coverage requires a 50 percent co-pay for psychotherapy and a 20 percent co-pay for medical management of psychotropic drugs.[2] Further problems in access arise from restrictions placed by Medicare on the certification of nonpsychiatrist providers (such as psychiatric nurses or social workers), who are more likely to make home visits.

Mandatory mental health services covered by Medicaid include a wide array of inpatient and outpatient services. However, most states place limits on coverage. For example, the median reimbursement rate for one psychotherapy visit was $53 in 1993, about one half of the average fee.[2] Perhaps not surprisingly, a small minority of mental health providers accept Medicaid, thereby restricting access to care.

TABLE 18.2 Age and Sex Differences in Use of Mental Health Services, by Type of Service, United States, 1987

Population Characteristic	Total Population (in thousands)	Ambulatory Care: Rates of Use			
		All (%)	Mental Health Specialty (%)	Prescribed Medicines (%)	Inpatient Hospital (%)
Total	239,393	5.2	2.7	4.1	0.4
Males	115,861	4.3	2.2	2.7	0.4
Under 19	34,501	3.9	2.1	1.1	0.2
19-39	40,406	4.6	2.6	1.5	0.5
40-54	18,890	5.5	3.0	3.3	0.7
55-64	10,350	3.5	1.3	5.8	0.4
65 and over	11,714	3.1	0.9	7.5	0.5
Females	123,532	6.1	3.1	5.4	0.4
Under 19	33,067	3.2	1.9	0.5	0.2
19-39	42,241	7.5	4.5	3.1	0.4
40-54	20,025	8.7	4.6	8.1	0.5
55-64	11,617	5.9	2.1	9.9	0.3
65 and over	16,581	5.5	1.2	14.8	0.6

SOURCE: Agency for Health Care Policy and Research, National Medical Expenditure Survey—Household Survey. Freiman M, Cunningham JP, Cornelius L: *Use and Expenditures for the Treatment of Mental Health Problems.* AHCPR Pub. No. 94-0085. Rockville, MD: Public Health Service, 1994.

Table 18.3 shows that type of insurance coverage plays a role in use of mental health services among older Americans. In particular, Medicaid coverage is associated with the highest rates of use.[a] According to Freiman et al.,[39] this may be due to somewhat more generous coverage of mental health treatment by Medicaid or to the greater likelihood that the older persons with chronic mental illness are covered by Medicaid.

Findings from multivariate analyses of factors affecting use of mental health services by older adults in the NMES data reveal a set of factors concordant with the risk factors for poor mental health among older women: Widowhood, chronic health problems, and disability days were significantly associated with use.[41]

Similar to the findings of the ECA and NMES surveys, the FEP study of over 400,000 federal employees over age 55 insured by Blue Cross/Blue Shield in 1983 revealed that Black and White women had higher rates of use of outpatient mental health services than Black and White men, respectively.[40] Interestingly, a race-by-sex effect was found:

TABLE 18.3 Use of Mental Health Services, by Variants of Medicare Coverage, United States, 1987

	Ambulatory Care: Rates of Use				
	Total Population (in thousands)	*All (%)*	*Mental Health Specialty (%)*	*Prescribed Medicines (%)*	*Inpatient Hospital (%)*
Medicare only	3,823	5.7	2.1	10.9	0.9
Medicare and private insurance	23,576	5.0	1.6	12.5	0.6
Medicare and Medicaid or other public insurance	2,824	14.6	6.3	20.4	2.4

SOURCE: Agency for Health Care Policy and Research, National Medical Expenditure Survey—Household Survey. Freiman M, Cunningham JP, Cornelius L: *Use and Expenditures for the Treatment of Mental Health Problems.* AHCPR Pub. No. 94-0085. Rockville, MD: Public Health Service, 1994.

The rates of service use by Black women were still lower than those of White men.

WOMEN'S GREATER USE OF MENTAL HEALTH SERVICES: DOES THIS CONFER AN ADVANTAGE?

Higher rates of outpatient mental health services use by older women appear to confer an advantage not experienced by older men. However, it is important to note that this gender gap occurs in the general medical sector rather than in the specialty mental health sector (see Table 18.1). Since appropriate recognition and treatment of mental health problems are problematic in this sector,[14,23] it cannot be concluded that women's mental health needs are being met appropriately.

Of course, if older women have greater need for these services, higher levels of use are appropriate. As shown in Table 18.1, rates of disorder are somewhat higher for older women compared with older men, so it is possible that greater need is driving greater use. On the other hand, some have argued that gender differences in prevalence are not substantial and that older women are not at greater risk. Leaf and Bruce[46] found that the effects of gender were not significant in multivariate analyses predicting service use after controlling for the effects of psychiatric symptomatology and other factors. Resolution of this issue requires further epidemiologic studies measuring both the prevalence of mental disorders and service use. In the meantime, there are other potential explanations for this gender gap.

Studies of nonelderly populations have shown gender differences in help-seeking behavior and provider attitudes that may partially explain why women are higher users of mental health services. Compared with men, women are more likely to use general medical services, to perceive an emotional problem and seek help for it, and to be recognized as having emotional problems by physicians.[47,48] The threshold for a mental disorder diagnosis is lower for women than for men, particularly when diagnosed by primary care physicians, who may perceive men's problems with alcohol as nonpsychiatric.[49]

While it is difficult to disentangle the effects of greater need, propensity to use services, and propensity to diagnose older women's problems as mental disorders, all are likely to explain greater service use by women. Regardless of cause, these higher utilization rates still fall well below estimates of need. The implications of unmet need can be profound, including a decline not only in functioning and in quality of life, but in life expectancy. In addition to morbidity risk, depression has been linked to increased risk of mortality among older adults in the community[50,51] and in nursing homes.[52]

MENTAL HEALTH TREATMENT IN LONG-TERM AND INSTITUTIONAL CARE

Estimates of unmet need in long-term care are much higher than those for community-dwelling older persons. Analyses of data from the 1985 National Nursing Home Survey revealed that only 4.5 percent of elderly residents received any mental treatment in a one-month period, while two thirds of the nursing home population had a mental disorder diagnosis in their records.[53] A total estimate of unmet need in nursing homes is 91.4 percent.[38]

Concern about this problem and the burgeoning costs of long-term care led to the passage of Public Law 100-203, known as the 1987 Omnibus Budget Reconciliation Act (OBRA), in which Congress mandated treatment of mental illness in nursing homes. Under provisions of the law, nursing homes are required to screen both applicants and current residents for mental disorders. Residents in need of "active treatment" (excluding those with dementia) are to be identified and treated in the nursing home or discharged to an appropriate psychiatric facility. According to Larson and Lyons,[54] slightly more than one half of current nursing home residents would be exempt from OBRA regulations; of these, 57 percent have a diagnosis of senile dementia. Though not yet a reality, strict enforcement of OBRA regulations could lead to the discharge of elderly patients with a mental illness to community living without adequate care.[54]

Semi-institutional housing alternatives—known as board and care homes, rest homes, assisted living homes, and adult foster care homes—represent a growing source of care for older persons who need assistance with daily activities but do not need full-time nursing care.[55] Unfortunately, little is known about these settings; they vary from small, family-run homes to large institutions regulated to varying degrees by state and local agencies.[56] One national survey reporting on use of psychotropic medications in board and care homes highlighted the problem of inadequate medical follow-up.[57]

The scarcity of data about use of institution-based mental health services by elderly persons prevents extensive examination of gender differences in rates; most surveys do not provide age-by-sex breakdowns in rates of use. However, the available data indicate few gender differences in rates of mental health service use in either the acute or long-term care institutional sectors. A study of nursing home residents by Burns et al.[53] found almost identical rates of use by men and women. For use of specialty psychiatric hospitals, the NMES found virtually identical admission rates for men and women over age 65[41] as did the FEP analyses of federal employees over age 55.[40]

Of course, identical population-based utilization rates still indicate greater overall use by older women since they are more numerous in the older population. Even a casual glance at nursing homes and other residential facilities for elderly persons reveals a predominance of women residents—about 70 percent.[58]

Different issues emerge when addressing the needs of older women with serious mental illness (SMI) whose onset of mental illness occurred when they were younger. A number of authors have examined the needs of elderly persons with SMI[59-62] and of women with SMI in particular.[63] About 90 percent of all institutionalized elderly persons with SMI reside in nursing homes; only 8 percent are in state and county psychiatric hospitals.[61] Women comprise 71 percent of the SMI population in nursing homes, about the same as their general proportion in the nursing home population.[58]

Current cohorts of older women with SMI have typically experienced stays in public psychiatric hospitals and inadequate community-based care. Many end up in nursing home placement where adequate mental health treatment is rarely available. Furthermore, treatment and rehabilitation in their younger years likely encouraged traditional female roles and de-emphasized autonomy[42,63,64] and involved prescriptions for more drugs and for higher dosages of neuroleptics than men.[43] The results are greater dependency, higher risk of tardive dyskinesia, and reduced ability to benefit from mental health treatment when it is available.

Not all older women with SMI reside in nursing homes—perhaps one of the most enduring images of these women is that of the homeless "bag lady." Research on homeless elderly persons with SMI is relatively rare and has thus far concentrated more on men than on women.[65,66] We do know that shelter beds for homeless women are fewer in number than those for men and that women's shelters tend to be more restrictive and less tolerant of deviant behavior.[63] In short, many homeless women's shelters remain uninviting to older women with SMI.

BARRIERS TO OLDER WOMEN'S USE OF MENTAL HEALTH SERVICES

Like their younger counterparts, older adults use mental health services well below even conservative estimates of need for these services. Indeed, unmet need is highest for those over age 65,[23,34] and older women are no exception.

A number of factors have been put forth to explain underuse of mental health services by older adults. System barriers include the nonavailability of mental health services as well as fragmentation of the existing services delivery system, low levels of Medicare reimbursement for mental health treatment, a scarcity of trained geropsychiatric providers, and negative provider attitudes toward treating elderly persons. Discussions of nonsystem barriers typically focus on a reluctance to use mental health services among elderly persons.[1,34,67]

Services for elderly persons are fragmented across a number of sectors, including social services, area agencies on aging (AAAs), community mental health centers (CMHCs), general hospitals, and nursing homes. Even when geriatric mental health services are available and accessible, their use may be inhibited by poor integration of systems of detection and referral. Of particular concern is the lack of interface between aging programs, the primary care sector, and the mental health system. A survey of CMHCs showed that less than one fourth had interagency agreements with AAAs, and few AAAs consider mental health services a priority issue.[68]

Many hospitals and nursing homes are ill-prepared to provide mental health treatment to their patients. While 28 percent of general hospitals had separate psychiatric units in 1990, this proportion is expected to decrease as cost-saving reductions in inpatient care continue.[69]

Data from the 1985 National Nursing Home Survey reveal that 68 percent of nursing homes reported having access to the services of a mental health specialty provider.[70] However, reports of the availability of a mental health professional obscure a wide range of possibilities. A national survey of 369 nursing homes conducted in 1992 found that while 90 percent reported that a psychiatrist was "available" to their facility, only 2.3 percent had a psychiatrist on staff and 29.2 percent had a psychiatrist under contract. Seven percent reported having a psychiatric nurse on staff or under contract and 24.8 percent had a clinical social worker on staff or under contract.[71]

Cost barriers related to low reimbursement for mental health services by Medicare, Medicaid, and private insurers are a persistent problem for older women in need since Medicare requires a 50 percent co-payment for psychotherapy visits and a 20 percent co-payment for medication management visits. Even a relatively small co-payment may inhibit the pursuit of care. A survey by Fogel[72] found that of 97 residents of elderly housing who acknowledged suffering from depression and indicated a willingness to seek treatment at no cost, only 7 said that they would seek treatment for a $20 out-of-pocket cost.

The powerful confluence of ageist and sexist attitudes may subtly (and not so subtly) pervade mental health services delivery to
older women. Resistance to treating elderly persons and the absence
of trained mental health providers have been noted by many
authors.[3,11,22,38,71,73-75]

Fogel[72] reported that all of the mental health professions have developed professional organizations or subsections dedicated to care of elderly persons and that advanced training programs have grown in
number in recent years. However, the stigma of working with elderly
persons and comparatively low reimbursement rates affect recruitment
and training in these professions.[11,76] Hence, geriatric specialization in
these professions remains less attractive compared with other specialty
areas.[75,77,78]

Lack of accurate information about "successful aging" underlie
stereotypical attitudes about the inevitability and irreversibility of age-
related mental decline. With so many providers skeptical about the efficacy of mental health services for older women, the risk of neglect or
inappropriate treatment rises commensurately. These barriers to mental
health treatment particularly affect older women in primary care settings.

In addition to system-related barriers, a number of researchers have
noted that current cohorts of elderly persons are reluctant to employ
psychological terminology in expressing distress and to view use of
specialty mental health treatment as appropriate or necessary.[73,79,80]
Waxman, Carner, and Klein[81] found that only one third of an elderly
community sample reported that they would seek help from a mental
health professional for symptoms of depression. The remaining two
thirds reported that they would tell a friend or family member (42 percent) or would tell no one (21 percent). When asked from whom they
would seek help for psychiatric symptoms, 88 percent selected a general
physician.[81]

A survey of 476 New Jersey elderly persons by Feinson[74] found that
among an array of barriers and incentives to use of mental health services, the most strongly endorsed was a single incentive: the recommendation of the primary care physician. Seventy-two percent stated they
would be more willing to seek mental health care if their physician recommended it, followed by recommendations by family (59 percent) and
by the clergy (58 percent). Statistical analyses revealed no gender dif-

ferences in these findings, although no sex role-related barriers (such as family responsibilities) were assessed in the survey.

PSYCHOPHARMACOLOGY AND MEDICATION MANAGEMENT IN PRIMARY CARE

As with other issues dealing with medical and psychiatric treatment of older adults, use of psychotropic and other prescription drugs is largely a women's issue.[23] Women make 58 percent of all physician office visits but receive 73 percent of all prescriptions for psychotropic drugs (90 percent when the physician is not a psychiatrist). Male psychiatrists prescribe psychotropic drugs twice as often as female psychiatrists and are more likely to prescribe drugs for female patients than for male patients.[14]

It is in the primary care setting where medication management is most critical for older women. Despite a propensity to recognize women's distress and rely on psychotropic drug therapies,[82] few primary care physicians are meeting women's mental health needs.[23] Nondrug therapies and referrals are rarely recommended—as few as 10 percent of depressed patients are referred to mental health specialists.[83] Even prescriptions for psychotropic drugs such as antidepressants tend to be at dosages below therapeutic levels.[84,85]

For older patients in primary care, a psychotropic drug is typically one of several medications prescribed by the physician. Open physician-patient communication and management of potential drug interactions are critical but often neglected dimensions of patient care.[86]

RECOMMENDATIONS FOR FURTHER RESEARCH

Evidence of healthy resilience as well as risk points to the need for researchers to move beyond the "good news" about older women's health to ascertain if concomitant gains in mental health have been achieved. Although the ECA surveys demonstrated that the vast majority of older women are not suffering from mental disorders, we do know that a significant proportion experience subclinical states of depression and anxiety.[28] At the same time, declining rates of disability among those over age 65 provide a measure of optimism.

Future research is needed using both qualitative and quantitative approaches to examine successful coping strategies employed by women as they age. How do these "survivors" and "thrivers" meet the inevitable challenges of life? Is late-life resilience related to successful coping throughout the life course?[87-92] Innovative research designs such as life course and cohort perspectives[88-91] can reveal how and why some women adapt while others suffer from physical and emotional disabilities.

Older women are a heterogeneous group—differences in income, race, and ethnicity; life course experiences; and cohort membership can affect risk for mental and emotional problems. While it is plausible that earlier adversity in life contributes to hardiness and survivorship,[7,91] the needs of poor and minority women can hardly be assumed to be less than those of their middle-class counterparts. For these women, "triple jeopardy" may pose risks difficult to overcome.[12] Thus, the hardiness of being a survivor and the general availability of Medicare insurance may not offset the very real threats of poverty, crime, and poor access to medical care in old age. Until further research is conducted, the risks of triple jeopardy warrant further attention.

Several suggestions for clinical services research emerge from this chapter. Appropriate management of mental health problems in primary care—including the use of psychotropic and other drugs—affects older women in large numbers. Until the 1990s, psychotropic drug trials almost invariably excluded women even though women were the predominant users once these drugs came on the market.[93,94] We have hardly begun to address gender differences in psychopharmacology even though it is known that estrogen levels affect response to psychotropic drugs.[95] Hormonal fluctuations and hormone replacement therapies (HRTs) during and postmenopause undoubtedly play a role in drug absorption and effects. In this context, it is plausible that physicians may be prescribing HRTs when psychotropic drugs are indicated or vice versa. Research is urgently needed in this area.

Researchers could also contribute by examining how existing initiatives to improve mental health treatment in primary care may be tailored to the needs of older women. The *Depression Guidelines*, recently published by the Agency for Health Care Policy and Research, were designed to enhance recognition and treatment of depression in primary care.[96] The efficacy of these guidelines for older patients who often somatize distress has not yet been established.

While the absolute number of women in need is much smaller when compared with primary care, the long-term care sector is a site where unmet need is substantial. Although a few innovative programs for mental health consultation in nursing homes were reported in the 1980s,[97,98] research on mental health services in nursing homes remains an area of neglect. The enforcement and impact of the OBRA regulations, changes in Medicaid reimbursement, use of psychotropic drugs and other medications—all are viable topics for future research.

Since the vast majority of older women reside at home, research is urgently needed on improving community-based mental health treatment to enhance the quality of life and reduce rates of institutional placement. In the late 1970s and early 1980s, a number of community demonstration projects for elderly persons were initiated to provide comprehensive care and prevent institutionalization. These included social and health maintenance organizations (S/HMOs), the On Lok project in San Francisco, and the National Long-Term Care Channeling Demonstration. These projects targeted few resources to evaluate mental health status and service needs.

Under the auspices of the NIMH, Community Support Program (CSP) initiatives were begun in several states in 1985 to coordinate services for elderly persons with SMI and serious cognitive impairment. While outcome evaluations of CSPs are not yet available from all states, findings from the Iowa project indicated improvements in geriatric mental health using an outreach and case management model of services delivery.[99]

Programs for Assertive Community Treatment (PACTs), which have proven effective in providing team and home-based services for persons with severe mental illness,[100] might also provide a model for designing such services for older persons in need.

IMPLICATIONS FOR MENTAL
HEALTH SERVICES DELIVERY

Gender bias and devaluation of older women in the health care system reflect larger societal attitudes.[23] As the good news about increasing robustness of the elderly population disseminates to providers as well as the general public, stereotypical notions of gender and aging may be replaced by realistic assessments of need based on known risk factors. For older women in general, the delay in onset of physical disability (and the risk of associated psychiatric comorbidity) until after age 75 points to a longer period of productive healthy life. From a systems delivery perspective, the concern lies with the minority of older women who are at risk as well as the growing numbers of impaired older women and their caregivers.

Although it is difficult to predict without more recent epidemiologic data, there is little reason to believe that need for mental health services by older women will increase beyond current estimates (except for expected increases due to overall growth of the elderly population). Of course, even stable estimates of need without increased use of mental health services mean that unmet need will be substantial for years to come. As described earlier, systems delivery barriers center on lack of provider training and reimbursement incentives; fragmentation of the aging, social services, and health care systems; and stigma associated with working with elderly persons. Both cost-cutting pressures and the growing recognition that specialty mental health providers cannot meet all needs[1,2] underscore the importance of focusing on the primary care sector as the "frontline" of mental health services delivery for older women.

It is likely that future cohorts of more educated and psychologically attuned older women (particularly the aging baby-boom generation) will make greater use of specialty mental health services. Of course, a greater propensity to use services will have little effect in reducing levels of unmet need if cost barriers continue to expand and clinicians are not adequately trained and motivated to provide such care.

THE IMPACT OF MANAGED CARE ON MENTAL HEALTH SERVICES DELIVERY FOR OLDER WOMEN

The introduction of managed care in the Medicare program raises additional concerns about access to mental health services for older women. Congressional interest in curbing growth in the Medicare budget has led to the provision of incentives for managed care corporations seeking to tap the Medicare market—Medicare HMOs currently cover 10 percent of the Medicare population and are gaining ground rapidly.[101]

One potential advantage to managed care plans is their elimination of the 50 percent co-payment for outpatient mental health care provided in the network. (Out-of-network use would still require a co-payment.) Dropping this discriminatory cost barrier may enhance access to services, but patients and their primary care physicians must be willing and able to seek appropriate in-network help for this incentive to have an impact.

Concerns raised about managed care in general become even more critical when dealing with an at-risk population such as elderly persons. With strong inducements to cut costs by limiting use, primary care gatekeepers may be discouraged from paying attention to mental symptoms and approving visits for mental health treatment. The already existing situation described earlier—neglect of mental health needs and reliance on psychotropic drugs—could be exacerbated under managed care.

The tendency of many HMOs to "carve out" their mental health benefits in subcontracts with private companies raises concerns as well. First, the incentive to cut costs in carved-out mental health plans remains unchanged. While many of these companies advertise toll-free hot lines to reduce barriers to initial access, the overriding concern of many such companies is with management of costs after patients enter treatment. While healthy older adults may see no disadvantage to this, disabled persons are ill-served by reductions in services. Second, carving out mental health coverage undermines coordination of care for the elderly population, who are more likely to have physical and mental comorbidities. With no financial incentives for services integration, private companies are unlikely to pursue innovative models of services delivery for elderly persons.

It is too early to know exactly how managed care will affect mental health services for the elderly population. Unfortunately, carrying out research on this may be difficult since managed care data are proprietary, differ considerably from plan to plan, and rarely include information on the full range of psychosocial needs of older women. Even successful efforts to cut mental health costs may yield little overall in savings. For example, mental health costs comprise only 2 percent of the total Medicare budget, amounting to only \$71 per annum per enrollee for all mental health and substance abuse services in 1990.[101]

CONCLUSION

This chapter attempts to summarize the available information on older women's mental health needs and service use. While there is good news from recent studies documenting robustness and well-being among older women, a significant number have unmet mental health needs that require changes in services delivery in primary care, hospital, nursing home, and community settings. Given the uncertainty surrounding the future of mental health services under managed care, there is an urgent need to focus the attention of researchers, providers, and policymakers on one of the fastest-growing segments of the population—aging women.

ENDNOTE

a. Sex-by-insurance type breakdowns were not available from the NMES report by Freiman.[39]

REFERENCES

1. Padgett DK, Burns BJ, Grau L, et al.: Mental health services use by older women: A review and proposed research agenda. Unpublished manuscript, 1995.
2. Glied S, Kofman S: *Women and Mental Health: Issues for Health Reform.* New York: Common Wealth Fund, 1995.
3. Rodeheaver D, Datan N: The challenge of double jeopardy: Toward a mental health agenda for aging women. *American Psychologist* 1988; 43:648-654.
4. Steuer JL: Psychotherapy with older women: Ageism and sexism in traditional practice. *Psychotherapy: Theory, Research and Practice.* 1982; 19:429-436.
5. Turner BF: Mental health and the older woman. In: Lesnoff-Garavaglia G (Ed.): *Handbook of Applied Gerontology.* New York: Human Sciences Press, 1987, pp. 201-203.
6. Porcino J: Psychological aspects of aging in women. (Special issue: Health needs of women as they age.) *Women and Health* 1985; 10:115-122.

7. Padgett DK: Aging minority women: Issues in research and health policy. *Women and Health* 1989; 14:213-225.

8. Roth S: *Attitudes Toward Death Across the Life Span.* Unpublished Ph.D. dissertation, West Virginia University, 1977.

9. Manton KG, Stallard E, Corder L: Changes in morbidity and chronic disability in the U.S. elderly population: Evidence from the 1982, 1984, and 1989 National Long Term Care Surveys. *Journal of Gerontology* 1995; 50b:S194-S204.

10. Rowe JW, Kahn RL: Human aging: Usual and successful. *Science* 1987; 237:143-149.

11. Gatz M, Pearson CG: Ageism revised and the provision of psychological services. *American Psychologist* 1988; 43:184-188.

12. Minkler M, Stone R: The feminization of poverty and older women. *The Gerontologist* 1985; 25:351-357.

13. Burkhauser RV: Protecting the most vulnerable: A proposal to improve social security insurance for older women. *The Gerontologist* 1994; 34:148-149.

14. Russo NF: *A Women's Mental Health Agenda.* Washington, DC: American Psychological Association, 1985.

15. Grau, L: Mental health and older women. *Women and Health.* 1989; 14:75-92.

16. Steinmetz SK: *Duty Bound: Elder Abuse and Family Care.* Newbury Park, CA: Sage, 1988.

17. Zarit SH, Todd PA, Zarit JM: Subjective burden of husbands and wives as caregivers: A longitudinal study. *The Gerontologist* 1986; 26:260-266.

18. Morris RS, Morris LW, Britton PG: Factors affecting the emotional well-being of the care-givers of dementia sufferers. *British Journal of Psychiatry* 1988; 153:147-156.

19. Harper DJ, Manasse PR, James O, et al.: Intervening to reduce distress in caregivers of impaired elderly people: A preliminary evaluation. *International Journal of Geriatric Psychiatry* 1993; 8:139-145.

20. Canetto SS: Gender and suicide in the elderly. *Suicide and Life-Threatening Behavior* 22:80-97.

21. Verbrugge LM: Pathways of health and death. In: Apple RD (Ed.): *Women, Health, and Medicine in America: A Historical Handbook.* New York: Garland, 1990, pp. 41-79.

22. George LK: Community and home care for mentally ill older adults. In: *Handbook of Mental Health and Aging.* 2nd ed. New York: Academic Press, 1992, pp. 793-813.

23. Padgett DK: Women's Mental Health: Some directions for research. *Journal of Orthopsychiatry* 1997; 67:522-534.

24. Blazer DG, Williams CD: The epidemiology of dysphoria and depression in an elderly population. *American Journal of Psychiatry* 1980; 137:439-444.

25. Nolen-Hoeksema S: Sex differences in unipolar depression: Evidence and theory. *Psychological Bulletin* 1987; 101:259-282.

26. George LK, Landerman R, Blazer DG, et al.: Concurrent morbidity between physical and mental illness. In: Carstensen LL, Neale J (Eds.): *Mechanisms of Psychosocial Influence on Physical Health, With Special Attention to the Elderly.* New York: Plenum, 1989, pp. 9-22.

27. Angel RJ, Angel JL: Mental and physical comorbidity among the elderly: The role of culture and social class. In: Padgett DK (Ed.): *Handbook on Ethnicity, Aging, and Mental Health.* Westport, CT: Greenwood, 1995.

28. Addonizio G, Alexopoulos GS: Affective disorders in the elderly. *International Journal of Geriatric Psychiatry* 1993; 8:41-47.

29. Regier DA, Goldberg ID, Taube CA: The de facto US mental health services system: A public health perspective. *Archives of General Psychiatry* 1978; 38:685-693.

410   EMPOWERMENT, SURVIVORS, AND AT-RISK POPULATIONS

30. George LK, Blazer DG, Winfield-Laird I, et al.: Psychiatric disorders and mental health service use in later life. In: Brody JA, Maddox GL (Eds.): *Epidemiology and Aging*. New York: Springer, 1988, pp. 203-234.
31. Leaf PJ, Livingston MM, Tischler GL, et al.: Contact with health professionals for the treatment of psychiatric and emotional problems. *Medical Care* 1985; 23:1322-1337.
32. Schurman RA, Kramer PD, Mitchell JB: The hidden mental health network. *Archives of General Psychiatry* 1985; 42:89-94.
33. Phillips MA, Murrell SA: Impact of psychological and physical health, stressful events, and social support on subsequent mental health help-seeking among older adults. *Journal of Consulting and Clinical Psychology* 1994; 62:270-275.
34. Shapiro S, Skinner ES, Kramer M, et al.: Measuring need for mental health services in a general population. *Medical Care* 1985; 23:1033-1043.
35. Kessler RC, Nelson CB, McGonogle KA: The epidemiology of co-occuring addictive and mental disorders: Implications for prevention and service utilization. *American Journal of Orthopsychiatry* 1996; 66:17-31.
36. Established populations for epidemiologic studies of the elderly. In: Cornoni-Huntley J, Blazer DG, Lafferty ME, et al. (Eds.): *Resource Data Book*. Vol. 2. Bethesda, MD: National Institute on Aging, 1990, pp. 90-95.
37. Parmalee PA, Katz IR, Lawton MP: Incidence of depression in long-term care settings. *Journal of Gerontology* 1992; 47:189-196.
38. Burns BJ, Taube CA: Mental health services in general medical care and in nursing homes. In: Fogel BS, Furino A, Gottlieb GL (Eds.): *Mental Health Policy for Older Americans: Protecting Minds at Risk*. Washington, DC: American Psychiatric Press, 1990.
39. Freiman MP, Cunningham PJ, Cornelius LJ: The demand for health care for the treatment of mental problems among the elderly. In: *Advances in Health Economics and Health Services Research*. Greenwich, CT: JAI, 1993, pp. 17-36.
40. Padgett DK, Patrick C, Burns BJ, et al.: Use of mental health services by Black and White elderly. In: Padgett DK (Ed.): *Handbook on Ethnicity, Aging, and Mental Health*. Westport, CT: Greenwood, 1995, pp. 144-163.
41. Freiman M, Cunningham JP, Cornelius L: *Use and Expenditures for the Treatment of Mental Health Problems*. AHCPR Pub. No. 94-0085. Rockville, MD: Public Health Service, 1994.
42. Carmen E, Russo NF, Miller JB: Inequality and women's mental health: An overview. *American Journal of Psychiatry* 1981; 138:1319-1330.
43. Eichler A, Parron DL (Eds.): *Women's Mental Health: Agenda for Research*. Rockville, MD: U.S. Department of Health and Human Services, 1987.
44. Birkett DP: *Psychiatry in the Nursing Home: Assessment, Evaluation, and Intervention*. Binghamton, NY: Haworth, 1991.
45. Burns BJ, Kamerow DB: Psychotropic drug prescriptions for nursing home residents. *Journal of Family Practice* 1988; 26:155-160.
46. Leaf PJ, Bruce ML: Gender differences in the use of outpatient mental health-related services: A re-examination. *Journal of Health and Social Behavior* 1987; 28:171-183.
47. Kessler RC, Brown RL, Broman CL: Sex differences in psychiatric help-seeking: Evidence from four large-scale surveys. *Journal of Health and Social Behavior* 1981; 22:49-64.
48. Cleary PD, Burns BJ, Nycz GR: The identification of psychiatric illness by primary care physicians: The effect of patient gender. *Journal of General Internal Medicine* 1990; 5:355-360.
49. Hohmann AA: Gender bias in psychotropic drug prescribing in primary care. *Medical Care* 1989; 27:478-490.

50. Bruce ML, Leaf PJ: Psychiatric disorders and 15-month mortality in a community sample of older adults. *American Journal of Public Health* 1989; 79:727-730.
51. Bruvill PW, Hall WD: Predictors of increased mortality in elderly depressed patients. *International Journal of Geriatric Psychiatry* 1993; 9:219-277.
52. Rovner BW, German PS, Brant LJ, et al.: Depression and mortality in nursing homes. *Journal of the American Medical Association* 1991; 265:993-996.
53. Burns BJ, Wagner HR, Taube JE, et al.: Mental health service use by the elderly in nursing homes. *American Journal of Public Health* 1993; 83:331-337.
54. Larson DB, Lyons JS: The psychiatrist in the nursing home. In: Copeland JRM, Abou-Saleh MT, Blazer DG (Eds.): *Principles and Practice of Geriatric Psychiatry*. New York: Wiley, 1994, pp. 953-959.
55. Eckert JK, Lyon SM: Board and care homes: From the margins to the mainstream in the 1990s. In: Ory MG, Duncker NP (Eds.): *In-Home Care for Older People: Health and Supportive Services*. Newbury Park, CA: Sage, 1992, pp. 97-114.
56. Mor V, Sherwood S, Gutkin C: A national study of residential care for the aged. *The Gerontologist* 1986; 26:405-417.
57. Avron J, Dreyer P, Connely K, et al.: Use of psychoactive medication and the quality of care in rest homes. *New England Journal of Medicine* 1989; 320:227-232.
58. Cicchinelli LF, Bell JC, Dittmar ND, et al.: *Factors Influencing the Deinstitutionalization of the Mentally Ill: A Review and Analysis*. Denver, CO: Denver Research Institute, University of Denver, 1981.
59. Aiken LH: Chronic mental illness. In: Fogel BS, Furino A, Gottlieb GL (Eds.): *Mental Health Policy for Older Americans: Protecting Minds at Risk*. Washington, DC: American Psychiatric Press, 1990.
60. Light E, Lebowitz BD (Eds.): *The Elderly With Chronic Mental Illness*. New York: Springer, 1991.
61. Burns BJ: Mental health services research on the hospitalized and institutionalized CMI elderly. In: Light E, Lebovitz BD (Eds.): *The Elderly With Chronic Mental Illness*. New York: Springer, 1991, pp. 207-215.
62. Cohen C: Integrated community services. In: Sadavoy J, Lazarus LW, Jarvik LF (Eds.): *Comprehensive Review of Geriatric Psychiatry*. Washington, DC: American Psychiatric Press, 1991.
63. Bachrach LL: Chronically mentally ill women: Emergence and legitimation of program issues. *Hospital and Community Psychiatry* 1985; 36:1063-1069.
64. Keskiner RA, Zalchman MJ, Ruppert EH: Advantages of being female in psychiatric rehabilitation. *Archives of General Psychiatry* 1973; 28:689-692.
65. Cohen C, Sokolovsky J: *Old Men of the Bowery: Survival Strategies of Homeless Men*. New York: Guilford, 1989.
66. Cohen CI: The chronic mentally ill elderly: Service research issues. In Light E, Lebowitz BD (Eds.): *The Elderly With Chronic Mental Illness*. New York: Springer, 1991, pp. 193-206.
67. Burns BJ: Prevention of mental disorders of old age. In: Copeland JRM, Abou-Saleh MT, Blazer DG (Eds.): *Principles and Practice of Geriatric Psychiatry*. New York: Wiley, 1994, pp. 1011-1017.
68. Light E, Lebowitz BD, Bailey F: Community mental health centers and elderly services: An analysis of direct and indirect services and service delivery sites. *Community Mental Health Journal* 1986; 22:294-302.
69. Redick RW, Witkin MJ, Atay JE, et al.: Availability of psychiatric beds, United States: Selected years, 1970-1990. *Mental Health Statistical Note* 1994; 213:1-7.

70. Hing E, Sekscenski E, Straham G: *National Nursing Home Survey, 1985*. Washington, DC: U.S. Government Printing Office, 1989.
71. Lombardo NE: *Barriers to Mental Health Services for Nursing Home Residents*. Washington, DC: American Association of Retired Persons, 1994.
72. Fogel BS: The United States' system of care. In: Copeland JRM, Abou-Saleh MT, Blazer DG (Eds.): *Principles and Practice of Geriatric Psychiatry*. New York: Wiley, 1994, pp. 923-930.
73. Butler RM, Lewis MI: *Aging and Mental Health*. St. Louis, MO: C. V. Mosby, 1982.
74. Feinson M: *Mental Health and Aging: What Are the Epidemiological Myths, Realities, and Policy Implications?* Jerusalem: Brookdale Institute of Gerontology, 1991.
75. Harper M, Grau L: State of the art in geropsychiatric nursing. *Journal of Psychosocial Nursing* 1994; 32:7-12.
76. Koenig HG, George LK, Schneider R: Mental health care for older adults in the year 2020: A dangerous and avoided topic. *The Gerontologist* 1994; 34:674-679.
77. Smoyak S: American psychiatric nursing: History and roles. *American Association of Occupational Health Nursing Journal* 1993; 41:316-322.
78. Gottlieb GL: Market segmentation. In: Fogel BS, Gottlieb GL (Eds.): *Mental Health Policy for Older Americans: Protecting Minds at Risk*. Washington, DC: American Psychiatric Press, 1990.
79. Goldstrom ID, Burns BJ, Kessler LG, et al.: Mental health services use by elderly adults in a primary care setting. *Journal of Gerontology* 1987; 42:147-153.
80. Grau L, Padgett D: Somatic depression among the elderly. *International Journal of Geriatric Psychiatry* 1988; 3:201-207.
81. Waxman HM, Carner EA, Klein M: Underutilization of mental health professionals by community elderly. *The Gerontologist* 1984; 24:23-30.
82. Ford DE: Recognition and underrecognition of mental disorders in adult primary care. In: Miranda J (Ed.): *Mental Disorders in Primary Care*. San Francisco: Jossey-Bass, 1994, pp. 186-205.
83. Rogers WH, Wells KB, Meridith LS, et al.: Outcomes for adult outpatients with depression under prepaid or fee-for-service financing. *Archives of General Psychiatry* 1993; 50:517-525.
84. Eisenberg L: Treating depression and anxiety in the primary care setting. *Health Affairs* 1992; 11:149-156.
85. Katon W, VonKorff M, Lin E, et al.: Adequacy and duration of antidepressant treatment in primary care. *Medical Care* 1992; 30:67-76.
86. Rost K, Roter D: Predictors of recall of medication regimens and recommendations for lifestyle change in elderly patients. *The Gerontologist* 1987; 27:510-515.
87. Datan N: Aging women: The silent majority. *Women's Studies Quarterly* 1989; 1:12-19.
88. Jackson JS, Antonucci TC, Gibson RC: Ethnic and cultural factors in research on aging and mental health: A life-course perspective. In: Padgett DK (Ed.): *Handbook on Ethnicity, Aging, and Mental Health*. Westport, CT: Greenwood, 1995.
89. Pearlin LI, Skaff MM: Stress and the life course: A paradigmatic alliance. *The Gerontologist* 1996; 36:239-247.
90. George LK: Missing links: The case for a social psychology of the life course. *The Gerontologist* 1996; 36:248-255.
91. Elder GH Jr: Perspectives on the life course. In: Elder GH Jr (Ed.): *Life Course Dynamics*. Ithaca, NY: Cornell University Press, 1985.
92. Jeffreys M: Social inequalities in health—Do they diminish with age? *American Journal of Public Health* 1996; 86:474-475.

93. Hamilton JA: Biases in women's health research. *Women and Therapy* 1992; 12:93-103.
94. Yonkers KA, Harrison W: The inclusion of women in psychopharmacologic trials. *Journal of Clinical Psychopharmacology* 1993; 13:380-382.
95. Hamilton JA, Parry B: Sex-related differences in clinical drug response: Implications for women's health. *Journal of the American Medical Women's Association* 1983; 38:126-132.
96. Depression Guideline Panel: *Depression in Primary Care: Vol. 1. Detection and Diagnosis.* Clinical Practice Guideline, No. 5, AHCPR Pub. No. 93-0550. Rockville, MD: U.S. Department of Health and Human Services, Public Health Service, Agency for Health Care Policy and Research, 1993.
97. Bienfeld D, Wheeler BJ: Psychiatric services to nursing homes: A liaison model. *Hospital and Community Psychiatry* 1989; 40:793-794.
98. Tourigny-Rivard MF, Drury M: The effects of monthly psychiatric consultation in a nursing home. *The Gerontologist* 1987; 27:363-366.
99. Buckwalter KC, Smith M, Zevenbergen P: Mental health services of the rural elderly outreach program. *The Gerontologist* 1991; 31:408-412.
100. Burns BJ, Santos AB: Assertive community treatment: An update of randomized trials. *Psychiatric Services* 1995; 46:669-672.
101. American Psychiatric Association: Medicare and mental health care: Problems and prospects for change. On-line report (http://www.psych.org/pub_pol_adv), August 1997.

Author Index

Subject Index

About the Contributors

Mary Jane Alexander, Ph.D., is a psychologist and research scientist at the Nathan S. Kline Institute for Psychiatric Research. She directs the Recovery and Special Populations Core at the Center for the Study of Issues in Public Mental Health. She does services research in co-occurring severe mental illness and addiction, and on the impact of early exposure to trauma on clinical profiles and cost of services.

Lyndra J. Bills, M.D., is a board-certified psychiatrist and Medical Director of The Sanctuary,® a specialized inpatient hospital program for the treatment of adults traumatized as children, located at Friends Hospital in Philadelphia.

Andrea K. Blanch, Ph.D., is currently Associate Commissioner for Programs for the Maine Department of Mental Health, Mental Retardation and Substance Abuse Services. She previously served as Director of Community Support Programs for the New York State Office of Mental Health.

Sandra L. Bloom, M.D., is a board-certified psychiatrist and founder and Executive Director of The Sanctuary,® a specialized inpatient hospital program for the treatment of adults traumatized as children, located at Friends Hospital in Philadelphia. She is President of the International Society for Traumatic Stress Studies. She is also President of the Philadelphia chapter of Physicians for Social Responsibility. She is author of *Creating Sanctuary: Towards the Evolution of Sane Societies*.

Barbara J. Burns, Ph.D., holds academic appointments at Duke University Medical Center as Professor of Medical Psychology, Department of Psychiatry and Behavioral Sciences; Associate Research Professor, Center for Health Policy Research and Education; and Senior Fellow, Center for the Study of Aging and Human Development. She is Research Fellow at the Cecil G. Sheps Center for Health Services Research at the University of North Carolina at Chapel Hill. She serves as Director of the Services Effectiveness Research Program in the Department of Psychiatry and Behavioral Sciences at Duke University and Co-Director of the Postdoctoral Research Training Program in Mental Health Services and Systems. Key research interests focus on the effectiveness of mental health services for adults with severe mental illness and children with serious emotional and behavioral disorders.

Elaine (Hilberman) Carmen, M.D., is Medical Director of the Brockton Multi-Service Center, a large, publicly funded community mental health center providing comprehensive services to a population of individuals with serious mental illness in southeastern Massachusetts. Her recent work has focused on the identification and treatment of survivors of physical and sexual abuse who are diagnosed with a major mental illness. She chaired the Massachusetts Department of Mental Health task force concerned with restraint and seclusion of persons who have been physically and/or sexually abused.

Judith A. Cook, Ph.D., is Associate Professor of Sociology in Psychiatry and Director of the National Research and Training Center on Psychiatric Disability at the University of Illinois at Chicago, in the Department of Psychiatry. Her research includes studies of outcomes among women with psychiatric disability, mothers with mental illness, women with HIV/AIDS, and bereaved mothers following the death of a child.

Sandra L. Forquer, Ph.D., is currently Senior Vice President, Western Region, for Options Healthcare, Inc., located in Norfolk, Virginia. She also serves as Executive Director for Colorado Health Networks, the Colorado Medicaid Capitation Project serving 43 of 63 counties. Prior to joining Options in 1995, she served as Deputy Commissioner for the New York State Office of Mental Health.

Paula Goering, R.N., Ph.D., is Associate Professor in the Department of Psychiatry and Faculty of Nursing at the University of Toronto. She is Director of the Health Systems Research Unit and of the Clarke Consulting Group, as well as Program Leader of a Mental Health Policy Research Group. She began her career as a Clinical Nurse Specialist and has maintained her interest in the care of those with severe mental illness while working as a researcher, planner, and consultant.

Lois A. Grau, Ph.D., is Director of the Health Care Organization and Administration Track of the New Jersey Graduate Program in Public Health and Assistant Professor in the Robert Wood Johnson Medical School, Department of Environmental and Community Medicine. Her current research addresses cross-cultural issues in elder abuse.

Dianne Greenley, M.S.W., J.D., is the Managing Attorney for Mental Health Advocacy at the Wisconsin Coalition for Advocacy, the state protection and advocacy agency for people with disabilities. She is a graduate of Stanford University, the Smith College for Social Work, and the University of Wisconsin Law School. She has been an advocate for the rights of persons with mental illness for over 20 years.

Cathleen Patrick Harman, Ph.D., held the position of Research Associate in the Department of Psychiatry at the University of Colorado Health Sciences Center when she wrote her contribution to this book.

Maxine Harris, Ph.D., is Clinical Director of Community Connections in Washington, D.C. She is also the author of several books and numerous articles on women's issues and innovative treatments for persons diagnosed with serious mental illness.

Ann Jennings, Ph.D., has been involved for over 12 years in the design and implementation of strategic planning to produce fundamental changes in the way mental health and related human services delivery systems view and treat persons with histories of trauma. Currently, she is Director of the Office of Trauma Services with the Maine Department of Mental Health, Mental Retardation and Substance Abuse Services, focusing on interpersonal violence, particularly on the relationship of childhood and ongoing sexual and physical abuse to mental illness and emotional disorders. She has formed a statewide coalition of survivor/recipients of mental health services, trusted professionals, public mental health service providers, and policymakers; conducted a comprehensive needs assessment; initiated statewide strategies in the trauma model; influenced departmental and court-mandated consent decree policies to further treatment responsive to the needs of trauma survivors; and designed and spearheaded the creation of a statewide system of trauma services in Maine.

Coni Kalinowski, M.D., is a community psychiatrist who has worked extensively in the field of psychosocial rehabilitation, serving people having psychiatric disabilities. She has designed and implemented integrated services teams using client-directed services approaches, and she provides training and consultation to people working to make their mental health systems more empowering of consumers. She is a proponent of client-directed prescribing of psychotropic medications. She is presently practicing in Santa Barbara, California, and is teaching at Antioch University.

Bruce Lubotsky Levin, Dr.P.H., FABHM, is Associate Professor of Child and Family Studies in the Louis de la Parte Florida Mental Health Institute at the University of South Florida (USF) and Associate Professor of Community and Family Health at the USF College of Public Health. He is also Adjunct Associate Professor of Health Services Research in the School of Public Health at the University of Texas Health Science Center at Houston. He serves as editor of the *Journal of Behavioral Health Services & Research* (formerly *Journal of Mental Health Administration*), and is senior editor of a text titled *Mental Health Services: A Public Health Perspective* (1996). He received his undergraduate degree at the University of Wisconsin and his graduate degrees at the University of Texas. His research interests include managed behavioral health services, mental health policy, and mental health insurance coverage.

Pamela McDonnell, M.P.A., is Program Analyst at the Office for Women's Services at the Substance Abuse and Mental Health Services Administration, National Institute of Mental Health, in Rockville, Maryland.

Carol T. Mowbray, Ph.D., is Associate Dean for Research and Associate Professor at the University of Michigan School of Social Work and Faculty Associate in the School's Center for Research on Poverty, Risk and Mental Health. She has developed and evaluated several community-based interventions focused on homelessness, dual diagnosis, vocational rehabilitation, and supported education. She is currently the principal investigator on a federally funded, longitudinal study of women who have mental illness and are coping with parenthood. She is active in the International Association for Psychosocial Rehabilitation at the state and national levels. She has edited two books and written numerous articles for professional journals on program evaluation and on women's mental health, among other topics.

Kristina Muenzenmaier, M.D., is currently Attending Psychiatrist on the Residency Training Unit, Bronx Psychiatric Center; Assistant Clinical Professor of Psychiatry, Columbia University; and organizer and member of the Trauma Committee at Bronx Psychiatric Center.

Joy Perkins Newmann, M.S.W., Ph.D., is Associate Professor of Social Work and Director of the Mental Health Services Research Training Program at the University of Wisconsin–Madison. Her current research focuses on gender, serious mental illness, and the treatment and recovery process with a special emphasis on the role that histories of abuse play in access to care and in course, quality, and cost of care.

Joanne Nicholson, Ph.D., is Clinical and Research Psychologist in the Department of Psychiatry, Center for Psychosocial and Forensic Services Research at the University of Massachusetts Medical School, where she is Associate Professor of Psychiatry. She directs the activities of the Child and Family Research Core within the center, and is the principal investigator of the three-year, NIDRR-funded Parenting Options Project. She has established an active, consumer-based program of research on parents with psychiatric disabilities and their families. She writes extensively on the challenges facing these families and provides training and consultation to professional and consumer groups.

Daphna Oyserman, Ph.D., is Associate Research Scientist at the Institute for Social Research–Research Center for Group Dynamics, University of Michigan. Her areas of research interest focus on the interplay between social identity, sociocultural context, and behavioral, motivational, and affective outcomes. She is a WT Grant Faculty Scholar, currently studying the impact of African American identity on outcomes for youths, including school persistence and vulnerability to depression. Additional NIMH funding research includes the School to Jobs intervention study.

Deborah K. Padgett, Ph.D., is Associate Professor in the Research Area at the Ehrenkranz School of Social Work, New York University. She received her doctorate in anthropology and completed postdoctoral fellowships in sociomedical sciences at the Columbia University School of Public Health and in mental health services research at Duke University, Department of Psychiatry. She is the editor of *Handbook on Ethnicity, Aging, and Mental Health* (1995), and the author of *Qualitative Methods in Social Work Research: Challenges and Rewards* (1998). She has published extensively on mental health needs and services use of elderly persons, culturally diverse ethnic groups, the homeless, and children and adolescents.

Darby Penney, M.S., is Director of Recipient Affairs at the New York State Office of Mental Health, where she is responsible for bringing the perspectives of consumers/survivors/ex-patients into the policy-making process. She is Chair of the National Association of Consumer/Survivor Mental Health Administrators. She has written and presented widely on issues including recipient perspectives on managed care, recovery from psychiatric disability, recipient involvement in planning and policy making, and coercion in the mental health system.

James Purcell, M.A., is Senior Policy Analyst with the New York State Council on Children and Families. He was previously Associate Commissioner of the New York State Department of Social Services, responsible for child welfare and domestic violence programs. He has a master of arts degree from the State University of New York at Albany.

Anne Rhodes, R.N., M.Sc., is a doctoral candidate in epidemiology at the University of Toronto. She recently finished a research fellowship within the Mental Health Systems Program in psychiatry. Her research interests pertain to gender, mental health systems, and psychiatric epidemiology.

Priscilla Ridgway, M.S.W., has over 25 years of experience in the mental health field encompassing direct services, consumer advocacy, program administration, policy development, planning, and research. She achieved national recognition for her role in designing innovative housing approaches, strategic planning, and consumer housing preference needs assessment methods while working within the Center for Psychiatric Rehabilitation at Boston University. She is currently a doctoral student at the University of Kansas, School of Social Welfare, Lawrence, Kansas. Employed at the Kansas Mental Health Research Laboratory, she is conducting inquiry into best practices in housing and employment and the emerging recovery paradigm among persons with psychiatric disabilities.

Patricia Perri Rieker, Ph.D., a medical sociologist, is Professor of Sociology at Simmons College and Associate Professor of Psychiatry at Harvard Medical School. Her current research focuses on the recovery of life qualities after traumatic experiences. Her most recent book is a co-edited collection of original essays titled *Mental Health: Racism and Sexism*.

Alba Rueda-Riedle, M.A., is a Ph.D. candidate in the Psychology Department at Wayne State University in Detroit, Michigan, and a research associate at the School of Social Work, University of Michigan, Ann Arbor. Her areas of specialization are social and developmental psychology. Her interests focus on cross-cultural research, particularly with regard to gender issues, as well as women's health and social roles, including drug abuse and drug abuse prevention. Currently, she is studying the influence of sociocultural factors on women's functioning as parents and women's perceptions of themselves as mothers.

Daniel G. Saunders, Ph.D., is Associate Professor at the University of Michigan's School of Social Work, where he teaches courses on direct practice and domestic violence. He is Co-Chair of the University of Michigan Task Force on Violence Against Women and Co-Director of the university's Interdisciplinary Family Violence Research Program. He was co-founder of a shelter for battered women and founder of a program for men who batter. His research on domestic violence focuses on abuser types and treatment, the traumatic aftermath of violence and victimization, and the attitudes and responses of professionals. His publications have appeared in numerous books and journals.

Susan D. Scheidt, Psy.D., is Associate Clinical Professor at the University of California, San Francisco, with a joint appointment in the Department of Medicine and Psychiatry at San Francisco General Hospital (SFGH). Her career thus far has focused on individuals with serious mental illness in inpatient settings. Currently, she is Attending Psychologist and Director of Training at the Division of Psychosocial Medicine, SFGH. Her main professional interests include brief psychotherapy with low-income, multicultural clients, including individuals with chemical dependency problems, and behavioral medicine.

Herbert J. Schlesinger, Ph.D. is the Alfred J. and Monette C. Professor of Psychology, Emeritus, Graduate Faculty of Political and Social Sciences, New School for Social Research; Adjunct Professor of Psychology in Psychiatry, Cornell University Medical College; Attending Psychologist, New York Hospital; Training and Supervising Analyst, Columbia University Center for Psychoanalytic Training and Research; and Lecturer, Department of Psychiatry, College of Physicians and Surgeons, Columbia University. His research interests include the effects of outpatient mental health treatment on use of medical services, and use of mental health services by age, sex, and ethnic subpopulations, and under different health care systems and reimbursement systems.

Alexa Simpson, M.P.H., M.F.A., has over 20 years of training and experience in both Western and Eastern approaches to wholeness, health, and creativity. She is an Interior Designer, Health Educator, Corporate Stress Management Consultant, Clinical Hypnotherapist, and Certified Yoga Teacher. She is the founder and director of Yoga for Life, in Benicia, California, and the author of *The Transformation Journal* (1996).

Susan Stefan, J.D., is Professor of Law at the University of Miami School of Law. Prior to 1990, she was an attorney at the Mental Health Law Project (now the Bazelon Center for Mental Health Law) in Washington, D.C. Her most recent publications include "Issues Relating to Women and Ethnic Minorities in Mental Health Treatment and Law," in Sales and Shuman, Eds., *Law, Mental Health and*

Mental Disorder (1996) and "Reforming the Provision of Mental Health Treatment," in Moss, Ed., *Man-Made Medicine* (1996). She is currently working on a book on legal remedies for discrimination against people on the basis of mental disability for the American Psychological Association Press.

J. K. Sweeney, M.S., is Associate Researcher in the School of Pharmacy, University of Wisconsin–Madison. Her research is in the area of mental health services and expenditures.

Gillian Van Dien, M.S., worked at the University of Wisconsin, School of Social Work, at the time she wrote her contribution to this book.

Bonita M. Veysey, Ph.D., is Senior Research Associate at Policy Research Associates, Inc., an independent research company in Delmar, New York. Dr. Veysey has conducted national research projects in the area of criminal justice/mental health services. Her primary interest is the specific needs of women with substance abuse and mental disorders in the criminal justice system, and she has consulted with correctional facilities regarding the need for services for female offenders. Dr. Veysey holds a Ph.D. in sociology from the State University of New York at Albany.

Gary Wheeler, M.A., is a shipwright who has a master's degree in psychology with further postgraduate work in human development. He is an accomplished designer and inventor, referring to himself as "an inventor of the obvious." He lives aboard his 36-foot wooden sailboat in San Francisco, California.

Friedner D. Wittman, Ph.D., M.Arch., trained as an architect with emphasis on developing facilities for health and social services, and with experience as a commissioned officer in the U.S. Public Health Service Corps, has taught at the University of California, Berkeley, School of Architecture, and is Program Director of the Community Prevention Planning Program at UC Berkeley's Institute for the Study of Social Change. In his private practice, he has designed over 30 facilities specifically planned for persons with substance abuse and/or mental health problems. He is President of CLEW Associates, a Berkeley-based consulting firm, from which he continues to develop environmental approaches to the prevention of alcohol and drug problems, as well as render architectural programming and design consultation for facilities that provide social services.